The Guide to Interpersonal Psychotherapy

T0355219

The Guide to Interpersonal Psychotherapy

Updated and Expanded Edition

MYRNA M. WEISSMAN

JOHN C. MARKOWITZ

GERALD L. KLERMAN

OXFORD
UNIVERSITY PRESS

OXFORD
UNIVERSITY PRESS

Oxford University Press is a department of the University of Oxford. It furthers
the University's objective of excellence in research, scholarship, and education
by publishing worldwide. Oxford is a registered trade mark of Oxford University
Press in the UK and certain other countries.

Published in the United States of America by Oxford University Press
198 Madison Avenue, New York, NY 10016, United States of America.

© Oxford University Press 2018

First Edition published in 2007

Library of Congress Cataloging-in-Publication Data
Names: Weissman, Myrna M., author. | Markowitz, John C., 1954– author. |
Klerman, Gerald L., 1928–1992, author.
Title: The guide to interpersonal psychotherapy / Myrna M. Weissman,
John C. Markowitz, Gerald L. Klerman.
Other titles: Clinician's quick guide to interpersonal psychotherapy
Description: Updated and expanded edition. | Oxford ; New York :
Oxford University Press, 2018. | Revision of: Clinician's quick guide to
interpersonal psychotherapy. 2007. |
Includes bibliographical references and index.
Identifiers: LCCN 2017023276 (print) | LCCN 2017024722 (ebook) |
ISBN 9780190662608 (updf) | ISBN 9780190668808 (epub) | ISBN 9780190662592 (paperback)
Subjects: LCSH: Interpersonal psychotherapy.
Classification: LCC RC489.I55 (ebook) | LCC RC489.I55 C555 2018 (print) |
DDC 616.89/14—dc23
LC record available at https://lccn.loc.gov/2017023276

Printed by Marquis Book Printing, Canada

CONTENTS

Interpersonal psychotherapy (IPT) is one of the best-researched of the evidence-based psychotherapies. This book is designed as the "go to" manual for learning IPT for depression and its various adaptations for other disorders. It is also intended for clinicians who have had some exposure to IPT in workshops or supervision and want a reference book and a treatment manual for their practice. Researchers and clinicians who want to adapt IPT for a new diagnosis, age group, format, or culture may use this book as a foundation. We describe the elements, strategies, and techniques that define IPT. A range of mental health professionals may benefit from this book: psychiatrists, psychologists, social workers, nurses, school counselors, as well as workers in impoverished areas where few mental health treatment options may exist.

In the early 1970s, at the dawn of evidence-based psychotherapy research, Gerald L. Klerman, M.D., and Myrna M. Weissman, Ph.D., developed and, with colleagues, tested a short-term treatment for depression (Weissman, 2006). The success of their studies led to this treatment becoming known as IPT. The treatment was described in the original study manual, *Interpersonal Psychotherapy for Depression* (1984), and subsequently in the *Comprehensive Guide to Interpersonal Psychotherapy* (2000), the slimmed-down *Clinicians' Quick Guide for Interpersonal Psychotherapy* (2007), and the *Casebook of Interpersonal Psychotherapy* (2012). The current book, the descendent and update of those volumes, is the definitive IPT manual.

IPT has been repeatedly studied in randomized controlled trials. IPT studies have been published in major journals. These successes have led to its inclusion in treatment guidelines in Australia, Canada, Germany, Japan, the Netherlands, New Zealand, Norway, Scotland, Sweden, the United Kingdom, and the United States, and to its recognition and recommendation by the World Health Organization. Increasing numbers of practitioners have begun to learn the approach. In this context, several other IPT manuals have appeared. Some have been specialty manuals—elaborated adaptations of IPT for specific formats or treatment populations. Examples include a group treatment manual that the World Health Organization has adapted for dissemination worldwide (WHO, 2016) and manuals outlining IPT for depressed adolescents (Mufson et al., 2011), bipolar disorder (Frank, 2005), and posttraumatic stress disorder (Markowitz, 2016) (Sections III through V of this book review these and other adaptations). Other manuals have imitated the book you are holding, sometimes departing from the evidence-based approach on which IPT was built. This book contains the material that provided the basis for the very earliest and subsequent IPT research and training, and is the platform on which to build future IPT research and practice.

Many clinicians have heard or read about IPT, but are not quite sure what it is or how to do it. Because programs in psychiatry, psychology, social work, and other mental health professions have been slow to incorporate evidence-based psychotherapy into their required training (Weissman et al., 2006), most mental health clinicians have not received formal training in IPT. Only in the past decade have many begun to learn IPT, primarily through postgraduate workshops or courses or by reading the Weissman et al. 2000 or 2007 manuals. This book now updates those.

We present a distillation of IPT in an easily accessible guide. This book contains a modicum of background theory—we have restored some of the material cut from the 2007 edition—but is designed to be, like IPT itself, practical and pragmatic. The book describes how to approach clinical encounters with patients, how to focus the treatment, and how to handle therapeutic difficulties. We provide clinical examples and sample therapist scripts throughout.

Section I (Chapters 1 and 2) sets a framework for IPT in the modern psychotherapeutic world and briefly outlines the approach. Section II (Chapters 3–11) describes in detail how to conduct IPT for major depressive disorder. You will need to read this section to know the basics of IPT. If you are interested in learning some of the adaptations of IPT for mood disorders with special populations or circumstances, proceed to Section III (Chapters 12–18) and, for non-mood disorders, to Section IV (Chapters 19–23). Although most of the IPT research was based on DSM-III or DSM-IV diagnoses, we have rearranged the grouping of diagnoses to follow the DSM-5 taxonomy. Section V (Chapters 24–26) deals with structured adaptations of IPT (cross-cultural adaptation and group, conjoint, telephone, and online formats), some of which are also covered in earlier chapters that describe the use of these modifications. Section V also addresses further training and finding IPT resources.

We have kept the chapters relatively brief so that you can quickly turn to topics of interest. Each chapter on an IPT adaptation for a particular diagnosis briefly relates the symptoms of the disorder, the specific modifications of IPT for that disorder, and the degree to which outcome data support this application. Rather than clutter the clinical text with descriptions of studies, we refer interested readers to the International Society of Interpersonal Psychotherapy website (http://ipt-international.org/), which maintains a periodically updated bibliography of research. The busy clinician may read the flow chart in Chapter 2 (Table 2.1) and proceed directly to Chapter 4, "Beginning IPT."

There are limits to what a book can provide. At best, it can offer guidelines to enhance practitioners' existing skills. If this is a "how to" book, it presupposes that the clinicians who use it understand the basics of psychotherapy and have experience with the target diagnoses or specific population of patients they are planning to treat. This book does not obviate the need for clinical training in IPT, including courses and expert supervision (see Chapter 26). On the other hand, trainers in resource-poor countries in humanitarian crisis have done quick trainings for health workers of necessity (Verdeli et al., 2008).

We dedicate the book to the late Gerald L. Klerman, M.D., a gifted clinical scientist who developed IPT with Dr. Weissman, his wife. As lead author of the original 1984 manual, he developed IPT but unfortunately did not live to see its current research advances and clinical dissemination. We thank many colleagues throughout the years who pushed the boundaries of IPT by developing and testing adaptations, and whose work is cited throughout.

This book has been updated for 2017, but the field is rapidly changing. Updates on studies may be obtained through the International Society of Interpersonal Psychotherapy (https://www.interpersonalpsychotherapy.org/).

All patient material has been altered to preserve confidentiality.

ACKNOWLEDGMENTS

We thank our partners, Jim and Barbara, for their patience and support through the lengthy review process. We thank Myrna's late husband, Gerry Klerman, for his brilliant and enduring ideas and drive, which provide the bedrock of this book and which are now spreading around the world. We thank the numerous far-flung members of the International Society of Interpersonal Psychotherapy who contributed updates on their work. Thanks also to Rachel Floyd and Lindsay Casal Roscum, who provided technical support on the text revision in New York. This book would not exist had not our editors at Oxford University Press, Sarah Harrington and Andrea Zekus, met with us on an icily rainy afternoon in early February 2016 and urged us to revise the 2007 book. They have provided invaluable support along the way.

Myrna Weissman and John Markowitz

ACKNOWLEDGMENTS

Introduction

The Interpersonal
Psychotherapy Platform

Since the publication of the 2007 version of this book, enormous changes have occurred in psychotherapy and in IPT. While overall psychotherapy use has declined slightly in the United States (Marcus et al., 2010), there has been a marked increase in the use of evidence-based psychotherapy and of IPT. This growth is reflected in IPT's inclusion in national and international treatment guidelines, the proliferating training programs (Stewart et al., 2014; IAPT, www.iapt.nhs.uk; http://www.iapt.nhs.uk/workforce/high-intensity/interpersonal-psychotherapy-for-depression/), an explosion of international interest, and the evolution of the International Society of Interpersonal Psychotherapy (ISIPT; http://ipt-international.org/).

For example, in 2016 the World Health Organization, in collaboration with the World Bank, declared the need to emphasize mental health treatment in health care; their mhGAP program[1] sponsored dissemination of IPT for depression all over the world. Other programs sponsoring IPT training and use are Grand Challenges Canada;[2] the international Strong Minds program in Uganda and elsewhere in Africa;[3] the use of IPT for refugees and national disasters in Haiti, Jordan, and Lebanon; and more recently for primary care in Muslim countries (see Chapter 24). These projects have highlighted the universality of interpersonal problems and of the wish to heal them. It has been relatively easy to adapt IPT for different cultures and settings, as human attachments and the response to the trigger of their breakage are conserved across cultures and countries. Communication in relationships varies with culture, but the fundamental issues and emotional responses to them remain the same. Rituals of death may vary by religion and culture, but the experience of grief following the death of a loved one

1. http://www.who.int/mental_health/mhgap/en/

2. http://www.grandchallenges.ca/

3. http://strongminds.org/

is nearly universal. Thus the elements of IPT, the problem areas and interventions, transfer readily across cultures, ages, and situations.

Yet the vast increase in IPT training at many levels, and the range of cultures and situations for which IPT has been adapted, raise questions about its elasticity and authenticity: How far can one alter the model and still call it IPT?

We call this book the *platform* for IPT. By platform, we mean both a manifesto or "formal declaration of principles" (www.thefreedictionary.com/platform) and the technical definition of "a standard for the hardware of a computer system, determining what kinds of software it can run" (http://www.oxforddictionaries. com/us/definition/american_english/platform). This book provides the platform for the clinical and research use of IPT, defining its essential elements. Any adaptation must have these elements to be considered IPT. The book also defines incompatibilities with IPT: absence of defined time limits or an interpersonal focus, jettisoning of the medical model, therapist passivity, focus on personality or on transference or cognitions, and so forth.

We are pleased that so many investigators and clinicians find the elements of IPT useful and have adapted them for differing treatment populations, diagnostic groups, and treatment formats. We encourage such exploration and adaptation. But to call what they do IPT, adaptors must employ the basic elements or describe why a particular one may not be suitable. To depart from the model we describe, which has been the basis for the research that put IPT on the international map, is to depart from the evidence base that gives IPT clinical validity.

ELEMENTS OF PSYCHOTHERAPY

In an effort to develop evidence-based standards for psychotherapy, the Institute of Medicine (IOM) in 2015 called for research on a common terminology of the elements of individual psychotherapy across psychotherapies and across diagnoses. The term "elements" has entered the evidence-based psychotherapy literature to denote the core components of treatment methods. The IOM defined "elements" as therapeutic activities, techniques or strategies that are either nonspecific or specific (IOM, 2015). Nonspecific elements, often described as "common factors" (Frank, 1971; Wampold, 2001), are common across psychotherapies. These techniques help to build a trusting therapeutic alliance, enable the patient to express intimate material, and account for a great, shared portion of the therapeutic benefit of all talking therapies (Wampold, 2001). These nonspecific elements, such as establishing confidentiality, engaging the patient, warmth, empathy, nonjudgmental listening, trust, and encouragement of affect, are all part of IPT (see Chapter 3). Common factors may be a necessary component of any therapy and account for a significant proportion of treatment outcome. These techniques, which IPT (and ideally all) therapists use to facilitate more specific IPT strategies, are neither unique nor new.

We describe more specific elements in Chapter 10. Specific IPT strategies include (1) using the medical model, in which the therapist defines and describes the onset of symptoms and diagnosis, and gives the patient the "sick role"; (2) elic-iting an interpersonal inventory; (3) specifying a time limit for treatment; and (4) presenting early in treatment a formulation linking an interpersonal problem area (grief, role dispute, role transition, or interpersonal deficits) to the psychiat-ric diagnosis. IPT also uses strategies such as helping patients to connect mood fluctuations to daily interpersonal events, communication analysis, and explor-ing interpersonal options, as well as techniques shared with cognitive-behavioral therapy (CBT) and other treatments, such as role play.

Some of these "specific" IPT elements arise in other psychotherapies, some-times under other names. Nonetheless, the goals, the sequence, the emphases, and the explicit description of these elements to the patient as part of the thera-peutic strategy are unique to IPT. These elements hold across the numerous IPT adaptations for different diagnoses, age groups, formats, and cultures. Many are captured by therapist adherence measures used in research studies (e.g., Hollon, 1984). Most importantly, the research evidence based on nearly 100 clinical trials derives from these specific elements. As health care (at least in the United States) moves toward measurement-based practice, fidelity measures may become used to ensure that clinicians in general practice do in fact use these elements of IPT appropriately as the basis for reimbursement.

Proponents of the "elements" approach, who apparently consider all psycho-therapies fundamentally similar, have largely been cognitive-behavioral thera-pists who are comfortable with dismantling CBT into component parts. IPT, like other affect-based therapies (Milrod, 2015; Swartz, 2015), takes a more holistic approach. IPT may amount to more than the sum of its parts, and subtracting cru-cial elements may damage the treatment as well as depart from its evidence base. Hence we encourage researchers and clinicians to use IPT as an integrated whole and as a complete package, as defined in this book, making necessary adaptations defined for a specific patient population.

BOUNDARIES OF ADAPTATION

The adaptation of IPT for different disorders, symptoms, situations, and cultures has rapidly grown. Questions may arise about how much adaptation is reasonable while still retaining the title of IPT.

The basic specific elements of IPT we describe constitute the core of IPT. Researchers can modify these by adjusting time length, as in brief IPT, interper-sonal counseling, or maintenance treatment. As for psychotherapy more gener-ally, it remains unclear what the optimal length of IPT may be. Nonetheless, it is crucial to **define the time frame at the outset of treatment**: a fixed number of weekly sessions (or for maintenance, perhaps monthly) for a delineated dura-tion. The pressure of the time limit helps drive IPT forward. IPT ingredients can be adapted for different ages (for example, adolescent, prepubescent, and geriatric), and the researcher may tweak the approach for the target population. An adaption may change the format (e.g., group or couples IPT) or the target diagnosis (e.g., posttraumatic stress disorder [PTSD] or bipolar disorder). If the researcher shifts the diagnosis, the IPT focus on the relationship between syndrome and interpersonal context remains. Another basic principle and historical aspect of IPT is that such adaptations deserve testing to evaluate whether they work.

IPT adaptations for different cultures necessarily incorporate cultural sensitivities and customs. Examples include family participation in therapy sessions; disputes regarding the moving of a second wife into the home; concepts of death and ways of showing reverence to the dead; dealing with assertiveness; and avoiding direct criticism that might threaten the stability of *familismo* (Markowitz, 2009). Incorporating these differences as special issues again does not fundamentally change the clinical IPT paradigm linking mood to life circumstance. We thank the many IPT investigators who have contributed their adaptations to the field, many but hardly all of whom we cite in this book. Our overview is necessarily selective rather than exhaustive: too many IPT adaptations already exist to cover in this book, and we hope researchers will test many more.

More than one therapeutic approach may benefit patients with a particular diagnosis, and no one treatment works all the time. The availability of a range of evidence-based psychotherapies and somatic treatments (such as pharmacotherapy) that can benefit patients serves the public health interest. A therapeutic problem is how to respond to some clinicians' eagerness to combine different treatment approaches they like without violating the integrity of IPT as validated in clinical trials. We caution against casual therapeutic eclecticism, for two reasons:

1. Research evidence shows that thematic adherence—good therapist fidelity—is associated with better outcomes (Frank et al., 1991).
2. A patient in a time-limited therapy should leave treatment with a coherent understanding of how to respond to symptoms.

A therapist who mixes too many methods may look brilliant to the patient, seemingly having a (different) answer to every situation, but will leave the patient confused about how to handle life stressors after therapy ends (Markowitz & Milrod, 2015). Therapist adherence to a single, clear approach is more likely to communicate a useful model for responding to symptoms.

Nonetheless, it may be helpful on occasion to augment IPT with other treatment elements. When doing so, the clearest and likely most helpful way to proceed is to explicitly add a separate module to the IPT core. For example, motivational interviewing may help to encourage patients to engage in therapy or to diminish substance use (Swartz et al., 2008). Perhaps the best example of this is Ellen Frank's adding to IPT (for depression) a behavioral component to regulate levels of arousal and to preserve sleep for bipolar patients, an amalgam she terms Interpersonal and Social Rhythm Therapy (IPSRT; Frank, 2005). The innovator will need to consider whether mixing elements from different psychotherapies creates potential theoretical or practical treatment contradictions, and if so how to address them. The modular approach keeps IPT and the added module distinct in their indications and potentially in the evaluation of their efficacy.

We fully support referring IPT patients to other evidence-based therapies, medication (which shares the medical model and hence can be easily combined with IPT), and/or an alternative psychotherapy, if IPT has not produced clinical progress or it becomes clear to patient and therapist that IPT is not the most appropriate treatment. The goal of therapy is that the patient achieve remission.

A final boundary issue is that other evidence-based psychotherapies might add IPT elements as modules, for example the interpersonal inventory or an interpersonal problem area. Developers of such approaches should not tinker with IPT and market it under a different name, which would only blur the field of psychotherapeutic evidence.

TRANSDIAGNOSTIC ISSUES

Another term that has arisen since 2007 is "transdiagnostic," describing psychotherapies and their elements that work across diagnoses. To some degree the rise of this term reflects the divergent adaptations of CBT, some of which are more cognitive and some more behavioral, for a range of differing disorders. Many of these specific CBT adaptations—for example, exposure and response prevention for obsessive-compulsive disorder—have shown impressive efficacy. The problem is that the approaches can so differ that therapists who are expert in one manualized CBT approach may be unskilled in a second one; this has led to a yearning for a single, unified approach that treats multiple diagnoses. IPT, by contrast, has always been "transdiagnostic." The core elements of IPT were developed to treat adults with major depressive disorder (MDD), but they all fundamentally apply wherever they have been tested, for example to bipolar disorder, social anxiety disorder, dysthymic disorder, and bulimia, across age groups and cultures. IPT for primary substance use does not appear efficacious (see Chapter 19).

There seems to be a near universality across cultures to attachment, interpersonal issues, social support, and their relation to psychopathology. A clinician should have familiarity with the target diagnosis when moving from treating MDD to using IPT for another disorder, but the basic IPT approach should fundamentally remain. In using IPT, regardless of diagnosis, the therapist needs to define the target disorder (or symptoms) and its onset, and to identify the focal interpersonal problem area in the patient's current life. The relationship between onset of diagnosis and interpersonal problem area should be maintained.

While we have emphasized diagnosis in treatment studies, IPT in primary care has targeted symptoms, and in resource-poor countries has targeted distress, successfully using the same linkage between focal interpersonal problem area and symptomatology. "Distress" usually includes symptoms of depression and/or anxiety, although other symptomatology is possible.

HOW DOES IPT WORK?

Exactly how any psychotherapy works is unknown. A therapeutic alliance is necessary; the "common factors" (Frank, 1971) play an important role; and specific factors may add to those. We describe below the theoretical (Bowlby, Sullivan, attachment theory) and the empirical (life events research) framework underlying IPT. Here we describe how the elements of IPT link to the framework (Fig. 1.1) and explain the mechanisms of change or how IPT may work.

The genetics underlying depression and all psychiatric disorders remains unknown, although considerable research has provided glimpses of understanding. Most psychiatric disorders run in families with moderate heritability (Guffanti et al., 2016), their expression moderated by the environment or families in which the individual lives. The recognition that the environment influences gene expression—the field of epigenetics—is growing in importance. Situations of environmental stress that threaten attachment, such as the death of a loved one, may be considered the proximal triggers (what IPT classifies as interpersonal problem areas) that can lead to phenotypic change, or symptom onset. IPT attempts to clarify the relationship between symptom onset (change in phenotype) and its trigger (the interpersonal problem area), propelled by the pressure of time-limited treatment. Much of the work in IPT involves helping patients to see the relationship between their environmental triggers and the changed phenotype, then encouraging them to find interpersonal responses to ameliorate the crisis (which is why we have made the arrows in Fig. 1.1 bidirectional).

Sometimes symptoms arise without dramatic environmental triggers and lead to interpersonal difficulties (role disputes or transitions). IPT is ultimately less interested in causality than in the connection between the two.

The nonspecific elements facilitate the relationship, establish trust, and provide some of the therapeutic effects of IPT. IPT uses "common factors" like affective arousal and success experiences (Frank, 1971) particularly effectively, helping patients to tolerate affect and use it as information to create interpersonal successes. The techniques include standardized methods for facilitating dialogue and evoking affect. The interpersonal inventory helps identify both the problem area (trigger) and potential social supports and dangers in the environment that the patient can manage to reduce symptoms.

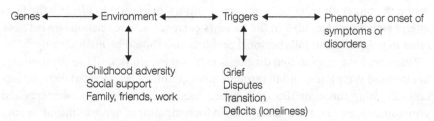

Figure 1.1. A Stress-Diathesis Model.

The diagnostic review, medical model, and psychoeducation in IPT help to clarify symptoms and their onset and to comfort patients about their prognosis and the range of available treatments. The time limit focuses the treatment, sets goals, pressures the work forward without formally assigning homework, and ensures that the therapist and patient consider alternative treatment options if the symptoms do not improve within a reasonable interval. The early work in acute treatment helps patients make the crucial recognition that their interpersonal encounters evoke strong feelings that, rather than being "bad" or "dangerous," provide interpersonal information (e.g., anger means someone is bothering you) they can reflect upon and use to handle their environment. The middle phase of IPT focuses on helping patients to do so. The focus is on the current "here and now" environment, not on the reconstruction of the patient's remote past to understand the current problem. Treatment focuses on the interpersonal meaning of the patient's emotions and how the patient can translate them into action to improve her life. The termination phase summarizes understanding of the process and what the patient has achieved, bolsters autonomy, and concludes acute treatment.

HISTORICAL, THEORETICAL, AND EMPIRICAL BASIS OF IPT

> One of the greatest features of the brain is that it responds to the environment.
>
> —KLERMAN, *circa 1973*

IPT was developed before the explosion in neuroscience and genetics research in psychiatry and before the notion of epigenetics gained prominence. It was developed in the context of refining assessment of new medications for psychiatric disorders and the development of tools to study the environment.

IPT grew from Gerald L. Klerman's belief that vulnerability to depression and other major psychiatric disorders had a biological basis. This was not a mainstream idea in the 1960s, when psychoanalytic thinking and theory dominated psychiatry. Klerman and other rising psychiatric leaders in those days were trained in psychoanalysis. While Klerman received analytic training, he began his research career at the National Institute of Mental Health (NIMH). He was a psychopharmacologist when he began the first large-scale study testing the efficacy of medication (in this case, amitriptyline) and psychotherapy for maintenance treatment of depression (Klerman et al., 1974; Weissman et al., 1981).

The psychotherapy, first called "high contact" in this trial (in contrast to a "low contact condition"), became IPT (Klerman et al., 1984; Markowitz and Weissman, 2012). It was added to the medication trial as a treatment arm in order to mimic clinical practice, as psychotherapy was widely used but had not been defined in manuals suitable for clinical trial testing. We defined high contact/IPT in a manual for the study to ensure reliable training of therapists. The need to test the new psychiatric medications led to the development of rating scales and other tests on which Klerman capitalized for the study of psychotherapy.

The effect of the environment on the brain was a basic tenet of Klerman's thinking. During medical school, he had also studied sociology. As a resident in psychiatry he wrote about the effect of the ward atmosphere and family visits on patients' symptoms. Klerman saw that the brain responded to the environment. Therefore, psychotherapy could work through understanding both the toxic and supportive aspects of the environment in the patient's current life and close interpersonal relations, and relating these to the onset of symptoms. When Weissman joined Klerman in this work, she had just completed social work training, well before earning a Ph.D. in epidemiology. Her training in addressing current, practical social and interpersonal problems and functioning in the "here and now" fit naturally into the development of IPT.

The writings of Adolf Meyer and Harry Stack Sullivan, founders of the interpersonal school, which emphasized the effect of the patient's current psychosocial and interpersonal experience on symptom development, provided compatible theories for this practical therapy. By applying these ideas to depression, three component processes were identified (Klerman et al., 1984):

1. Symptom formation involving the development of depressive affect and the neurovegetative signs and symptoms. This component was hypothesized to be the primary target of medications.
2. Social and interpersonal relations involving interaction with others in social roles. Such relationships may be based on learning from childhood and other experiences, as well as current social reinforcement. This component led to the classification of the IPT focal problem areas. It was hypothesized that the prime target of psychotherapy would be reflected in social functioning.
3. Personality, involving enduring traits such as expression of anger, guilt, self-esteem, interpersonal sensitivity, and communication. These traits may predispose to depression, but it was hypothesized that neither psychotherapy nor medication would greatly affect them. However, successful symptom reduction and social functioning may reduce negative personality traits.

For a more comprehensive historical discussion of the evolution in psychiatric thinking from Freud and the interpersonal school, see Klerman et al. (1984).

Attachment Theory

Bowlby's work on attachment (1969) influenced IPT. Sadness and depressed mood are part of the human condition and a nearly universal response to disruption of close interpersonal relations. Bowlby argued that attachment bonds are necessary to survival: the attachment of the helpless infant to the mother helps to preserve the offspring's biological survival. The continued presence of secure attachment figures helps a child to explore her physical environment and make social and group contacts, and to feel safe and supported in it. Many psychiatric disorders result from inability to make and keep affectional bonds. Disorders often have an onset with the disruption of an attachment bond (Milrod et al., 2014).

Bowlby used these observations to develop a general approach to psychotherapy that included examining current interpersonal relations and how they developed over the life span based on experience with various attachment figures. These ideas appear in IPT problem areas: grief, role disputes, role transitions, and interpersonal deficits of attachment, with the focus mainly on current relationships, not necessarily their past origins. IPT makes explicit the relationship between the symptoms/diagnosis onset and the proximal attachment disruptions. Attachment theory has stimulated a body of empirical research especially on mother–infant attachments (e.g., Fearon et al., 2006), as well as on offspring of depressed parents, attachment disruption of adults (Lipsitz & Markowitz, 2013), and epidemiological studies of social support, social stress, and life events. Related research addressed the importance of social supports as a compensation for loss and conflict (Brown & Harris, 1978). As more sophisticated rating scales were developed, this field became more empirically based.

Studies showing the onset of symptoms and disorders in association with stress, life events, and the long-term consequences of childhood maltreatment (Brown & Harris, 1978; Caspi et al., 2003) have emerged. Accelerating this work, the psychiatric epidemiology revolution beginning in the 1980s provided data on rates, risks, and onset of psychiatric disorders in large community samples (e.g., Kessler et al., 2005). Tools for examining the brain, such as the electroencephalogram (EEG) and magnetic resonance imaging (MRI), have been widely used in psychiatry for studying possible mechanisms. Few studies, however, have yet used such assessments to study IPT outcome (Brody et al., 2001; Martin et al., 2001; Thase et al., 1997).

Psychopharmacology Revolution

The development of IPT was influenced by the availability of new psychopharmacological agents and the need to systematically assess their efficacy in clinical trials. The use of the medical model; taking a medical history; making a diagnosis using systematic, serial assessments; and educating the patient had not been a psychotherapy tradition through the 1960s but developed as an essential part of medication trials. At that time, many practitioners considered medication and psychotherapy antithetical (Armor & Klerman, 1968; Klerman, 1991; Rounsaville et al.,1981), but these medicalized elements have now become more routine in psychiatry. The medical model was incorporated into the IPT initial phase assessment of symptoms—then a radical idea for psychotherapy—and social functioning assessments were encouraged, with flexibility as to which rating scales were used.

Testing IPT in controlled clinical trials, as one would test medication, was essential from the treatment's inception. The first IPT manual (Klerman et al., 1984) was not written until two further clinical trials showed efficacy, comparable to requirements for establishing the efficacy of medication. Clinical trials for adaptations were also required. This proved important when two early clinical trials showed that IPT was not efficacious for treating substance abuse (Carroll et al., 1991; Rounsaville et al., 1983).

Klerman advocated for research standards in psychotherapy that were comparable to those in pharmacotherapy research. He suggested that there be an equivalent of the Food and Drug Administration for psychotherapy (London & Klerman, 1982). Klerman felt that psychotherapy strategies should be specified in a manual with scripts to guide training and communication to ensure that psychotherapy procedures were comparable across therapists. He and Aaron Beck were friends and most respectful of one another. IPT and CBT developed in parallel until Klerman's untimely illness and death, which slowed IPT's development until recently.

EFFICACY AND EFFECTIVENESS

The efficacy of individual IPT for adults with major depression, which forms the platform for the manual, has been tested in many controlled clinical trials (Cuijpers et al., 2011). There are more than 100 clinical trials of IPT (Barth et al., 2013; Cuijpers et al., 2008, 2011, 2016). Based on careful reviews, the efficacy of IPT is well established compared to CBT, medication, and for other forms of mood and non-mood disorders. The efficacy for adaptations of major depression in different formats, age groups, and subtypes is presented in relevant chapters of this book.

An Outline of IPT

As an acute treatment, IPT has three phases: a beginning, a middle, and an end. Each phase lasts a few sessions and has specific tasks. A fourth phase may follow acute treatment: namely, continuation or maintenance treatment, for which therapist and patient contract separately (see Chapter 7). Table 2.1 (located at the end of this chapter) outlines the phases and strategies of IPT for major depression presented in Chapters 2 through 9. Most of the adaptations of IPT for other disorders or treatment populations follow a similar outline, with specific adaptations indicated in each chapter.

INITIAL SESSIONS

As treatment begins, the therapist works to establish a positive treatment alliance by listening carefully; eliciting affect; helping the patient to feel understood by identifying and normalizing feelings; and providing support, encouragement, and psychoeducation about depression. At the same time, the therapist has a sequence of tasks specific to IPT. Defining and diagnosing depression, exploring the patient's interpersonal inventory of current relationships to find potential social supports and interpersonal difficulties, providing the sick role, defining an interpersonal focus, and linking the focus to the depressive diagnosis in a focal formulation are key steps that set the stage for subsequent phases of the treatment. These initial steps also tend to provide early symptomatic relief.

Here are the steps for diagnosing depression:

1. Review the depressive symptoms or syndrome. Assess the patient's symptoms and their severity. Use a symptom presentation from the DSM-5 or ICD-11 to help the patient understand the diagnosis. Use a scale such as the Hamilton Rating Scale for Depression (Hamilton, 1960), the Beck Depression Inventory (Beck, 1978), QIDS (Rush et al., 2003), or PHQ-9 (Kroenke et al., 2001) to help the patient understand the severity and the nature of her symptoms. The Ham-D and the PHQ-9 appear in the appendices of this book. Explain what the score means, and alert the patient that you will be repeating the scale regularly to see

how treatment is progressing. (For a fuller range of depression and other rating scales, see APA & Rush, 2000.)

2. Give the syndrome a name: *"You are suffering from major depression."* Explain depression as a medical illness, and explain its treatment. Depression is an *illness*, a *treatable* illness, and *not the patient's fault.* Despite its symptom of hopelessness, depression has a good prognosis. Explain that you will be repeating the depression scale periodically so that both you and the patient can assess her progress.

3. Give the patient the **sick role**: *"If there are things you can't do because you're feeling depressed, that's not your fault: you're ill."* However, the patient has a responsibility to work *as* a patient to get better.

4. Set a **time limit**. Explain to the patient that IPT is a time-limited treatment that focuses on the relationship between interactions with other people and how she is feeling. You will be meeting for X weekly sessions (define the number: generally eight to sixteen sessions in as many weeks), and the patient has a good chance of feeling better soon.

5. Evaluate the patient's need for medication. Prescribing medication may depend on symptom severity, comorbidity, the patient's treatment preference, and other factors. Many patients may recover from major depression with IPT alone. (If you do not prescribe medications, consider having the patient consult with someone who does.)

6. Relate depression to an interpersonal context by reviewing with the patient her current and past interpersonal relationships. Explain their connection to the current depressive symptoms. Determine with the patient the **interpersonal inventory**:
   • Nature of interaction with significant persons: How close does the patient get to others? How does she express anger?
   • Expectations of the patient and significant persons; differentiate them from one another and discuss whether these expectations were fulfilled
   • Satisfying and unsatisfying aspects of the relationships
   • Changes the patient wants in the relationships

7. Identify a **focal problem area**: grief, role disputes, role transitions, or interpersonal deficits.
   • Determine the problem area related to current depression, and set the treatment goals.
   • Determine which key relationship or aspect of a relationship is related to the depression and what might change in it.

8. Explain the IPT concepts and contract. Outline your understanding of the problem, linking illness to a life situation in a **formulation**:

You're suffering from depression, and that seems to have something to do with what's going on in your life. We call that (complicated bereavement, a role dispute, etc.). I suggest that we spend the next X weeks working on solving that difficult life crisis. If you can solve that problem, your depression is likely to lift as well. Does that make sense to you?

9. Agree on treatment goals and determine which problem area will be the focus. Obtain the patient's explicit agreement on the focus.
10. Describe the procedures of IPT. Clarify the focus on current issues, stress the need for the patient to discuss important concerns, review the patient's current interpersonal relations, and discuss the practical aspects of the treatment (length, frequency, times, fees, policy for missed appointments, and confidentiality).

INTERMEDIATE SESSIONS: THE PROBLEM AREAS

With the patient's agreement to your formulation, you will enter the middle phase of treatment and spend all but the final few sessions working on one of the four IPT problem areas: grief, role dispute, transitions, or deficits. During this time, remember to:

- Maintain a supportive treatment alliance: Listen and sympathize.
- Keep the treatment centered on the focus, as your treatment contract specified you would.
- Provide psychoeducation about depression where appropriate to excuse the patient for low energy, guilt, and so on.
- Pull for affect (do not be afraid to let it linger in the room).
- Focus on interpersonal encounters and how the patient handled them:
  - What the patient felt
  - What the patient said (content)
  - How the patient said it (emotional tone)
- If things went well, congratulate the patient, and reinforce adaptive social functioning.
- If things went badly, sympathize and explore other options.
- In either case, link the patient's mood to the interpersonal outcome.
- Role play interpersonal options.
- Summarize the sessions at their end.
- Regularly (e.g., every three or four weeks) repeat the depression measure to assess symptom severity.

TERMINATION

The third phase of IPT ends the acute treatment. Review with the patient the progress of the previous sessions. If the patient has improved, ensure that she takes credit: "*Why are you better?*" Discuss what has been accomplished and what remains to be considered. Address termination several weeks before it is actually scheduled. If the patient remains symptomatic, consider a further course of treatment, such as maintenance IPT, the addition of medication, a different medication, or a different kind of psychotherapy.

Table 2.1 IPT OUTLINE

Therapist's Role

Be the patient's advocate (not neutral).
Be active, not passive.
Therapeutic relationship is not interpreted as transference.
Therapeutic relationship is not a friendship.

Initial Sessions

1. Diagnose the depression and its interpersonal context.
2. Explain depression as a medical illness and present the various treatment options.
3. Evaluate need for medication.
4. Elicit interpersonal inventory to assess potential social support and problem areas.
5. Formulation: Relate depression to interpersonal context (derived from interpersonal inventory).
6. Explain IPT concepts, contract.
7. Define the framework and structure of treatment and set a time limit.
8. Give the patient the sick role.

Intermediate Sessions				
	Grief/Complicated Bereavement	Role Disputes	Role Transitions	Interpersonal Deficits
Goals	1. Facilitate the mourning process. 2. Help the patient re-establish interests and relationships.	1. Identify the dispute. 2. Explore options, and choose a plan of action. 3. Modify expectations or faulty communications to bring about a satisfactory resolution.	1. Facilitate mourning and acceptance of the loss of the old role. 2. Help the patient to regard the new role in a more positive light. 3. Help the patient restore self-esteem.	1. Reduce the patient's social isolation. 2. Encourage the patient to form new relationships.
Strategies	Review depressive symptoms/ syndrome. Relate symptom onset to the death of the significant other. Reconstruct the patient's relationship with the deceased.	Review depressive symptoms/ syndrome. Relate the symptom onset to an overt or covert dispute with significant other with whom the patient is currently involved.	Review depressive symptoms/ syndrome. Relate depressive symptoms to difficulty in coping with a recent life change. Review positive and negative aspects of old and new roles.	Review depressive symptoms/ syndrome. Relate depressive symptoms to problems of social isolation or lack of fulfillment.

| Strategies | Describe the sequence and consequences of events just prior to, during, and after the death.

Explore associated feelings (negative as well as positive).

Once affect emerges, tolerate it in the room. | Determine the stage of dispute:

1. Renegotiation (calm the participants to facilitate resolution)
2. Impasse (increase disharmony in order to reopen negotiation)
3. Dissolution (assist mourning)

Understand how nonreciprocal role expectations relate to the dispute:

What are the issues in the dispute?

What are the differences in expectations and values?

What are the options?

What is the likelihood of finding alternatives?

What resources are available to bring about change in the relationship?

Are there parallels in other relationships?

What is the patient gaining?

What unspoken assumptions lie behind the patient's behavior?

How is the dispute being perpetuated? | Explore the patient's feelings about what is lost.

Explore the patient's feelings about the change itself.

Explore opportunities in the new role.

Realistically evaluate what is lost.

Encourage appropriate release of affect.

Encourage development of social support system and of new skills called for in new role. | Review past significant relationships, including their negative and positive aspects.

Explore repetitive patterns in relationships.

Discuss the patient's positive and negative feelings about the therapist, and encourage the patient to seek parallels in other relationships. |

(continued)

Table 2.1 CONTINUED

Termination Phase

1. Explicitly discuss termination.
2. Acknowledge that termination is a time of (healthy) sadness—a role transition.
3. Move toward the patient's recognition of independent competence.
4. Deal with nonresponse:
   - Minimize the patient's self-blame by blaming the treatment.
   - Emphasize alternative treatment options.
5. Assess the need for continuation/maintenance treatment.
   - Renegotiate the treatment contract.

How to Conduct IPT

What Is IPT?

OVERVIEW

IPT is a time-limited, specified psychotherapy developed initially for patients with major depressive disorder (MDD) and later adapted for other disorders as well. Designed for administration by experienced and trained mental health professionals, it has also been taught clinically to less trained personnel. IPT has been used with and without medication (see Klerman, Weissman, Rounsaville, & Chevron, 1984; Weissman, Markowitz, & Klerman, 2000); for a brief history of IPT, see Weissman (2006). The description of IPT presented here illustrates the treatment of patients with MDD because that is its best established and most widely employed use. IPT for depression provided the basis for other adaptations. The approach applies across a range of age groups with MDD and to many other disorders. Adaptations for other age groups and subtypes of depression and for non-mood disorders are described in Sections III and IV.

Depression usually occurs in the context of a social and an interpersonal event. Some common events are:

- a marriage breaks up
- a dispute threatens an important relationship
- a spouse loses interest and has an affair
- a job is lost or in jeopardy
- a move to a new neighborhood takes place
- a natural or unnatural disaster leads to dislocation
- a loved one dies
- a promotion or demotion occurs
- a person retires
- a medical illness is diagnosed
- circumstances lead to loneliness and isolation

Understanding the social and interpersonal context of the development of the depression may help to unravel the immediate precipitants for the symptoms. This can be the first step in helping the patient to understand depression as an illness and to develop new ways of dealing with people and situations. Developing these new social skills can treat the current episode and reduce future vulnerability.

There are several appropriate treatments for depression. A range of effective medications and several empirically validated psychotherapies exist. Often medications and psychotherapy are used in combination. It is in the best interest of the depressed patient to have a variety of beneficial treatments available, with scientific testing prerequisite to claims of such benefit. IPT easily meets that criterion of proof.

IPT can be an important alternative to medication for patients seeking to avoid antidepressant medications, such as pregnant or nursing women, elderly or ill people who are already taking multiple medications and have difficulties with side effects, depressed patients about to undergo surgery, and patients who just do not want to take medication. Psychotherapy may also particularly benefit patients who find themselves in life crises and need to make important decisions, such as what to do about a failing relationship or a jeopardized career, or who are struggling to mourn the death of a significant other. This in no way devalues the importance of medication as antidepressant treatment. Medication may be especially helpful for patients who need rapid symptomatic relief; have severely symptomatic, melancholic, or delusional depression; who do not respond to psychotherapy; or who simply do not want to talk about their problems with a therapist. This eclectic view of treatment is part of the pragmatic clinical philosophy of IPT.

CONCEPT OF DEPRESSION IN IPT

IPT is based on the idea that the symptoms of depression have multiple causes, genetic and environmental. Whatever the causes, however, depression does not arise in a vacuum. Depressive symptoms are usually associated with something going on in the patient's current personal life, usually in association with people the patient feels close to. Indeed, if an environmental or interpersonal event does not trigger the depressive episode, then the onset of depression will breed interpersonal problems, so patients generally present with depression and interpersonal difficulties that the IPT therapist can link. The IPT therapist does not really care which comes first, because the goal is not to find a *cause* for the depressive episode, but rather to link mood to interpersonal state. It is useful to identify and learn how to deal with those personal problems and to understand their relationship to the onset of symptoms.

The IPT therapist views depression as having three parts:

1. *Symptoms.* The emotional, cognitive, and physical symptoms of depression include depressed and anxious mood, difficulty concentrating, indecisiveness, pessimistic outlook, guilt, sleeping and eating disturbances, loss of interest and pleasure in life, fatigue, and suicidality.

2. *Social and Interpersonal Life.* Depression affects the social network and ability to get along with other important people in the patient's life (e.g., family, friends, work associates). Social supports protect against depression, whereas social stressors increase vulnerability for depression. Interpersonal dysfunction follows from depression and may also present a vulnerability for depression. If you don't know how to say "no" to others, or to express your needs, life goes poorly and may push you into a depressive episode. Once depressed, the ability to express your feelings to others deteriorates.

3. *Personality.* People have enduring patterns for dealing with life: how they assert themselves, express their angers and hurts, and maintain their self-esteem; whether they are shy, aggressive, inhibited, or suspicious. These interpersonal patterns may contribute to developing or maintaining depression. Depressed individuals frequently describe longstanding passivity, avoidance of confrontations, and general social risk avoidance; these depressive tactics may lead to depressing outcomes.

Some therapists begin by trying to treat a person's personality difficulties and see personality as the underlying cause of depression. The IPT therapist does not try to treat personality and, in fact, recognizes that many behaviors that appear enduring and lifelong may be a reflection of the depression itself. Patients may seem dependent, self-preoccupied, and irritable while depressed, yet when the depression lifts, these supposedly lasting traits also disappear or recede (Markowitz et al., 2015a). This is the notorious clinical confusion between depressive *state* and personality *trait.*

The thrust of IPT is to try to understand the interpersonal context in which the depressive symptoms arose and how they relate to the current social and personal context. The IPT therapist looks for what is currently happening in the patient's life, the "here and now" problems, rather than problems in childhood or the past.

The goal is to encourage coping with current problems and the development of self-reliance outside of the therapeutic situation. The brief time limit of the treatment rules out any major reconstruction of personality. Many patients feel much better once their depression lifts. A time-limited, time-specified psychotherapy can help therapists and patients focus on goals and provide patients with the hope that they will feel better within a short period of time. Although IPT has been used for as long as three years as a maintenance treatment (Chapter 9), most psychotherapy in practice is brief. There is nothing to preclude a renegotiation of the time—adding continuation or maintenance to acute treatment—at the expiration of the acute time-specified treatment. On the other hand, if IPT has not been helpful at the end of its time-limited intervention, it may be appropriate to reconsider the treatment plan.

For psychiatric disorders, the most important environment consists of close personal attachments. These connections, their availability, and their disruption (or threat of disruption) can powerfully influence the emergence of symptoms (phenotypic expression), especially in genetically vulnerable individuals.

Situations in which these disruptions can be found and where symptoms may erupt have been defined as the focal problem areas in IPT. These are:

- grief (complicated bereavement)
- interpersonal role disputes
- interpersonal role transitions
- interpersonal deficits (isolation; paucity of attachments).

You can use IPT with patients who develop symptoms in association with any of these situations. Almost any depressed patient will fall into one of the four categories; the first three—life event–focused categories—are preferable to the last. We cannot readily alter genetic vulnerability, but we can improve social functioning, and through it, the environment. Symptoms can improve with the clarification, the understanding, and—especially—the management of these interpersonal situations associated with symptom onset. Psychotherapy can be crucial to this change. Evidence shows that the IPT paradigm works for major depression in patients of all ages and is applicable to other psychiatric disorders as well.

GOALS OF IPT

The goals of IPT are (1) to reduce the symptoms of depression (i.e., to improve mood, sleep, appetite, energy, and general outlook on life) and (2) to help the patient deal better with the people and life situations associated with the onset of symptoms. In fact, the patient is likely to achieve both goals. If the patient can solve an important interpersonal crisis (e.g., a role transition), this not only will improve her life but also should alleviate the depressive symptoms.

The IPT therapist focuses, within a time-limited treatment, on:

- current problems
- people who are important in the patient's current life
- linking interpersonal problems to symptom onset
- the patient's affect (both positive and negative feelings)
- helping patients to master present problems by recognizing their emotional responses to those situations; understanding these responses as helpful rather than "bad" feelings; and finding ways to effectively express them to address crises, gather social support, and develop friendships and relationships.

The IPT therapist does not:

- interpret dreams
- allow treatment to continue indefinitely
- delve extensively into early childhood

- encourage free association
- encourage dependence on the treatment or therapist
- focus on cognitions

The therapist views the patient as a person in distress, suffering from a treatable illness, and having symptoms that can be dealt with in the present. The IPT therapist wants to know:

- when the symptoms began
- what was happening in the patient's life when they began
- current stressors
- the people involved in these present stressors
- disputes and disappointments
- the patient's means of coping with these problems
- the patient's strengths
- the patient's interpersonal difficulties
- whether the patient can talk about situations that evoke guilt, shame, or resentment.

The IPT therapist:

- elicits affect, including negative affects like anxiety and anger
- helps the patient to explore options (rather than offering direct advice, this is often best accomplished by asking questions that allow patients to describe their own options)
- provides psychoeducation and corrects misinformation about depression
- helps the patient to develop resources outside the office.

The IPT therapist does not focus on why the patients became who they are. The goal is to find a way out of the problems, not the route in. Thus, IPT does not focus on:

- childhood
- character
- psychodynamic defenses
- the origins of guilt, shame, or resentment (these are understood to be symptoms of depressive illness)
- fantasy life or insight into the origins of the behavior.

UNDERSTANDING HOW THE DEPRESSION BEGAN

To develop an understanding of how the depressive episode began and the current context in which it arose, the patient might answer the following questions:

1. What problems are you facing at the moment?
2. Who are the people who are important to you these days? Who are potential social supports, and from whom may you have become estranged?
3. When did you start feeling depressed, sad, blue?
4. What was going on in your life when you started to feel depressed? Have any upsetting events occurred? Has anyone close to you died?
5. Are you involved in disputes or disagreements with other people in your life right now? How are you dealing with these disputes?
6. What are your current disappointments? How are you dealing with them?
7. What situations make you feel guilty, ashamed, or angry?
8. What are your stresses?
9. What do you see as the things that you can do well (or were able to do well before you got depressed)?

FACTS ABOUT DEPRESSION

These facts, well known to most mental health professionals, may help to educate the patient about depression:

- Major depression is one of the most common psychiatric disorders, affecting 3 to 4 percent of individuals at any time.
- Depression is more common in women than in men. (This is reassuring for women patients but is not something therapists should necessarily emphasize to men, who may feel diminished by hearing it.)
- Depression is otherwise an equal opportunity disorder. It occurs across countries, levels of education, and occupations. It affects rich and poor and people of all races and cultures.
- Depression (like other medical illnesses) runs in families and has serious consequences for family life.
- Depression often begins in adolescence and young adulthood and may recur throughout life.
- There are many effective treatments for depression, including medications and certain psychotherapies. Sometimes these treatments are combined.
- Depression tends to be a recurrent disorder. Some patients will need treatments for long periods. Others will have one bout and never have another period of symptoms.
- No one treatment works for all individuals or all types of depression. If one treatment does not work after a sufficient time, the therapist and the patient ought to consider another. (Indeed, if IPT has not helped after the initial time period, the therapist and the patient should consider switching or augmenting it.)

Something to consider telling a patient:

Fleeting moments of feeling sad and blue or depressed are a normal part of the human condition. Such passing mood changes tell individuals that something is upsetting in their lives. Clinical depression is different: it is persistent and impairing and includes a range of symptoms.

There are different types of depression, and it will help your patients for you to provide a precise diagnosis: MDD, dysthymic (persistent depressive) disorder (Chapter 17), or bipolar disorder (Chapter 18).

MAJOR DEPRESSIVE DISORDER

MDD, the most common of the depressions, includes a sad or dysphoric mood and loss of interest or pleasure in all or almost all of one's usual activities or pastimes. This mood persists for at least several weeks and is associated with other symptoms that occur nearly every day, including disturbance in appetite (loss of or increase in appetite); changes in weight; sleep disturbance (trouble falling asleep, waking up in the middle of the night and not being able to return to sleep, waking up early in the morning and feeling dreadful); and a loss of interest and pleasure in food, sex, work, family, friends, and so on. Agitation, a sluggish feeling, a decrease in energy, feelings of worthlessness or guilt, difficulty in concentrating or thinking, thoughts of death, a feeling that life is not worth living, suicide attempts, or even suicide are other symptoms of depression. According to the fifth edition of the *Diagnostic and Statistical Manual of Mental Disorders* (DSM-5), patients who express at least five of nine symptoms, persisting for several weeks and resulting in an impaired ability to care for self or family or to go to work and carry out daily life, and excluding other physical causes such as hypothyroidism, meet the criteria for MDD (see Table 4.1 in the next chapter).

It has long been known that different forms of MDD exist, defined by particular groups of symptoms, and many subtypes have been suggested. The subtype with the most important treatment implications is **delusional depression**. Delusional, or psychotic, depression includes the usual depressive symptoms as well as psychotic distortions of thinking consistent with depressive themes such as guilt, self-blame, a feeling of inadequacy, or a belief that one deserves punishment. People with delusional depression may feel that the depression came on because they are bad or deserve to be depressed. Delusional depression is infrequent. When it occurs, it requires medication or electroconvulsive therapy and usually cannot be treated by any psychotherapy alone, including IPT.

DYSTHYMIC DISORDER/PERSISTENT DEPRESSIVE DISORDER

Renamed persistent depressive disorder in DSM-5, the main feature of dysthymic disorder is a chronic disturbance of mood (i.e., sad or blue feelings, loss of interest in activities, low energy), but the symptoms lack sufficient severity to meet the criteria for MDD. Nonetheless, they are constant. They must persist for at least two years to be considered dysthymic disorder but frequently last for decades. Such individuals often mistake this chronic depression for their "melancholic" personality and may not seek treatment, seeing the problem as a personality trait that cannot be changed. Yet the chronicity of dysthymic disorder sometimes makes it more debilitating than episodic major depression, and it is treatable. IPT has been adapted to these symptoms and tested in patients with dysthymic disorder (Browne et al., 2002; Markowitz, 1998; Markowitz, Kocsis, Christos, Bleiberg, & Carlin, 2008; Markowitz, Kocsis, Bleiberg, Christos, & Sacks, 2005).

BIPOLAR DISORDER

Bipolar disorder includes manic states in addition to depression. Mania is a predominant mood that is elevated (feeling high, euphoric), expansive, or irritable. Accompanying this mood are excess activity, racing thoughts, a feeling of power, excessively high self-esteem, decreased need for sleep, distractibility, and impulsive involvement in activities that have a high potential for painful consequences, such as excessive spending or sexual activities. Bipolar disorder may also involve psychotic symptoms. IPT has been adapted and has shown benefit as an adjunct to medication for patients with bipolar disorder. Patients with bipolar I disorder require medication.

MILD DEPRESSION

Many persons have mild or subsyndromal depression (e.g., symptoms such as sleep problems or loss of interest that do not reach the threshold criteria for MDD). These states are referred to by different names, such as minor depression, depression not otherwise specified, mixed anxiety/depression, and adjustment disorder with depressed mood. People with these milder symptoms often do not seek treatment or are seen by their family doctor, a primary care practice, or a practitioner in a health maintenance organization (HMO) (see Chapter 16). If these symptoms persist, they should not be ignored, as they are impairing and can interfere with the patient's quality of life and productivity. Moreover, minor depressive symptoms increase the risk for developing MDD.

IPT has been increasingly used outside of the United States for patients in health clinics who have mild depressive and/or anxious symptoms. They may not meet criteria for a major disorder but report distress. Some of these patients face chronic severe stressors. Although IPT has generally emphasized the importance of a medical model, in such circumstances, as for Interpersonal Counseling (Chapter 16), the term "symptoms" or "distress" may be used instead of depression.

Beginning IPT

This chapter describes the technical aspects of how to begin IPT, including how to assess depression and complete the tasks of the first sessions. Clinicians who are experienced in assessing depression can skip this section. We first describe the tasks of the opening sessions and explain how to carry them out. The order may vary slightly depending on the patient's clinical presentation, but by the end of the first phase, as the therapist, you should ensure that every task has been covered. You should strive to keep the initial phase of IPT brief, seeking to reach the middle phase as soon as possible.

TASKS OF THE INITIAL VISITS

During the first three (or, if possible, fewer) visits, the IPT therapist takes a clinical history, collecting information about the patient's symptoms and current interpersonal situation. This allows you to make a psychiatric diagnosis and to select an interpersonal focus for the treatment. If the patient has not had a recent physical examination, especially if the patient is over the age of 50, recommend one to rule out physical explanations for depressive symptoms (e.g., hypothyroidism).

During the first visits the therapist:

1. Reviews the depressive symptoms and makes a diagnosis
2. Explains depression as a medical illness and describes the various treatment options
3. Evaluates the need for medication
4. Reviews the patient's current interpersonal world (the "interpersonal inventory") in order to diagnose the context in which the depression has arisen
5. Presents a formulation, linking the patient's illness to an interpersonal focus
6. Makes a treatment contract based on the formulation, and explains what to expect in treatment

7. Defines the framework and structure of treatment, including a time limit

8. Gives the patient the "sick role."

REVIEW THE SYMPTOMS AND MAKE THE DIAGNOSIS

Numerous scales have been developed to measure depressive symptoms (Rush et al., 2007). Among them, the Hamilton Rating Scale for Depression (Ham-D; Hamilton, 1960; see Appendix A) is a clinician-administered scale that has been used the longest and most widely, including in most studies of IPT. Many clinics now use self-report paper-and-pencil or computerized scales such as the Beck Depression Inventory (Beck, 1978) or PHQ-9 (Kroenke et al., 2001) in initial patient screening. The Ham-D does not diagnose depression but is a useful guide to help determine the specific symptoms and degree of suffering that depressed patients experience.

The Ham-D assesses symptoms that patients have experienced over the course of the previous week. In general, a total Ham-D score of 7 or less is considered normal, not depressed. A score of 9 to 12 indicates mild depression, usually not reaching the threshold of major depressive disorder (MDD). A score of 13 to 19 is consistent with moderate depression. A score of 20 or more indicates moderate to severe depression. A score of 30 or higher is clearly severe depression.

Antidepressant medication is likely to be helpful for any elevation in depressive symptoms, but patients with scores in the high 20s or in the 30s may require medication as part of their treatment in order to ensure an optimal outcome. This is not to say that IPT will not benefit patients with such high scores, but combined treatment may be preferable to monotherapy.

Whatever scale you use, plan to repeatedly administer it to your depressed patients over the course of IPT. Showing the patient symptoms on a standardized scale helps her to realize that what often feels like something personally bad and toxic is in fact a long-defined syndrome: the Hamilton scale has been around longer than many of the patients you may use it with. These outside sources thus contribute to psychoeducation and to making the disorder discrete and ego-alien. Repeating the scale periodically helps you and the patient to measure the progress of treatment. Simply seeing the symptoms listed on a scale may help to convince the patient that they are symptoms, not personal flaws. The frequency with which you repeat the scale is less important than doing it regularly: for example, every three or four weeks until the patient reaches remission (Ham-D < 8).

We recommend using the DSM-5 (American Psychiatric Association, 2013) or ICD-10 criteria to formally diagnose major depression, again giving the patient the opportunity to distinguish disorder from self. Emphasize that this is a treatable condition that is not the patient's fault. Table 4.1 lists the DSM-5 criteria for major depression.

Table 4.1 DSM-5 CRITERIA FOR MAJOR DEPRESSION

American Psychiatric Association Diagnostic Criteria (DSM-5) for Major Depression

---

A. At least five of the following symptoms are present during the same two-week period nearly every day. At least one of the symptoms is either (1) depressed mood or (2) loss of interest or pleasure.
  1. Depressed mood most of the day, nearly every day
  2. Diminished interest or pleasure in all or almost all activities, most of the day
  3. Significant weight loss or weight gain when not dieting, or decrease or increase in appetite
  4. Insomnia or hypersomnia (oversleeping) nearly every day
  5. Psychomotor agitation or retardation nearly every day (observable by others)
  6. Fatigue or loss of energy
  7. Feeling of worthlessness or excessive or inappropriate guilt
  8. Diminished ability to think, concentrate, or make a decision
  9. Recurrent thoughts of death or suicide, a suicide attempt, or a specific plan for committing suicide

B. The symptoms cause clinically significant distress or impairment.

C. The episode is not attributable to the physiological effects of a substance or to another medical condition.

D. The occurrence of the major depressive episode is not better explained by schizoaffective disorder, schizophrenia, schizophreniform disorder, delusional disorder, or other specified and unspecified schizophrenia spectrum and other psychotic disorders.

E. There has never been a manic episode or a hypomanic episode.

Reprinted with permission from the Diagnostic and Statistical Manual of Mental Disorders, Fifth Edition, *(Copyright © 2013). American Psychiatric Association. All Rights Reserved.*

ANXIETY, ALCOHOL, DRUGS

It is important to assess substance use as a potential confound or comorbidity compounding depression. Ask patients about the frequency and severity of alcohol use and the presence of related symptoms (hangovers, blackouts, seizures) and other drug use.

EXPLAIN THE DIAGNOSIS AND TREATMENT OPTIONS

Once you have established that the patient has MDD, explain to the patient what depression is. While recognizing the patient's suffering, be clinically optimistic about the future. You might say something like:

I understand that you're feeling awful. Depression is a treatable illness, and your chances of getting better are very good. You've said that you're feeling hopeless, but that hopelessness is a symptom of depression, not your true prognosis.

Your clinical hopefulness does not mean that you should discount the patient's current suffering. It is also important to explain to the patient any comorbid diagnosis and how this may influence treatment.

We suggest that you first explain which of the patient's symptoms are part of the depressive diagnosis (e.g., sleep, guilt). Then educate the patient about depression in general:

Depression is a common disorder. It affects 3 to 4 percent of adults at any one time. Depression may feel like a hopeless condition, but that hopelessness is a symptom of the depression—it's not your prognosis. Even though you are suffering now, depression does respond to treatment. The outlook for your recovery with treatment is excellent. There are many effective treatments available— many different medications and different psychotherapies—so you do not need to feel pessimistic even if the first one does not work.

Most people with depression recover quickly with treatment, and some even recover without treatment, although that may take longer. The prognosis is good, even though some people may need continuing treatment for extended periods in order to prevent recurrence. Once you receive treatment, you should return to normal functioning when the symptoms disappear.

THERAPIST NOTE

Dysthymic, chronically depressed patients may actually improve with treatment to better functioning than what they have for too long considered "normal."

While you are depressed you may not feel like socializing or doing things that you usually do. You may need to explain this to your family members. However, you are going to be actively engaged in treatment and will be working hard toward recovery. The expectation is that, as you recover, you will resume your normal activities and should get back to normal, if not better. In fact, there is every reason to hope that you will be better than before, although it may be hard to believe this now, when you're feeling down and helpless and hopeless.

The underlying message is that depression is a disorder over which the patient does not have full control, but from which the patient is likely to recover without serious residual damage. Treatment will hasten recovery.

Depression is *not* a failure, a punishment for past misconduct, or even a deliberate act. It is not something the patient has willed. In fact, it is important to emphasize that:

- Depression is a treatable medical illness.
- Depression is not the patient's fault.
- No one wants or tries to be depressed.

With many patients, it may be useful to recognize that suffering from depression represents a kind of vulnerability, in the same way that having diabetes or hypertension represents other types of vulnerability.

EVALUATE THE NEED FOR MEDICATION

Although an extensive literature supports the use of medication and psychotherapy alone and in combination in the treatment of depression (Cuijpers et al., 2013; Karyotaki et al., 2016), empirical studies have not determined when one approach will be superior to another for an individual patient. The recommendation of medication for a particular patient generally depends on the severity of symptoms, the patient's preference, the history of treatment response, and medical contraindication. If the patient has severe sleep and appetite disturbance, agitation, retardation, loss of interest in life, difficulty in thinking coherently; if there are no medical contraindications; and if the burden of depressive symptoms is severe, medication should probably be recommended, either alone or in combination with psychotherapy. As medication tends to work faster than psychotherapy, high suicide risk is a particular indication for medication—in addition to psychotherapy—for depressed patients. Indeed, high suicide risk may indicate the need for combined psychotherapy and pharmacotherapy. Pregnancy and lactation may be relative contraindications for medication. If you are not a physician, consider consulting with a psychiatrist about the need for medication with a depressed patient.

The presence of a life stress that brought on the depression does not preclude the use of medication, either with or without psychotherapy. If the patient is already taking medication but depressive symptoms persist, IPT can be added as an augmentation strategy. Because IPT and pharmacotherapy share a medical model of depression as an illness with both biological and environmental features, IPT is neatly compatible with antidepressant medication.

REVIEW THE PATIENT'S CURRENT PROBLEMS
IN RELATIONSHIP TO DEPRESSION
(INTERPERSONAL INVENTORY)

Once you have determined that your patient has clinical depression, explore what is going on in the patient's current social and family life that may be associated with the onset of the symptoms. In preparation for the subsequent sessions of IPT, you and the patient will choose one (or at most two) focal interpersonal problem areas to work on. The choices, again, are *grief, role dispute, role transition*, or *interpersonal deficits*. Choosing a problem area helps you and the patient to focus the therapy on the depression and the events surrounding it, rather than digressing into unstructured discussion on any topic that might surface.

Review who the *key people* are in the patient's life to get a full picture of her interpersonal connections. Explore the quality of important relationships:

- How close to people does the patient get? Can she confide intimate feelings and express needs or disagreements?
- To whom can the patient turn for support (even if she has withdrawn and is not using social supports at present)?
- Does the patient express anger when another person bothers her ("I don't like it when you . . .")? How effectively? How much comfort does the patient have in expressing her wishes ("I want . . .") and needs? These are typically difficult maneuvers for depressed patients.
- What beneficial and maladaptive patterns can you find in the patient's interactions with important others?

There are different ways to obtain this information, but the goal is to define the current primary problems temporally and emotionally related to the onset or maintenance of depressive symptoms. When reviewing important ties that may have relevance to the patient's symptoms, keep a broad perspective. Consider the family, roommates, friends, coworkers, and other members of the social circle (Weissman, 2016).

It is useful to begin with a review. Some of the following questions may be helpful:

What was going on in your life and what was happening around the time you started feeling bad—at work, at home, with your family and friends? Had anything changed?

It is best to leave these questions open-ended. Some withdrawn patients may require more specific prompting:

When you started to feel depressed, what was happening in your life? Was there a disappointment in a relationship? Did your marriage begin to have problems? Were you and your children or parents in a dispute? Did your child leave home? Did you start a new job? Did someone move in with you? Did you yourself move? Was it the anniversary of someone's death? Were you put in situations where you had to meet new people and establish relationships?

Such life circumstances are often associated with depression. Try to determine—and help the patient try to understand—what might have triggered the onset of this depressive episode. Even if you can find no precipitant for the depressive episode, upsetting life situations are likely to emerge as consequences of the depressive episode itself. Strains in relationships (role disputes) and life changes—such as ending a relationship or job (role transitions)—may follow the onset of depressive symptoms. These still qualify as possible focal areas for IPT, inasmuch as IPT focuses on the connection between one's life situation and mood rather than causality.

Asking these questions may help you to find a social and an interpersonal context for the patient's depression. Your aim will be to link the patient's interpersonal situation (a spouse's affair, a mother's death, a move to a different city) to the onset of symptoms in a brief contextualizing narrative that makes sense to both the patient and you. Patient self-report forms have been developed to assess problem areas (Weissman, 2005).

The problem areas on which IPT therapists focus treatment fall into four groups, as listed in Table 4.2.

Obviously these problem areas are not mutually exclusive, and you may find that what the patient thought was the central problem is merely the tip of an iceberg. Use the initial sessions to ensure that you have focused on a pivotal, emotionally meaningful area for the patient and that you have ruled out surprises that might otherwise arise later in treatment. Choosing a good focus is essential to an organized and focused therapy for patients whose depression may cause disorganization, distractibility, and poor concentration.

Most depressed people have more than one interpersonal problem area. For the purpose of organizing the therapy and helping to treat a major depressive episode, however, you should focus on one (or at most two) during the course of the treatment. One is preferable. To choose multiple foci risks diluting the treatment so that there is no real focus at all. We recognize that selecting only one is not always easy, especially for clinicians without prior experience in time-limited therapies. However, our experience is that, with some practice, most clinicians are able to correctly select the main focus. Research has found that IPT therapists agree in choosing a primary focus (Markowitz et al., 2000).

Table 4.2 IPT PROBLEM AREAS

Problem Area	Life Situation
Grief	*Complicated bereavement* following the death of a significant other or close relative (Chapter 5)
Role dispute	*Struggle*, disagreement with spouse, lover, child, other family member, friend, or coworker (Chapter 6)
Role transition	*Life change*: graduation, a new job, leaving one's family, divorce, going away to school, a move, a new home, retirement, medical illness, immigration (Chapter 7)
Interpersonal deficits	*No acute life events*: none of the above. Paucity of attachments, loneliness, social isolation, boredom. (This category does *not* necessarily mean the patient has a personality disorder.) (Chapter 8)

In working on complicated grief over the death of a loved one, you may help the patient to handle role disputes with other family members while still focusing the overall treatment on the grief. It is preferable to keep things simple, keeping sorrow as the overarching topic, rather than to give the patient a laundry list of interpersonal problems. Sometimes the patient's problems may change during the course of treatment (particularly, of course, in the maintenance phase). For example, a woman who comes in saying, "My children are my big problem" may later, as she gets to know you, bring up the more pressing area of distress: her spouse's extramarital affair. (Again, it is best to try to uncover this at the start.) The idea is to identify the most recent and most disturbing stresses at the outset.

Some patients initially concentrate on the physical symptoms of depression, such as sleep and appetite disturbance, because they feel these to be the most distressing. They may not believe that there is a connection between their life circumstances and these symptoms, or they may either secretly or openly fear having some undetected physical illness. Although this is often only a fear, depressive symptoms can appear in the context of a variety of physical illnesses, and depressive patients tend to neglect their physical health. Hence a physical examination often helps to clarify the diagnosis.

Tell the patient:

Over the next few weeks, we'll try to understand the interpersonal situation(s) that may be related to some of the symptoms that are making you uncomfortable. Solving those problems situations is likely to help you feel better.

PRESENT THE FORMULATION

In the first few sessions, you need to establish the diagnosis of depression and identify the patient's interpersonal problems. Next, tie together the depressive diagnosis and its interpersonal context in a treatment formulation, providing a potential focus for the IPT treatment. A formulation might sound like this:

You've given me a lot of helpful information in the last two sessions. May I give you some feedback to see whether you think I understand your situation? . . . We've already established that you are suffering from an episode of major depression, which is reflected in your Hamilton Rating Scale for Depression score of 25. (As we've discussed, depression is a treatable illness and not your fault.) From what you've told me, your depression seems related to what has been going on in your life recently, namely:

- *The death of your mother, a terrible blow that you have had trouble adjusting to. We call this grief, or complicated bereavement. [or]*
- *Your struggle with your husband about whether to move/have another baby/give up your career. We call this a role dispute. [or]*

- *Your life has turned upside down since you moved/changed jobs/got married/got divorced/were diagnosed with leukemia. We call this a role transition. [or]*
- *Your social isolation, lack of friends, loneliness, or boredom. [To tell patients they have "interpersonal deficits" risks sounding insulting.]*

This kind of interpersonal situation has a proven association with depression. What causes depression is unknown, and it probably has multiple causes, but it is often related to life problems like the ones you've described.

I propose that, for the next X weeks, we focus on helping you solve your [complicated bereavement/role dispute/role transition/social isolation]. If you can solve that problem, not only will you improve your life situation, but your depressive symptoms are likely to improve as well. Repeated research studies have shown this to be the case. Does this plan make sense to you?

This formulation is a key juncture, the bridge between the initial phase and the rest of treatment, whose focus it determines. Choosing the focal point requires clinical acumen. Again, your goal is to choose a plausible, simple focus based on the patient's history, an organizing narrative to which the patient can relate and which helps the patient to feel understood (Markowitz & Swartz, 2006).

Present the formulation early in the therapy, no later than the third session, so that sufficient time remains for the middle and termination phases of treatment. The early, explicit formulation, which defines the focus for the rest of the treatment, is a powerful organizing feature of IPT.

MAKE THE TREATMENT CONTRACT AND EXPLAIN WHAT TO EXPECT

Note that the formulation concludes with a proposed treatment contract. You ask whether the patient agrees with this formulation and is willing to work on it for the next X weeks. Practical and financial considerations determine the precise number of sessions to recommend (generally eight to sixteen weekly sessions). Predetermine a fixed number (e.g., twelve weeks), not a range, and aim to make these *consecutive* weekly sessions in order to maintain treatment momentum. An important function of the time limit is to pressure the patient (as well as the therapist), combatting depressive passivity and moving the therapy forward. Thus, more sessions are not necessarily more helpful.

Your presentation of the formulation thus constitutes a treatment contract. You may use this opportunity to explain again the relationship that often occurs between symptoms and problems in life. The patient's agreement on this focus seals the contract. You need to obtain an explicit agreement on this crucial point. Thereafter, if the patient should digress from the focus, you can bring the treatment back to this agreed-upon theme. This treatment focus should be seen as a collaborative effort. Although patients usually accept the presented focus, if the patient disagrees with it, you should explore what the patient sees as an alternative interpersonal focus and might well agree to pursue that.

THE SICK ROLE

Another facet of the initial phase of IPT is to give your patients the "sick role," excusing them from blame for the depression and for what the depression prevents them from being able to do. You can often helpfully make analogies to other medical illnesses:

> *No one is at her best when suffering from an illness. If you had appendicitis or the flu, you wouldn't blame yourself for being unable to perform at your best. Depression is no different, in some ways even worse.*
>
> *The symptoms of depression may prevent you from dealing with other people as successfully as usual. We will try to discover what you want and need from others and learn what options you have and how to get them. We will also talk about what options are unrealistic and not possible. This is a good time to experiment with handling situations: we can discuss afterward what's gone right or gone badly. On the other hand, if you can't do certain things because you're feeling too depressed or exhausted or hopeless, that's too bad (we'd like to see how you handle such situations), but don't beat yourself up—you're not to blame for being ill. We expect that over the course of treatment you will regain the ability to do all of those things. You're fighting an illness, but it's a treatable illness.*

After giving the patient an initial understanding of how you see the problem and agreeing on the focus of treatment, emphasize the following:

- *We will be focusing on your life as it is now.*
- *Therapy will focus on your relationships with important people in your life.*
- *We will discuss these relationships and your feelings. If you feel that the direction of the sessions is not useful or that I'm doing something that's bothering you, please let me know. I won't be offended, and your feelings are important.*

Discuss the expected duration and frequency of the treatment, including how often you will be meeting. The usual time is once a week for about fifty minutes for a period of three to four months. Set a firm time limit, and hold to it so that both you and the patient have a timeline by which to measure progress. Depressed persons who recover from an episode but require maintenance treatment to prevent recurrence may subsequently contract to continue treatment for extended periods at a reduced session frequency.

A couple of additional things to mention to the patient:

- *Anything you tell me will be kept in confidence. The only exceptions are legal ones (like child abuse or your intending to harm or kill someone). Otherwise, I won't talk to anyone about our treatment without your permission.*
- *In the therapy we will discuss feelings and situations that concern you and may be related to your depression. I am interested not only in what happens to you in between sessions but also in your feelings about these events. You can select the topics that are the most important to you since you are the one who knows best what things bother you.*

ENTERING THE INTERMEDIATE SESSIONS

Following the diagnosis, identification of the problem areas, agreement on the formulation, and establishment of the treatment contract, the work of IPT begins on the problem area: grief, interpersonal disputes, transitions, or (in the absence of any of the first three) interpersonal deficits.

Begin each session after the first one by reviewing the patient's last week. The archetypical opening question is:

How have things been since we last met?

If the patient begins by discussing mood ("I've been feeling awful"), ask about the interpersonal context:

I'm sorry to hear that. Did anything happen this past week that might have contributed to your feeling that way?

Conversely, if the patient answers the initial question by reporting an event ("I had a terrible day at work"; "It was my birthday Tuesday and I got drunk"), link it to mood:

Sorry to hear that. How did that make you feel?

With two questions, then, you should be able to elicit a recent incident about which the patient has feelings. The next step is to explore the incident and the patient's feelings about it. What happened? How did the patient feel about what happened? What did the patient want or expect to happen? What were the specifics of the encounter? Try to recreate a transcript of the encounter, including the patient's actual words and tone of voice, her feelings as the interchange transpired, and the other person's reactions.

For example, if the patient reports a disagreement with a spouse, family member, or coworker, you would want to dissect the incident. At each juncture, ask:

What did you say then?
How did [the other person] respond?
Then how did you feel?

By reconstructing such incidents, pulling for both the patient's feelings and behaviors in interpersonal situations, you gain a better understanding of how the patient's life is proceeding and how she is handling crucial encounters.

If the patient has handled such an event well and is feeling a little better, it is important to note the connection between capable interpersonal functioning and improved mood. Moreover, you want to reinforce adaptive functioning:

Great work! No wonder you're feeling a little better.

If things have gone badly, as is more often the case early in treatment when the patient is most depressed, a similar but inverse approach applies: you want to help the patient understand the connection between bad events and worsening mood and depressive symptoms. Further, it is a chance to examine what has gone wrong in the interpersonal setting and how the patient might handle a similar situation the next time it arises:

Well, that sounds painful. I'm sorry to hear about it. But let's try to figure out where things went wrong . . . That strategy doesn't seem to be working. What other options do you have? What could you do in that situation if (as is likely) it were to happen again?

Listen for disjunctions—dissonances between the patient's feelings and actions. If the patient felt angry but said nothing, was the feeling of anger understandable and warranted, and did that silence contribute to an unsatisfactory encounter? It's important to validate the patient's feelings, particularly negative affects such as anger or sadness that depressed patients may see as bad or shameful. Yet if the patient dismisses such feelings as "bad" rather than understanding them as useful social information, she will probably not act on them, and the encounter will likely leave her feeling worse. Your role is to help the patient recognize that negative affects are normal and useful (rather than bad) and are key to handling encounters with other people:

Everyone feels angry when someone is bothering them. That's how you know that they're bothering you.

Having normalized these affects, what can the patient do with them? What other options might she have for handling such a situation? Depressed patients will frequently state that they have no options for managing a situation. Feeling hopeless, they will say they've "tried everything" or "nothing works." This is rarely true. The patient's previous efforts may have been half-hearted, and she may well have overlooked viable options because of discouragement, a sense that there was no reason to be upset by such a behavior, and so on. With some gentle questioning and encouragement, you can often get the patient to come up with feasible options. It is best to let the patient come up with the ideas, so that she feels competent and can take credit for the development, rather than suggesting them yourself (which makes you look good and the patient feel incompetent).

If someone is bothering a patient and she says nothing, feeling the resultant anger is just part of her problem, and this has negative interpersonal consequences. People expect other people to tell them when to back off. If the patient is silent when bothered, ignoring her reaction and trying to put other people's needs first, the other people may not even know they're bothering her—and are likely to keep repeating the offending behavior. Tolerating our negative feelings (anger, sadness, anxiety) and finding a way to verbalize them clarifies the situation, communicates interpersonal understanding, and generally relieves tension. The patient who can say, "Please don't do that. I don't like it when you do that," is likely to feel better and to find that she has greater control over her interpersonal environment.

But this takes practice. After exploring options and finding a new, potentially feasible strategy, you can then role play this with the patient:

> What would you like to say to [that person]?
> How did [the way you just said] that sound to you? Did you say what you wanted to get across? What did you think about your tone of voice?

Repeat the role play until the patient feels more comfortable with the intervention. The session usually ends with a summary of what has been covered and how it relates to the patient's depression.

This loosely structured sequence is the heart of the IPT intervention. The therapist focuses consistently on mood and interpersonal interaction, helping the patient to see the link between them, reinforcing adaptive interpersonal functioning, and helping the patient to explore and gain comfort with new options where old strategies have not been working. Given this emphasis in the therapy, it is hardly surprising that research has shown IPT helps patients to develop better psychosocial functioning.

INVOLVEMENT OF OTHERS

Although IPT is usually conducted as an individual psychotherapy, you may ask other family members to participate in one or two sessions if you and the patient feel that it would be helpful. With adolescents or children (Chapter 14), parents are always invited to participate in the initial sessions. Involvement of family members also occurs in situations of family, husband–wife, and/or parent–child disputes that have come to an impasse (see Chapter 25 on conjoint therapy). In some cultures, family members expect to participate in multiple sessions (Chapter 24; Weissman, 2016).

5

Grief

It has been recognized since antiquity that the death of a significant other is not only painful but can devolve into a form of depression. A century ago, Freud characterized this distinction between mourning and melancholia (Freud, 1917). The death means the loss of a close person, a relationship, a potential social support, and the dissolution of interpersonal bonds. Losing someone close can rip the fabric of an individual's life, creating an interpersonal void. We are supposed to notice such events, and the signal of interpersonal loss comes as a strong emotional reaction.

NORMAL GRIEF

Many of the symptoms that normally follow the death of a loved one resemble depression. In a normal grief reaction, the person feels sad and may lose interest in usual pleasures, have trouble sleeping, lose appetite and energy, and feel distracted even in carrying out routine tasks. These symptoms typically resolve over the course of a few months as the person processes the loss, thinking through remembered experiences with the deceased. This period of grief or mourning is a normal, useful, adaptive process and should be encouraged, not pathologized.

Further, if a patient is markedly dysfunctional or just wants to talk, the therapist need not discourage this. The availability of friends, family, and religious supports surrounding death can be comforting, but some patients lack these supports or feel isolated from them and want help during the period. As IPT benefits patients with major depression–level complicated grief, it is also likely to benefit patients with milder symptoms, including painful normal grief.

COMPLICATED GRIEF

Grief is a painful emotional experience, and some individuals find their emotional response too overwhelming to deal with. The death of a significant other tops the life event stress scales (e.g., Holmes & Rahe, 1967). Perceiving the feelings of mourning as dangerous, too painful to contemplate, they try to "keep busy" with other activities, numbing themselves in the hope that the feelings will subside. They may avoid their feelings by occupying themselves with funeral arrangements and taking care of other mourners rather than mourning themselves. The sadness of the loss may feel dangerous. If the relationship has been a conflicted one, for instance the death of a formerly abusive parent, the patient may feel guilty about feeling angry at the deceased ("What a terrible person I am to be angry at the dead, someone who can no longer defend herself!"). These patients suffer from not grieving. Avoiding the emotions leads the person to try to go through life containing them, distancing herself from emotional life, and consuming great emotional energy. This postponing and avoidance of grief is characteristic of complicated bereavement, a long-recognized form of major depression.

Less commonly, you may encounter a patient who has become in essence a professional mourner, whose entire life is devoted to the remembrance of the dead. A child's room may have been left as it was when he committed suicide years before, the pizza still rotting in its cardboard box. Such patients have adopted a mourner's role and feel any deviation, any indulgence in personal pleasure, as a betrayal of the memory of the deceased. These patients, too, will meet criteria for major depressive disorder, although their presentation is more typically an agitated depression than the constricted state of patients who are attempting to avoid their feelings

DSM-5 AND GRIEF

The DSM-5 (American Psychiatric Association, 2013) defines three types of grief: prolonged grief disorder, persistent complex bereavement disorder, and complicated grief. To add to the complexity, DSM-5 also notes traumatic grief as occurring when longing for or preoccupation with the deceased is persistent and the loss is seen as a trauma with intrusive images. The relationship between these different definitions, their similarities, and their predictive validity are open to debate (Maciejewski et al., 2016). They lie on the cusp of, and to varying degrees overlap with, mood disorders and posttraumatic stress disorders (PTSD).

The IPT manuals have always used "complicated grief" or "complicated bereavement" to define a major depressive episode associated with the death of someone close to the patient. This definition recognizes that some depression-like symptoms often accompany a death (normal mourning), but that if the symptoms reach the diagnostic threshold, or if a patient—often lacking family, religious, and other supports—seeks help for distress even without attaining the diagnosis of depression, IPT may be indicated. Lacking adequate data on the various DSM-5 grief subtypes, we take no other position about when to consider IPT.

GRIEF AS A PROBLEM AREA IN IPT

Therapists select grief as an IPT problem area when the onset of depressive symptoms is associated with the death of a significant other and the patient is struggling to come to terms with that loss. The loss of a close attachment is emotionally hard to bear. The significant other might be a spouse, partner, child, parent, other relative, friend, or even a dear pet. Note that in IPT, grief means complicated bereavement postmortem; life losses that are not deaths are defined as role transitions. It is important to take a careful history to see whether the onset of depressive symptoms relates to a death, as some patients may not make this connection. Some patients may also present with physical symptoms rather than sadness, which may connect to the illness from which the deceased died.

A complicated grief reaction may be diagnosed when grief is severe and the severe phase lasts longer than two months, or when a loved one has died and the patient has not experienced the normal mourning process. Telltale signs include the patient's failure to mention the dead person or to discuss the circumstances around the death. Depressive symptoms such as excessive guilt and suicidal ideation are not usually seen in normal grief and suggest the presence of complicated grief.

Signs of complicated grief present in patients who have suffered multiple losses and have not gone through a grieving period, who have avoided circumstances around the death such as mourning at the funeral or going to the grave, who fear developing the same illness as the deceased, who try to preserve the environment of the dead person, who lacked family or other social support during the period of bereavement, and who are still not functioning at work or with family at least two to three months after the death. The death has often brought their life to a halt: patients feel adrift, lost, and hopeless.

GOALS IN TREATING A GRIEF REACTION

It is important to convey to the patient that complicated grief is a form of depression that can and should be treated. Treatment is not a sign of disrespect for the deceased. The two goals of treating a complicated grief are:

- **To facilitate mourning** (catharsis). You can facilitate the mourning process by encouraging the patient to think and feel about the loss in detail, and by discussing the sequence and consequences of events prior to, during, in the immediate aftermath of, and since the death. What does the patient miss about the deceased? About their relationship?
- **To (re)establish interests and relationships** that can to some degree substitute for the person and the relationship that have been lost. The death has often left a vacuum in the patient's life, a loss of relationship and of direction that the patient may not feel capable of filling.

Overall Strategies

IPT provides three strategies for working with patients with complicated grief:

1. Educate about grief and depression.
2. Facilitate catharsis through letting the patient experience her feelings about the loss. Elicit the feelings through detailed discussions about the deceased, the death, and the relationship.
3. Find new activities and relationships to substitute for the loss and provide a direction forward in life.

Taking the History

Chapter 4 describes the opening phase of IPT, including diagnosing the target disorder, taking an interpersonally focused history, and providing a formulation. To collect the data from which to provide a formulation of complicated bereavement or grief, when assembling an interpersonal inventory, it is important to ask:

Has anyone close to you died?

If so:

I'm sorry to hear that. How did you handle that loss? What feelings did you have?
Did you attend the funeral? What was it like?
Where were you when you found out about X's death? (Did you feel you did something wrong?)
Do you feel you've been able to mourn that loss?

It may be difficult for the patient to answer these questions or painful to recall details. In treating grief, encouraging the patient to review picture albums and memorabilia, visit familiar places that evoke memories, go to a place of worship (where appropriate), or call friends or family and talk with them about the deceased can help. The goal is to elicit discrete vignettes that evoke feelings and to give the patient a chance to reflect on the feelings and what they meant, and to realize that—however powerful—they are tolerable.

Recalling the deceased and the lost relationship will likely evoke strong feelings. Many patients fear that the power of their grief might overwhelm them: that they will crumble, that if they once begin to cry they will never be able to stop. The IPT therapist's role is to encourage patients to tolerate their feelings, which feel powerful but are not as dangerous as they imagine, and are likely to subside if accepted.

Feelings are powerful but not dangerous. In fact, they may do the most harm if you try to hold them in.

Because many depressed individuals feel overly guilty, the therapist should inquire into the circumstances of the death. Many patients will feel they did something wrong, or should have done something differently: "If only I had stayed in the hospital room just then ..." or "If only I had left the hospital room to give him some space ..."—a circumstance now too late to rectify. Giving the patient a chance to air these feelings may help. Whereas in CBT, a therapist might ask a patient to weigh the evidence about a guilty belief, an IPT therapist lets the patient sit with and reflect on the feelings, eventually pointing out that guilt is a depressive symptom. (If the patient has more complex, potentially more justified feelings of guilt, after having truly neglected someone in need, or participating in an assisted suicide, you and your patient should explore guilt more fully.)

Some patients feel guilty about improving, seeing it as a betrayal of the deceased. They fear that if they recover from the grief (i.e., the depressive episode), it means they did not love the deceased as much as they had believed. To their way of thinking, if they really loved the person, the loss would be so great that they could never recover.

The interpersonal formulation, delivered within the first three sessions of treatment, should link the depressive disorder to the interpersonal problem area:

> You have suffered the death of someone close to you, which we know is the most painful kind of loss there is. You've understandably had some difficulty getting over it, and you've developed the symptoms of what we call complicated grief, which is a form of depression. It's a treatable problem, and it's not your fault. I suggest we spend the next X weeks working on what Michelle's death meant to you, what you miss about her, and how you can find a way to go on from there. To some degree this means coming to terms with the strong feelings you understandably have about her death. They feel powerful, but they're not really dangerous, and they should subside a good deal as you handle them. Does that make sense to you?

The principal techniques to use here are nondirective exploration and direct elicitation of affect (see Chapter 10).

Treatment Strategies

The early sessions of treatment for complicated grief focus on affect. Many patients will present an idealized version of what was a complicated or fraught relationship. A goal of treatment is therefore to gently elicit the patient's feelings, to give her a chance to reflect upon them, and to normalize them. The goal is to take the narrowly idealized, distanced and abstracted, two-dimensional view of the deceased and the lost relationship, and expand it into a more nuanced, balanced picture so that the patient can fully integrate the loss.

When first reviewing the patient's lost relationship with the deceased person, patients commonly recall their pleasant times together; they usually feel most comfortable (if sad) discussing these. Yet clearly patients also will have felt angry, disappointed, hurt, or unhappy about some characteristics of the deceased and their relationship. The patient may feel abandoned by the loved one or guilty about some aspect of the relationship, particularly about something the patient did or failed to do near the time of the death. At the same time, many patients with complicated bereavement fear the strength of their feelings and so try to avoid them. Strong negative emotions may include not only sadness but anger—and yet patients often feel that hating a dead person is a terrible thing and makes them a terrible person. How the therapist handles negative emotions toward the deceased may vary by culture (see Chapter 24).

Thus, you may start by inquiring about what was good about the relationship:

> *What do you miss about your mother? What were some of her good qualities? What do you miss about your relationship with her?*

Once the patient begins to reminisce, avoid the temptation to change the subject if emotions become powerful. Let the patient sit with and reflect on her feelings.

After exploring the positive aspects of the relationship (which may take a session or more), encourage the patient to openly express her less positive feelings, as they are normal: "*No two people get along all of the time. You must have a complex range of feelings about someone you cared so much about.*"

You can tell the patient that negative feelings may be followed by positive emotions and attitudes toward the loved one. This is no different from what would happen if the person were still alive: one would generally discuss upsetting things with that person, and that would make both of them feel better.

Patients with severe grief reactions may get irritated at any hints to discuss ambivalent feelings about the deceased, especially those patients with early caretaking deficits (insecure attachments) for whom the deceased provided an adult secure attachment. Tell the patient:

> *It's normal to feel upset and confused when you talk about the loss, but you will feel better again. I will be encouraging you to talk about your life with [the person], how your life has changed since the loss, and what the ups and downs have been. I will be encouraging you to talk about the things you did not like, as well as those you did like, about the relationship.*
>
> *Gradually, you will be able to sort through these emerging feelings and build a three-dimensional picture of your relationship with [the person you lost] that includes [the person's] good and bad points, as there are in all relationships.*
>
> *If you have difficulty in going through this grieving process, it might be helpful to discuss memories with friends or family. You might want to review picture albums or revisit places that were meaningful in your relationship. This can help you recollect the past. If you have old friends you have not seen since [the person] died, you might meet these people and review your past times together or even go over the albums with them. We can then discuss how those events go.*

Try not to be overly directive or didactic in relating this. The less you say in steering the patient in this direction of grieving, the better.

CATHARSIS

Many patients fear that if they begin to cry or mourn, they will not be able to stop and that the wave of grief will overwhelm them. It is important to reassure them that this will not happen. Once the patient begins to focus on the deceased person, the positive and negative aspects of their relationship and of that person, the hitherto controlled patient often begins to cry. A wave of affect rolls through the office. This makes many therapists anxious and raises the temptation to interrupt the patient. *Don't do it!* Your role as therapist is to help the patient learn that *emotions, while powerful, are not dangerous.* As the feelings are expressed, their force will diminish. Patients are then likely to feel calmer and more in control—sad, but less depressed. Once patients express strong emotion about the deceased, it is important to be calmly quiet and let them talk out their feelings. The main techniques used here are encouragement of affect and clarification.

REESTABLISHING INTERESTS AND RELATIONSHIPS

Once the patient has begun to process the grief, you can help her to fill the emptiness the death has often created. It is important not to proceed to this step until the patient has had a chance to deal with the grief feelings and to address the loss. You can say:

> *Social supports are important and protect against depression. It's often good to feel connected rather than carrying around your feelings all alone. Later in the therapy, when you're feeling a little better, you may want to try to call or go out to dinner with a friend, just to see how it goes. Your discussion of these experiences, good and bad, and your feelings around them are things we can discuss.*
>
> *As you begin to talk and think about the person who has died and to relive some of the experiences of the relationship and the loss, you are likely to feel better and should gradually begin to take on some of the old activities that gave you pleasure before the death. Although it may be hard to imagine this now, you may begin to look for ways to resume relationships and meet new friends who can also bring happiness to your life. We can talk about the practical efforts you are making and the feelings that surround these new steps.*

Sometimes a patient will have given up her social life or job in order to care for a dying family member. This may stir an uncomfortable resentment that the patient feels guilty for having: what a terrible person I am to be angry at a dying mother! After the death, the patient not only has lost the loved one but finds that her broader life has atrophied. The loss thus often leaves a patient feeling lost and directionless. Although one can't replace a parent or a best friend, it is possible to find new relationships and activities that provide satisfaction and give life a new sense of purpose. Sometimes the patient might volunteer at a hospital or cancer society in honor of the deceased.

If the patient undertakes a new activity or relationship, it is helpful to review afterward:

- *What did you do?*
- *What parts did you enjoy?*
- *What parts were difficult?*
- *Would you do it again?*
- *What else might you like to do?*
- *If some part of the activity, some interaction, was difficult, how else could you handle that in the future?*

Depressed patients who have an unresolved grief reaction may fear abandonment in new relationships. Any prospective new (or revived) relationships deserve discussion, including fears about them. Similarly, discuss activities that make the patient feel comfortable and those she fears. Encourage the patient to risk undertaking new activities and to use the therapy to discuss experience and reactions. Exploring interpersonal options (*"What might help you to feel better during this time?"*) and role playing them (*"How would you approach her? What might you say?"*) often facilitate this process.

As therapy progresses, the sessions will gradually shift from discussions of the deceased to issues surrounding these new efforts. The deceased person will be seen in a less emotionally charged way. Mourning continues for years: *the goal of IPT is not to end mourning but to ease it and to get the patient on the right path.* The patient will of course continue to remember the deceased but may feel less preoccupied with the loss.

Some patients present with chronic complicated bereavement: they have become professional mourners, dressed in black, their lives dedicated to the memory of the deceased. Any potentially pleasurable activity feels like a betrayal of the memory of their loved one. Friends and family who tell them to "get over it" simply don't understand their plight.

For such patients, the IPT therapist needs to underscore the severity of the loss:

This has been such a terrible loss to you that it's taken over your life for the last seven years. You feel like you'll never get over it.

While recognizing this dedication to the deceased, you need to find a way to reassure the patient that it's possible to honor the memory <u>and</u> to live one's life. Thus the treatment would begin as with the other form of complicated grief, asking about the death, what the patient loved about the deceased and the relationship, and gradually proceeding to less wonderful aspects of the relationship. As the patient tolerates the feelings and they diminish somewhat in intensity, you can gradually move into finding other activities and relationships:

> *You seem to feel guilty if you catch yourself enjoying an activity. But does that mean you'll ever forget your lost Jimmy? It is possible to have more than one feeling at a time, to honor his memory and to live your life.*

The techniques used here include communication analysis, decision analysis, and role play.

An adaptation of IPT for prolonged acute grief disorder, with or without depression, has been developed. This classification of grief is similar to a new diagnostic category of traumatic grief. The adaptation has been used when the longing and preoccupation with the deceased are persistent. The loss of the attachment figure is seen as a traumatic loss with intrusion images. Shear and colleagues have added elements of exposure-based PTSD treatment to IPT, including structured revision exercises and motivational enhancement to help patients reengage with their lives without the deceased (Shear et al., 2005, 2016).

CASE EXAMPLE: A HUSBAND'S DEATH

Mitzi is a 56-year-old schoolteacher and the mother of two grown children. Her life collapsed when her 60-year-old husband, Roy, died suddenly of a stroke. Their marriage had suffered some rockiness over finances and Roy's past extramarital affair. Nevertheless, the two were looking forward to enjoying their lives together now that their children were grown and they had finally saved enough money for vacations and relaxation. Mitzi, in her usual way, handled the funeral arrangements, comforted the children, consoled her husband's aged mother, and carried on as the backbone of the family. Although her husband's death occurred just before Thanksgiving, in the interest of family unity she decided to continue their Thanksgiving traditions. Two weeks after Roy's death, she returned to her teaching job and resumed playing tennis. She missed Roy and was weepy, but she felt that she had to carry on and to keep busy, both for her elderly mother-in-law and for the children.

A year later, the one problem that had developed after her husband's death, Mitzi's inability to get a full night's sleep, worsened. She also began to lose interest in teaching and felt that she could not go on. Convinced that she had an underlying medical problem (maybe cancer or heart disease), she consulted doctors and began to miss work. She could no longer carry through with Thanksgiving plans. She started to lose weight. Her friends felt she had aged five years in the past twelve months.

Mitzi entered IPT after a fourth medical checkup failed to find anything physically wrong with her. Her doctor noted that her loss of sleep, weight, energy, and interest in her work and family were symptoms of depression. Although she entered treatment, she denied that she was depressed and remained convinced that she had an undetected physical illness. In the initial sessions, it became clear that Mitzi fit the criteria for major depression despite her interpretation of her symptoms as physical illness. The therapist did not dispute this with her but began to inquire what had been going on in Mitzi's life and when her symptoms began. The therapist assessed her symptoms using the Hamilton Rating Scale for Depression (Hamilton, 1960) and found that her score was 27—in the severely depressed range.

Her husband's death immediately became the focus of attention: the sudden, unforeseen circumstances of his death, her inability to mourn, and her immediate resumption of activities to avoid mourning. It was also clear that Mitzi's symptoms had worsened around the anniversary of Roy's death—several weeks before Thanksgiving—when her mild sleep disturbance worsened and resulted in fatigue, failure to go to work, and, finally, inability to organize the family's Thanksgiving.

The therapist diagnosed major depression associated with complicated bereavement, emphasizing that depression was an illness with prominent physical as well as emotional and cognitive symptoms. Mitzi was able to agree with this diagnosis. Therapy progressed with a detailed discussion of the life she and her husband had shared. Each session began with details of her daily activities, usually a discussion of how she used to do the same things with her husband and how his loss felt to her. With the therapist's encouragement, Mitzi began to go through the picture albums of their shared life, which she had buried in a closet after Roy died. She cried frequently and acknowledged that she was really focusing on his death now, a year later, for the first time.

Over time, she revealed her anger at Roy for not taking vacations, which had cost them the chance to relax and have fun together. They had now missed any chance to vacation together. Toward the end of treatment, Mitzi arrived with a brochure. She and a close female friend were planning a cruise to the Bahamas. The end of therapy included a discussion of what it would be like to be a single woman on a cruise, as well as her enthusiasm for the trip and her guilt that her husband would not be able to share this activity. Her final Ham-D score was 5—within the normal range.

CASE EXAMPLE: HIDDEN DEATH

Linda, a 30-year-old college-educated and very attractive woman, had run through several therapies and therapists. Her affect shifted between bland and confrontational. She seemed out to challenge any help to prove it useless. When she presented for IPT she was mildly depressed (Ham-D = 15) and had been taking antidepressant medication for several months. Linda described her life as empty and meaningless. She had recently taken a new job as an administrative chief, a slight promotion from her previous position, but she said her main motivation for the move was to meet new people and feel less socially isolated. Her depression had increased when she found no improvement in her social life after two months at the new job. She came home and ate alone after work. Weekends were long and painful.

Linda described her previous therapists as unhelpful and poorly trained, and it seemed clear after two sessions that she would soon add her IPT therapist to that category. Her interpersonal inventory revealed no current close friends, few acquaintances, and no disputes. Her father was dead, her mother lived across the country, and she had limited contact with her and her younger sister, who lived near the mother. They were not estranged, Linda said; they just didn't keep in touch. Linda's current situation sharply contrasted with the rich life, full of social activities, she reported having had about four years before.

Finding a problem area proved difficult. At first it seemed that her transition into the new work situation might be a focus, but that proved a dead end: Linda found little difficulty in the change other than its failure to restart her social life. In the absence of other life events, interpersonal deficits (loneliness) seemed the next alternative: an absence of life events and problem areas. The therapist tried again to understand the onset of symptoms and the social context, in other words to find a life event.

She again asked Linda about the time four years before when she had friends, eliciting the friends' names and the nature of their relationships. During this third session, with some reluctance, Linda described her former boyfriend John. They were planning a four-week summer trip to Europe to hike and bike. They were both about to take on new jobs and wanted to use this interlude to rest, relax, and get to know each other better. They planned to get engaged after the trip and tell their families. Then one day, John and Linda spent time at her apartment. He was planning to drive back to his own apartment 20 miles away to pack, and they were to meet again at the airport the next afternoon. The next day, however, John never appeared. After frantic calls, Linda learned that John had been hit in a head-on collision, had been taken by ambulance to a hospital, and had died that night.

Linda met John's family for the first time at the funeral. She described the subsequent days as a blank blur. She began her new job as planned and said her life changed. She would wake in the middle of the night in terror. She stopped seeing friends. She couldn't cry. She felt that she wished she could join John. Although she had made a determined effort to block out the pain and any memories of this event, the focus of complicated grief had now become apparent.

With the therapist's gentle encouragement that it was better to process than to try to ignore the feelings of this terrible loss, Linda reluctantly and increasingly tearfully began to describe John, how they met, their relationship, and how they designed their planned vacation. She described the terrible meeting with the parents at the funeral. They knew little about her and blamed her for the accident. Had she given him something to drink at dinner? Why was she encouraging him to take a month-long vacation when he could have been working? She also noted that their mutual friends had drifted away with his death. She feared what his parents might be saying about her. They evidently needed someone to blame for this senseless accident.

Linda's emotions during the session ranged from wailing to fury to sadness. She was well into the grieving process that she had never undergone. After four more sessions, she decided to call some of their closest mutual friends and was surprised and pleased to learn they were happy to hear from her and didn't understand why she had turned away from them. At week eight she decided she could visit her mother and sister, whom she had not seen or returned calls from since John's death.

Acute treatment terminated at twelve weeks as planned. The quality of the interactions with the therapist had changed remarkably. Linda was no longer confrontational and began to consider new ways to meet people with similar interests, hiking and biking, and had begun to see one or two old friends. She expressed sadness at termination and thanked the (competent) therapist for her expertise. She was asymptomatic (Ham-D = 4). Linda decided to continue monthly maintenance for six months to help consolidate the gains she had made in her mood and social life.

6

Role Disputes

DEFINITION

Relationships require compromise. Individuals inevitably differ in their needs and distastes. In good relationships, two people recognize their own and their partner's needs and aversions, discuss them, and negotiate an arrangement that both find satisfactory. Relationships thrive through equitable compromise. Psychiatric disorders can disrupt or make it difficult to negotiate such relationships. Conversely, disputed relationships may generate depressive symptoms or episodes. IPT defines an *interpersonal role dispute* as a situation in which the patient and an important person in the patient's life have *differing expectations* about their relationship. This leads to either an open or a tacit struggle. The depressed individual is invariably losing out in this conflict, which may be either a source or consequence of a depressive episode.

An example is a wife who expects her husband to take care of her financially but who has had to hold a job herself to help pay the bills. The spouse, on the other hand, may expect the wife to share financial responsibility. The pair have *nonreciprocal expectations*. Or a boss may expect a worker to put in extra time without recompense, a tacit assumption that the worker may resent but feel powerless to confront. One partner in an intimate relationship may become involved in a second relationship, overt or hidden, and the aggrieved other partner may suffer from the change in intimacy. In each case, the two parties have different—and conflicting—expectations of the relationship. A patient's depression can be linked to unhappiness about the balance of these expectations in the relationship, and its solution lies in their renegotiation. The patient typically feels unable to effectively confront the other person, to assert her needs or to express displeasure.

Disputes usually become the focus of IPT when disagreements have stalled, become repetitive, or stalemated, offering seemingly little hope of improvement. The parties often feel they have reached an impasse. This situation may make the patient (or both parties) feel out of control, thus threatening the relationship. Depression can make it difficult for the patient to recognize the options available to pull the relationship out of a rut or to resolve a dispute. Even recognizing the option, the patient may feel inadequate to employing it: for example, confronting the other person and saying, "I need this" or "I feel like you're not listening to me." The therapist's goals are to diagnose the seriousness of the dispute and then to help the patient to reach some resolution. A role dispute is one of the most common problem areas for depressed patients seeking outpatient treatment.

Role disputes frequently coexist with role transitions. A change in job, birth of a child, or geographical move (role transition) may strain a marital relationship, causing a role dispute over responsibilities at home. Conversely, a difficult relationship with a coworker (role dispute) may lead to bad work decisions, triggering a demotion or unwise career choice (role transition). In order to keep the treatment organized, try to focus treatment on only one problem area, depending on which one seems most important to the patient.

GOALS OF TREATMENT

For a role dispute, the goals of treatment are to help the patient identify the disagreement, choose a plan of action, and modify communication or expectations or both to resolve the difference of opinion. Although the patient is likely to present the situation as impassible and impossible, some solution often exists. The therapist must help the patient to consider what options exist to attempt a renegotiation of the relationship. If renegotiation proves successful, which is the outcome in the vast majority of cases, the patient will have learned a social skill (e.g., better self-assertion, a more effective way of expressing anger to defend oneself) and a better understanding of the dynamics of the relationship, and will have resolved the conflict. Even if attempts to resolve the dispute prove unsuccessful, the patient will have learned to better communicate her feelings during a disagreement. Further, the initially guilty patient may come to recognize that the problem with the relationship does not lie entirely with her: the patient has at least made a good-faith effort to try to change things, and it may be the partner's unwillingness to change that is the problem. When the relationship cannot be successfully renegotiated, examining the options also helps the patient to decide whether staying in the troubled relationship is the best alternative.

Role disputes emerge from taking a careful history and collecting an interpersonal inventory. Sometimes the patient announces it in her chief complaint: "I've been depressed since I discovered my partner's having an affair." If not, the key initial question is:

Are you having disagreements or a dispute with someone? (Is there someone important with whom you haven't been getting along?)

If so, and if this dispute distresses the patient, the next step is to determine the stage of the disagreement. It is helpful to have a sense of how the patient generally handles anger and hurt in her dealings with other people. Does she recognize the connection between an interpersonal dispute and the rise of emotions like anger, frustration, or disappointment? The following questions will help:

- *How do you feel when you want something and he doesn't agree? What do you do with that feeling?*
- *How do you fight?*

Ask for blow-by-blow examples: "*What did you say? What did she say? How did you feel then? Then what did you say?*" and so on. This reconstruction of interpersonal encounters will give you a better sense of how the patient functions interpersonally, what may be going wrong in the relationship, and where the patient ignores or suppresses emotional responses to the other party.

STAGE OF THE DISPUTE

Identify the stage of the dispute. Is the dispute in a state of renegotiation, impasse, or dissolution? Are the patient and the significant other communicating at all, and if so, how?

Renegotiation

Renegotiation means the parties are in active contact about their differences:

- *Are you and [the other person] aware of the differences between you?*
- *Have you been trying to change things, even if unsuccessfully?*

Sometimes it emerges that the patient simply needs to express her needs and lacks the social skills to do so: "If I were to ask for a raise, I'd just get fired." Depressed patients tend to put their needs second to the needs of others, and may need your encouragement to recognize a modicum of healthy selfishness. Once she has accepted her desire as reasonable, the patient may benefit from role play in order to express her need to another person (e.g., to ask the boss for a raise).

Impasse

An impasse exists when discussion between the patient and the other person has stopped. There is smoldering, low-level resentment and hopeless resignation but no attempt to renegotiate the relationship. The individuals involved may deal with each other using the "silent treatment":

- *Have discussions between you and [the other person] about important issues stopped?*
- *Some disputes are quiet. You feel misunderstood and angry, but you don't talk about it. You are at an impasse.*

In renegotiation, as discussed above, the therapist emphasizes learning new ways of communicating a solution. If the situation has reached an impasse, the therapist may attempt to bring the issues between the parties out in the open. This can result in increased disharmony, at least at first, as the patient brings long-suppressed disagreements and disputes back out into the open. Arguments may ensue. The objective, however, is to develop better ways of dealing with the conflict, better communication, and effective compromise. This may help the patient understand how differences in expectations in the relationship may be related to her symptoms.

Dissolution

Dissolution may be appropriate when the relationship is irretrievably disrupted by the dispute and one or both parties actively strive to terminate it through divorce or separation, by leaving an intolerable marriage or work situation, or by ending a soured friendship. Dissolution is usually not the first option, but it remains an option if the patient cannot renegotiate a relationship to her satisfaction:

- *Are the differences between you so large or unsolvable that you want to end the relationship?*
- *Some relationships end because of irreconcilable differences. If you feel you've reached that point, how can you dissolve the relationship with the least harm?*

A dissolution triggers a role transition (Chapter 7), in this case the loss of a relationship. You can then help the patient to deal with the sadness and/or guilt associated with the loss of the relationship and also with accepting it as the best alternative. In this role transition, the patient must mourn the loss of the relationship and recognize opportunities in the new role.

THERAPIST NOTE

In some cultures, dissolving a marriage may be impossible or irreparably damaging. In such circumstances, you and the patient can explore new ways to maintain the relationship with minimal distress.

MANAGING ROLE DISPUTES

Regardless of the phase of the dispute, it is important to help the patient realize the degree of influence she had on the final outcome. Depressed individuals doubt they have control over their environments, yet in fact they can exercise some control. Even when the outcome is less than ideal, patients feel generally better when they recognize the result is partly due to their own efforts, rather than somebody else's. An accurate sense of agency is more empowering than the depressive feeling of helplessness.

In order to manage a role dispute, patients need to recognize their own feelings about what they want and don't want, feelings about the relationship and the other person, and what might constitute a reasonable compromise. Many depressed people have great difficulty with relationships because they tend to put the other person's needs before their own. Some patients feel selfish asserting their own needs. Anger feels like a "bad" emotion or one that will drive others away. IPT therapists validate these feelings as *normal* responses to interpersonal situations:

- *Everyone has needs, and it's important to assert them; otherwise, other people won't know what you want. If you're selfish all of the time, people don't like that, but if you never tell other people what you want or need, they may not know these things, and you are unlikely to get them. That is not fair to you and may at times create resentment for not being understood or cared for. This often spoils relationships in the long run.*
- *People expect others to stand up for what they want. If you don't, who will speak for you?*
- *Anger is a useful, normal signal that someone else is bothering you. You seem to have some reasons to feel angry. If you don't tell someone what is annoying you, that person is likely to continue doing it.*
- *It's particularly hard to express these feelings when you're depressed, but doing so may help to improve your situation in this dispute, and that may relieve your depression.*

The usual sequence of events is to:

- **Elicit the patient's feelings** in her description of an interpersonal encounter: "*What were you feeling?*
- **Validate and normalize them** (except, for example, inappropriate guilt, which can be identified as a symptom): "*Is it reasonable that you were feeling angry?*"
- **Explore options**: "*Looking back, what could you have done in that situation? What might you do when it arises again? Have you expressed those feelings to your spouse?*"
- Then **role play** to help the patient put those feelings into a statement and tone of voice in order to communicate it to the other person.

Negotiation requires expressing wishes directly ("*I would like . . .*") and objecting to the excessive demands of others ("*I don't like it when . . .*"; "*Please stop . . .*"). If the patient reopens negotiations with the other person, a clearer understanding of the nature of the dispute emerges. As the therapist, you will also help the patient to consider the consequences of many different alternatives before taking action. Note that the role play is not assigned as formal homework, but role play in session primes the patient to return to daily life and try out a potential new skill. The time pressure of brief therapy then pushes the patient to take the risk of trying something new, changing a dysfunctional pattern.

To work out a resolution requires airing the needs and wishes of both the patient and the other party. Sometimes in a marital dispute it is useful for the partner to also enter treatment. You might support the patient in a separate nego-tiation for marital therapy, in which both the partner and the patient see a ther-apist together in conjoint marital therapy (see Chapter 25). More often, IPT of role disputes functions as a kind of unilateral marital therapy in which the patient works on the marriage with coaching from the therapist. The advantage to this approach is that, because much of the work on the marriage takes place outside the office rather than in the therapist's presence, the patient can take credit for the gains achieved. This sort of "success experience" and embodiment of agency may bolster a patient's sense of mastery over a relationship and sense of independent autonomy as treatment termination approaches.

A theme in many marital disputes is that the patient feels left out and does not share activities with the spouse. On the other hand, the patient may be mak-ing little attempt at involvement and may expect the partner to know what she wants without being told. In these situations, you can blame depressive symptoms (social withdrawal, low energy, loss of pleasure) for the patient's difficulty in get-ting involved. Help the patient to recognize and speak clearly about specific things she wants (but has not been getting) from the spouse and to develop more direct and satisfactory ways of communicating with the partner. Exploring options and role play are key techniques for preparing the patient for such confrontations:

- *I'm interested in how you feel about these things, what you would like, and how you would like to get them. And what is [the other person's] point of view?*
- *How much of what you'd like to do have you actually told him?*

At times it may be appropriate to encourage the patient to directly discuss with the partner what the patient sees as the dispute, to listen to the other side, and to describe how they talk to one another:

Are you reluctant to approach each other? How do you handle differences? Can you handle them in a nondestructive way?

In the wake of such an exchange, (1) congratulate the patient for having had the courage to risk the encounter; (2) note the link between any mood shift and the handling of the interchange; (3) reinforce the adaptive maneuvers the patient used; and (4) commiserate and explore alternative options if things have not gone well.

If the patient engages in discussions with the other person about the dispute, you may ask afterward:

- *How did you and [the other person in the dispute] communicate with each other?*

- *How did the discussion proceed? What did you say? What did he/she say? How did you feel then? Then what did you say?*
- *What was the outcome?*
- *What did you like about the way you handled it?*
- *What didn't seem to work?*
- *Are you glad you had the discussion?*
- *What do you see as the next step? What options do you have?*

CASE EXAMPLE: OVERBURDENED AND UNAPPRECIATED

Joan, a 42-year-old college graduate with three teenage children, had recently started a new, part-time administrative job. Her depression involved a role dispute with her husband, Harry. She felt that he did not help her around the house, criticized her cooking and manner of dress, and generally made her feel terrible. Because her return to work was a response to Harry's concern of several years that she contribute to their income, Joan had expected he would give her more attention. Harry had felt that they could not afford to send the children to college on one income and that he had assumed a disproportionate burden. Joan, on the other hand, felt he had never appreciated the time and energy it took to raise the children: feeding, clothing, dressing, and transporting them, arranging play dates and recreational activities, and checking homework assignments. As all this already constituted a full-time job, outside employment would only increase her burden.

Her new job, as predicted, made her feel overworked and unappreciated. Although she relieved financial pressure by bringing in extra income, the marital relationship deteriorated further. Their sexual relationship came to a halt, and they barely spoke to one another. Their marriage had reached an impasse. Joan felt sad, listless, and resentful around the house and argued more with her children. She started to have problems falling sleep, found herself overeating, and had gained eight pounds in the preceding three months. Harry, who had exacting opinions about Joan's physical appearance, then criticized her about the extra weight. Her initial Hamilton Rating Scale for Depression score was 22—moderately to severely depressed.

Therapy began with a discussion of Joan's symptoms and their onset. It was clear that the symptoms had started after she began working and that the heart of the dispute lay in her feeling unappreciated and overworked. The therapist encouraged her to discuss these feelings with her husband, and they role played this during a session. When Joan later broached the topic at home, the discussion resulted in far better communications in which Harry was able to express some of his own feelings of disappointment in the relationship, as well as his positive feelings about the home and the security Joan had created for him. They spontaneously planned to spend at least two nights a month together doing something just for fun. Their sexual relationship improved, and Joan's depression began to lift. By the end of the twelve-week treatment, her Ham-D score had fallen to 7—within the normal range.

CASE EXAMPLE: FIGHTING BACK

Lindsay, a 29-year-old married Catholic social worker, presented in tears with the chief complaint: "My life is miserable." He reported years of intermittent milder depression that had worsened in the previous six months. When his therapist asked what might have been happening in his life to make him feel worse, he first mentioned work tension, but then ruefully revealed his concerns that his marriage was "failing." Jen, his wife of three years, had grown increasingly distant, sex had stopped for the past year, she no longer mentioned having the children they had both fantasized about, and she seemed preoccupied with text messages on her phone. Lindsay, whose approach to relationships was generally submissive and passive, went through Jen's credit card statements and found charges for expensive gifts, restaurant meals, and hotel stays of which he had been unaware. Guiltily, he broke into Jen's cell phone and found steamy text messages between her and someone named Edward.

Heartbroken at the prospect that Jen might be having an affair, and that his imagined "forever relationship" marriage could be crumbling so soon, Lindsay had kept silent for weeks. He felt depressed, anxious, and guilty (including guilty for having been spying on Jen); had difficulty falling and staying asleep; and began overeating and gaining weight. He reported passive suicidal ideation, although "I would never do anything [to hurt myself]." His Ham-D score was 28, indicating severe depression. He struggled to work with his patients and colleagues in a health-care setting.

The therapist gave Lindsay the diagnosis of a major depressive disorder and linked it to his marital crisis: "A marriage is supposed to provide more support than distress. No wonder you're upset if your wife is having an affair!" Lindsay agreed to a twelve-week course of IPT. The therapist explored his feelings about Jen, noting his difficulty in acknowledging anger. "I don't like that feeling," said Lindsay. "And who am I to get angry? She must see me as an inadequate husband, and that's why she's looking elsewhere." As this fairly religious couple had never agreed on an open relationship, the therapist explored Lindsay's feelings about the transgression of Jen's seeming affair. The therapist elicited his "irritation" (a word he tolerated better than "anger") in daily encounters with his wife, who continued to act in a distant and somewhat condescending matter. They then discussed whether this was a reasonable feeling: Jen seemed, at least, to have broken their marital vows.

The therapist asked: "What do you want to happen? What would make you feel happier?"

Lindsay said he would like to save the marriage, to make it better again.

"What options do you have to achieve that?" asked the therapist.

Lindsay's first answer was "none," but he decided it was worth trying to talk to Jen. The therapist agreed that communication about one's feelings was crucial to any good relationship. After several sessions of validation of his feelings of hurt and anger, and role playing the content and tone of their expression, Lindsay acted—although not as the therapist had anticipated. He confronted a difficult coworker: "I'm annoyed, even a little angry, that you didn't tell me about transferring that patient." Lindsay was somewhat surprised that these words came out, and surprised as well by the coworker's response, which was an unexpected apology.

After discussing this in session 7, Lindsay felt emboldened enough to confront Jen: "I'm not happy with the way our marriage is going, and I don't think you can be either."

Jen initially professed not to know what he was talking about, and Lindsay was tempted to let this go. Then, however, the dialogue grew: Lindsay said he was "angry and hurt at the way you've withdrawn from me." She softened, they both cried, and Jen confessed to having been troubled by her work situation and to have been seduced by a younger man there. Lindsay, prompted by role play rehearsal, found himself saying: "You shouldn't have done that. You owe me an apology!" Jen apologized and said she felt terrible for hurting someone she really did love, but did not commit to ending the affair.

Lindsay came to session 8 perplexed. On one hand, he felt validated in his feelings—he hadn't been imagining things, he had been able to express his anger, and he had even gotten an apology. (The therapist underscored and congratulated him on tolerating and expressing his feelings.) On the other hand, nothing was resolved, although his relationship with Jen did feel closer. Lindsay and the therapist discussed how he felt, whether it was reasonable, what he wanted to happen, and what options he had to achieve them. Lindsay role played telling Jen that he was angry but still loved her, their marriage was worth saving, and she should recommit to it.

Both again tearful, Jen agreed to do it and quickly submitted a request to transfer to a different office where she would no longer have contact with Edward. The marital sexual relationship resumed. Lindsay's Ham-D score fell to 6, denoting remission. As termination approached, the therapist asked him why he was so much better. Lindsay at first modestly credited the therapist for saving his marriage, but then spontaneously acknowledged his own active role in improving things. They discussed his toleration of negative emotions like anger, and his using them to assert himself to manage his relationships. At the six-month follow-up he remained euthymic, Jen seemed faithful, and she had become pregnant.

7

Role Transitions

DEFINITION

The IPT category of role transition is a broad and flexible one, often available to the therapist for treating patients who have not experienced the death of a significant other and do not report a charged role dispute. Depression associated with transitions occurs when a person has difficulty coping with a life change that affects her mood and requires different behavior or modifications in one or more close relationships. The change may be immediate, as in the case of divorce or becoming a single person, or more subtle and gradual, as with the loss of freedom following the birth of a child and becoming a parent. Retirement or changes in one's social or work role—especially changes that diminish social status—are other meaningful adjustments. Moving, taking a new job, leaving home, suffering from a severe medical disorder, alteration in economic status, and a change in the family due to illness (e.g., taking on new responsibilities due to the ill health of a spouse or parent) are other examples of life role transitions. Relocation and refugee status have increasingly become transition problems in countries around the world.

Many people do not fully enjoy life change even when the change is apparently a positive one, such as having a wished-for new baby or receiving a work promotion. Individuals who are vulnerable to depression may develop a depressive episode if confronted by a sufficiently disrupting or upsetting life change. Two aspects of a role transition may be upsetting. One is the loss of the old, familiar role, which may evoke a depressed nostalgia ("If only I could get back to that" or "Things were okay then") and reflect the disruption of social supports. The individual may also feel depressed and anxious about the unfamiliar new role, which can appear overwhelming and unpleasant. Thus the patient experiences the transition as dually negative.

The aims of treating depression associated with a role transition are to understand what it means to the patient: what the patient has lost, what the new situation demands, what might be gained, what expectations the person and others have in relation to that change, and how capable the person feels of meeting them.

Not all transitions are negative, but depressed patients tend to recognize the negative aspects rather than the benefits of the change. A sought-after promotion may produce conflicts about responsibility and independence. The person may have felt more comfortable in a more subordinate position or in a less demanding job, may feel guilty about having surpassed others, or may feel cut off from former colleagues whom the patient must now supervise and evaluate rather than fraternize with. Transitions may bring the loss of friends or close attachments and demand new skills. Role transitions may be even more difficult if they are unexpected and undesired.

The depressed patient is likely to recall the time before the change as idyllic, the change itself as traumatic, and the aftermath—the present and anticipated future—as dreadful, painful, and chaotic. Things feel out of control, in free fall (as illustrated in Fig. 7.1). This may reflect the patient's mood in the old and new roles more than the realities of the roles themselves. As the therapist, your goal is to help the patient not only to mourn what has been lost with the old role (e.g., being single, living in one's lifelong hometown, being healthy) but also to recognize the limitations and difficulties of that seemingly idyllic situation. Reciprocally, the therapist aims both to help the patient acknowledge what is difficult and painful about the change and the new role (e.g., being married, living in a new city, having an illness) and to recognize the potential advantages that may result from adaptation to the new role.

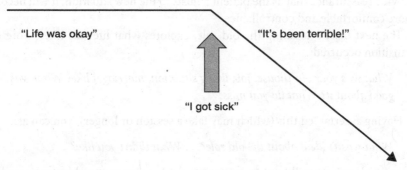

Figure 7.1. Role Transition.

Explore the patient's current situation to determine whether there is a problem with a transition: recent changes in the patient's life, how they affected her, the patient's feelings about the changes, important people who may have been left behind, and who has taken their place. Note that complicated bereavement (Chapter 5) is really a special case of a role transition, one involving the death of a significant other. The treatment strategies for grief and role transition are similar. IPT separates the two because death is an irrevocable transition, with distinct religious rituals available to assuage it; there are none for role transitions. The initial question to ask is:

What was going on in your life when you started to feel depressed? Had there been a big change in your life that might be related to the start of your depression?

GOALS AND STRATEGIES

Five tasks help the patient manage transition problems:

- Giving up the old role
- Mourning the old role: expressing sadness, guilt, anger, powerlessness, and fears about the loss
- Acquiring new skills, exploring opportunities for growth due to the change
- Developing new attachments and support groups
- Recognizing the positive aspects of the new role.

These tasks often overlap and the patient may achieve them only gradually. Whether or not the patient fully completes the transition in the course of an acute IPT treatment, she may achieve meaningful successes—sufficient to relieve the depressive symptoms and help her to feel mastery over the situation. You can help the patient to develop a map for what needs to be done and how to go about it.

Your first task is simply to name the role transition. Patients experience transitions as chaotic and out of control. Defining the problem as a role *transition* rather than chaos or free fall is reassuring: it gives a name to the circumstance. You can provide reassurance that as the patient adjusts to the new situation, it will become more comfortable and controllable.

The next task, evaluating the old role, explores what life was like before the transition occurred:

> What was your old [house, job, living situation, marriage] like? What was good about it? What do you miss?

Having ascertained this (which may take a session or longer), you can ask:

> What wasn't ideal about the old role?. . . What didn't you like?

Depressed patients will tend to exaggerate the benefits of the old situation while minimizing the negatives and the extent to which the previous situation was destructive or unpleasant. Conversely, they may see their new role as entirely bad, ignoring its benefits and potential benefits. For example, a failed, unhappy marriage may be idealized because the new role of divorcée or single parent feels unacceptable. Becoming a mother may feel like the loss of one's pre-parenthood identity. Giving up the old situation may be experienced as a loss and may trigger a mourning process. To facilitate this process, listen for and elicit the feelings that the transition evokes, such as guilt, disappointment, and frustration. As the patient experiences catharsis about the loss of the old role, you can help her to develop a more balanced emotional response to both the lost old role and the uncertain new role, recognizing the positive and negative aspects of each.

One role transition that we considered to be a test of the IPT approach involved treating depressed HIV-positive young men in the 1990s. This was before there were many effective treatments for HIV, and patients faced the prospects of a rapid, disfiguring, and shaming death. What was the "upside" of learning that you had a stigmatizing, sexually or drug-transmitted fatal illness in your twenties or thirties, that your immune system was reduced to a handful of remaining T-cells, and that you had a good chance of dying young? In a randomized, controlled trial, we found that IPT worked as well as medication and better than CBT and supportive therapies for such patients (Markowitz et al., 1998). The time pressure of having a potentially fatal, stigmatizing illness produced a pressure to get better fast: patients wanted to make the most out of however much precious time they had left, and were willing to take the risks to dramatically change their lives for the better.

As the patient deals with feelings about the loss of the past role, you can turn to the current situation:

> *What's upsetting about your current situation?*
> *What would make you feel better about it? . . . What options do you have to make it that way? . . . How could you do that?*

Resolving the role transition may require the patient to assert herself by expressing wishes or dislikes to others. This might involve asking for a raise or promotion at work, making friends in a new community, or saying "no" to others who are irritating the patient. Role play can help the patient to prepare to do this.

NEW SOCIAL OR WORK SKILLS

Developing new skills is an important part of the transition recovery process. The therapist is not a vocational counselor and does not necessarily assist in getting patients a different job, but will help them to explore the feelings that are keeping them from adjusting to the situation and acquiring new skills, new relationships, and new friendships. This may help patients to realistically assess their assets and skills for managing the transition. Discussing practical situations (e.g., finding an apartment, learning to navigate a new community, finding a job, meeting new people) can be useful. What options does the patient have? Where can she find supports? You can help the patient rehearse difficult situations, which may alleviate unrealistic fears that tend to arise when patients are depressed. Role play provides important practice for real life.

Making the transition to the new role—the new job, the new apartment, the new home, the role of single parent—may also mean creating new friendship patterns or support networks or developing different relationships with old friends. Because the rewards to be found in the new relationships or situations are unfamiliar, they may at first seem less desirable. The message to the patient is this:

> *Change is difficult, but it can be managed, and it may have more benefits than seem apparent when you're in the midst of a depression. Change is scary, but it can also be positive.*

In certain transitions, the patient may need to learn or exercise certain skills for the first time and may feel unprepared to perform them proficiently. Interestingly, there are positive features to be found even in objectively negative events, like a serious medical illness. Patients in IPT may come to see themselves as stronger, as survivors, with capabilities they didn't know they had, or they may learn to make the most of time, which now has an increased value in a shortened life span.

CASE EXAMPLE: A DREAM HOME

Jodi, a 38-year-old mother of two children, had recently moved to the suburbs and loved her new house. It was her dream house: a bedroom for each child, an extra bathroom so that she, her husband Marco, and the children did not need to fight over the sink every morning, a sunny breakfast room, a small garden, and good local schools. Coming from a poor family and having lived in a tenement, Jodi had finally made it. She and her husband would give their family the comforts that neither of them had been able to enjoy while growing up.

They had moved into their new home a year before. In the beginning they went through a flurry of decorating projects and adjustment to the luxurious new quarters. Over the last few months, however, the novelty had waned, and Jodi had started to feel almost desperate. Sad and blue, she cried often. How could she cry when she should be grateful for such splendor? Jodi felt alone and lonely. The move had entailed a much longer commute for Marco, the children had to travel by bus to a new school, and she didn't know the neighbors. A shy person, Jodi found it difficult to make friends. In her old neighborhood in the city, Marco had left for work at 8 a.m.; now he left at 6:30 a.m. and didn't return home until after 8 p.m.

Jodi missed walking to the local grocery store where everyone had known her, and meeting her old friends for coffee and a chat. She even had had to give up her part-time job in the city. To keep it, Jodi would have had to commute, necessitating the expense of a second car. Her dream was collapsing, yet she didn't feel she could complain to her husband because, after all, he had done this for her and the family. She should feel grateful. She didn't relate her depression to the move; she just thought she might be overtired from the stress of moving.

A review of Jodi's daily activities showed that she spent long hours by herself in the house. The IPT therapist helped Jodi to link her depressive episode to the move. Even though it had been a positive and desired relocation, the loss of friends and decreased availability of her husband were unforeseen problems. The therapist helped her see the connection and then find new ways to meet her need for companionship. Jodi gradually became more active in the new community and discussed her feelings with Marco. Although he could not change his work schedule, he sympathized with her problems and disclosed that he, too, missed some parts of the "old life."

The IPT therapist congratulated Jodi on reconnecting with her husband and mobilizing a needed social support. Upon realizing that he shared her feelings, Jodi felt better and grasped that she need not keep up the pretense that everything was perfect. With this improvement, she was able to make other changes in her life. She and her husband decided the expense of a second car would be worthwhile and would be paid for over time by Jodi's ability to continue her job. The car gave her a greater sense of control over her suburban environment and enabled her to drop off the kids at school. She became involved in the PTA and began to develop friends and social supports there. She emerged from twelve sessions of IPT euthymic, with a more balanced picture of suburban life. "I'm used to it now," she said happily.

Note that Jodi became estranged from her husband in the setting of her depression and this role transition. The IPT therapist could possibly have formulated the case as a role dispute but saw the marital tension as secondary to the larger picture of a role transition. The therapist also felt that framing the problem as a role transition would have greater plausibility and feel less threatening to Jodi than a marital role dispute. Accordingly, the therapist chose the role transition as the treatment focus but helped the patient to deal with her depression-induced withdrawal from her husband as part of treating the role transition.

CASE EXAMPLE: RETIREMENT

Phil, a vigorous 67-year-old, ran a small business he and his wife had started when they first married. Over the years, they had worked together, struggled, and finally made it profitable. He eagerly awaited retirement, when he would be able to do the things he had put on the back burner because of lack of time and money.

The previous year he had sold his store, invested his money, and planned how he would spend his time. Things did not work out as expected, however. Phil missed the daily chitchat with customers. He missed the structure of his work routine and, after a three-month vacation, was tired of traveling and wanted to return home. His wife devoted her time to cooking, gardening, their grandchildren, and volunteer work at the local hospital, but how would Phil spend his time? Over the past two months he had begun having trouble sleeping, lost his old zest and self-confidence, and started to lose weight. A physical exam showed him to be in good physical health. He even wondered what there was to look forward to. At night he took a much larger nightcap because of his insomnia and even started to drink occasionally during the day. Phil's general practitioner referred Phil to an IPT practitioner for psychotherapy.

A review of the timing of the onset of depression and his retirement quickly led to their connection: Phil saw that the symptoms were related to his retirement and not to a general deterioration of his health. He began to discuss his work. He talked about the customers he missed, how he would have coffee every day with the storeowner next door, and his pleasure at seeing a profit at the end of each month. In later sessions, he talked about the negative aspects of the work: the pressures of making payments, employee conflicts, and the demanding market.

As the therapy discussions progressed, Phil began planning to re-involve himself in activities he missed. He joined a golf club and volunteered in a chamber of commerce group, offering technical advice to small business owners in the community. His days became full once again, and his symptoms resolved.

CASE EXAMPLE: TROUBLE AT WORK

Ron, a 45-year-old accountant at a major firm, had graduated with a degree in accounting and an MBA. He joined his company at age 27, gradually working his way up to a managerial position. Over the last six months, his easygoing relationship with his boss seemed to deteriorate. Instead of having lunch together or informally dropping in and out of each other's offices, he found the boss's door remained closed. They rarely ate together. During large meetings Ron felt he was not called on to speak, and the meetings became quite formal. He believed something was going on and feared losing his job. He developed mid-insomnia, lost his appetite, became more irritable, and had more trouble concentrating and functioning at work. His Hamilton Rating Scale for Depression score was 20. It was clear that the depressive symptoms began with the changing relationship with his boss.

During their sessions, the therapist encouraged Ron to explore and role play options in order have a discussion with the boss about his place in the company and what he might expect. Ron set up an appointment. When they met, the nature of the company's financial difficulties became apparent, and Ron gradually started looking for employment elsewhere. He realized that the dispute had nothing to do with his own performance but with the changing economic climate. The company had lost large contracts, but not any of those with which he had been involved. During the course of the therapy, Ron practiced how he would handle potential termination negotiations with the boss. After discussing give-and-take strategies with his therapist, Ron tried them at his office and then reported to the therapist on his success or difficulty. His mood improved, and his Ham-D score fell to 11. Ron still felt somewhat anxious about his job instability but on the whole felt in better control of his environment. When therapy ended, he had reinforced his good relationship with his boss and had made contingency plans both for staying on in the restructured company and, alternatively, for exploring opportunities elsewhere.

CASE EXAMPLE: SINGLE AGAIN

Beth, a 37-year-old mother of one, has been divorced for a year and is relieved that her marriage is over. Besides having subjected her to physical violence, her ex-husband had neglected her and had had an affair. When she finally obtained the divorce, took her 8-year-old to a new apartment, and started a job, Beth felt that her life could begin again.

She had not anticipated, however, what it would be like to be a single mom. To whom could she turn when her child had a fever and needed to stay home from school? Although her husband had never provided much support, he had at least been there. Dating again, introducing her child to unfamiliar men, and handling sex were significant stresses and sometimes defeats. In her new role as a single mother, Beth faced a life and future that seemed more than she could possibly handle. She had developed typical depressive symptoms over the past few months and had a Ham-D score of 24.

In IPT, Beth first discussed her marriage: the problems and issues that led to the divorce and also the early years of the marriage, including the good times, such as when their son was born. She reviewed what she missed in the relationship and concluded that it was not her former husband but the somewhat protected role of being identified as a married woman. She came to realize that she had been making all of the decisions, supporting and taking care of herself and her son for the last seven years. She arranged for a better after-school program, which made her feel more confident about her son's well-being for the two hours between the end of his school day and her return from work.

Beth's major problem in the transition was dealing with new men in her life. She was afraid of making another "mistake," yet also feared being alone. In therapy she reviewed the men she had dated, her expectations, and her disappointments. Her therapist helped her to reduce the pressure she had placed on herself to find another intense relationship immediately and encouraged her to expand her social life and to include activities she enjoyed. Beth joined a tennis club and decided to take a five-day vacation with her son and sister. In therapy, she worked on building her assertiveness in relationships with men, tolerating anger, expressing her feelings more openly, and accepting that not all dates had to be successful and that it might take some time to find a stable romantic partner. Her depressive symptoms improved, and her Ham-D score declined to 9. She seemed more confident about her future and less pressured about "being alone."

Note that for both Ron and Beth, the story begins with an apparent role dispute. Role disputes and transitions frequently either coexist or lead into one another. Ron felt he was in a struggle with his boss; Beth was rebounding from a distressing marriage and divorce. Yet for both patients the principal issue was one of change—the boss was not in a personal struggle with Ron, and Beth's marriage was over. Since the key issue was the shift in their lives, rather than a struggle with someone in particular, *role transition* appears to have been the appropriate focus for the treatment.

8

Interpersonal Deficits (Social Isolation; No Life Events)

DEFINITION

Interpersonal deficits, loneliness, social isolation, or a paucity of attachments may be chosen as the focus of treatment if *none of the other interpersonal problem areas exist*. In a treatment designed to address life events, this category covers those patients who present without acute life events. The somewhat confusing term "interpersonal deficits" should be understood to mean "none of the above":

- No deaths (hence, no grief)
- Minimal relationships (hence, no role disputes)
- No life changes (hence, no role transitions)
- A paucity of attachments.

If any of the other problem areas can be found, do not use interpersonal deficits as a focus. The case example of "Hidden Death" in Chapter 5 presents elements that suggested interpersonal deficits, but careful assessment and increasing patient comfort with the therapist uncovered unresolved grief.

Patients treated for interpersonal deficits in IPT may have poorer outcomes than patients in other categories (Elkin et al., 1989; Markowitz & Swartz, 2007; Levenson et al., 2010) and might do better in an alternative treatment such as CBT or might require long-term treatment (although no data exist to support this statement). You should consider alternatives to IPT, such as a different psychotherapy or IPT plus medication for these patients, if the initial IPT treatment does not result in symptomatic improvement. Patients who fall into this category have few of the social supports that protect against depression, usually have impaired social skills, and feel uncomfortable in interpersonal situations. They tend to be isolated and lonely, and chronically so.

Whereas terms such as "grief," "role dispute," and "role transition" are useful labels to describe interpersonal situations to patients, "interpersonal deficits" risks sounding insulting. Therapists who treat patients using this focus should state that the patients are suffering from loneliness, isolation, or a lack of attachments or supports and that this isolation is contributing to their depression. The patient's interpersonal discomfort may be apparent in the therapeutic relationship—in her difficulty in maintaining a treatment alliance.

In part perhaps because of its ambiguous name, "interpersonal deficits" has raised more controversy and confusion than any other IPT term. Some therapists have tried to re-characterize it as "interpersonal sensitivities," a less wounding term; "interpersonal sensitivities" can sound like a personality difficulty, however, which is inconsistent with the IPT approach. Others have used the interpersonal deficits focus to treat patients who have multiple role disputes as opposed to a single, salient one. We agree that the term "interpersonal deficits" is inelegant, is inappropriate to state to patients, and conveys unintended hints of personality dysfunction. In some contexts we have called this problem area "loneliness" and "boredom" in order to destigmatize it. Nonetheless, IPT has used the term for more than forty years, and we opt to maintain it. Again, we see interpersonal deficits as the non–life event category of IPT, only for use in the relatively rare circumstance when the therapist can locate no life events in the patient's history. Multiple role disputes are more simply treated under the rubric of role disputes, where the "macro" paradigm of life event and mood as an overall formulation parallels the "micro" paradigm linking life and mood in each situation ("How have things been since we last met?").

Such interpersonally isolated people have problems establishing or sustaining intimate relationships or experienced severe disruption of important relationships as children. At least four types of patients may fall into this category:

- Individuals who are socially isolated, who lack relationships either with intimate friends or at work, and who have longstanding problems in developing close relationships
- Individuals who have an adequate number of relationships but find them unfulfilling and have problems sustaining them. (The quality of the relationships may be superficial. These people may have chronic low self-esteem despite seeming popularity or work success.)
- Chronically depressed or dysthymic individuals who have lingering symptoms that have gone untreated or been inadequately treated and whose symptoms interfere with relationships. (If chronic depression is the issue, the adaptation of IPT for dysthymic disorder may be worth attempting; see Chapter 17.)
- Individuals who have social anxiety disorder (also termed social phobia; see Chapter 21). Patients with social phobia may want to have, yet fear, relationships.

THERAPIST NOTE

IPT is a treatment based on life events. The interpersonal deficits focus differs from the others in lacking an acute focal life event. Although lack of relationships can be a major life stressor, it is often a chronic, not an acute, condition. This makes it less easy to use as a way of focusing the treatment. Again, it is preferable to use any of the other three categories if plausible life events can be found.

Many patients even with acute depression tend to experience it as a personal defect or personality trait. Some of these patients may appear personality-disordered to therapists as well, particularly those with "Cluster C" personality disorders, such as avoidant or dependent personality disorder that may simply reflect depressive symptomatology. Because it is difficult to accurately diagnose personality disorder in the setting of a (DSM-IV Axis I) disorder such as major depression, it makes sense to treat the depressive disorder first, as it usually responds to acute treatment, and to see what remains. Often treating the depression resolves the apparent personality disorder as well (Markowitz et al., 2015). Thus the IPT therapist withholds judgment and asks the patient to withhold judgment on personality until after treating the depression, explaining to the patient that it may all just be depression.

The tendency of patients to blame themselves as personal and/or personality "failures" increases with the chronicity of the depressive disorder. As patients who fall into the interpersonal deficits category may well have longer-standing symptoms, and are more prone to self-blame, there is all the more reason for the therapist to shift blame to the depression or life event rather than the patient. The label of interpersonal deficits/sensitivities lacks the life event on which to displace the blame.

THERAPIST NOTE

This section focuses on interpersonal deficits as a focal area for individual IPT treatment of major depression, but—as if this descriptor were not already confusing enough—the term has acquired a second meaning. Whereas for depression the descriptor "interpersonal deficits" is a focal area of last resort, in the *group IPT treatment of eating disorders*, it serves another function (see Chapter 20). Patients with eating disorders tend to limit their relationships to distanced superficiality, focusing on food rather than their emotions. One problem in adapting IPT for group therapy is the multiplicity of problem areas: some patients may be dealing with complicated grief, others with role disputes or transitions. To provide a common focus for group patients, IPT for eating disorders has frequently employed interpersonal deficits as a common bond. In this setting, it need not mean complete isolation and lack of relationships, but rather a difficulty in opening up and confiding in deeper emotional relationships.

GOALS AND STRATEGIES

The major task in this problem area is to reduce social isolation by improving the patient's skills in tolerating social anxiety, spending time with and talking to people; increasing the patient's self-confidence; strengthening the patient's current relationships and activities; and helping her to find new ones. This does not mean trying to transform a socially cautious person into a social butterfly—a prospect such a patient might find terrifying—but rather to modestly extend social functioning and build social supports.

If there are no important, meaningful current relationships in the patient's life, you may focus on past ones or—unusually, for IPT—on the relationship with you. The purpose of this is to help patients understand their problems in relationships and to practice forming new relationships. If you do spend time addressing the therapeutic relationship, do so as you would with any other interpersonal relationship. IPT does not interpret the transference, but rather helps the patient to relate emotions to interpersonal interactions in the here and now. Because this is a time-limited therapy, the work within the therapeutic relationship is a temporary step toward better social functioning in outside relationships. The three tasks are:

- To review past significant relationships, both good and bad
- To explore patterns of strengths and difficulties in these relationships
- To discuss the patient's feelings—positive and negative—about any current relationships (including possibly that with the therapist)

To learn about current friends and family, ask:

- *How often do you see them?*
- *What do you enjoy about seeing them?*
- *What problems come up?*
- *How can you find friends and activities like those you used to enjoy in the past or new ones that you might enjoy?*

You can anticipate difficulties in the therapeutic treatment with patients:

You have said it's hard for you to feel comfortable around other people. I expect that may happen here. If you feel shy and it's uncomfortable to talk to me, you can tell me so. If I should do anything that annoys you, please bring it up. I won't be trying to bother you, but it's exactly that kind of tension between people that we should be talking about and deciding how you can handle. Learning to talk openly about feelings in therapy may make it clear that your feelings, both positive and negative, aren't so dangerous to bring up, and that might make it easier for you in other relationships.

You might encourage the patient to work on isolation between sessions by re-contacting old friends (or possibly new ones) and seeking out social situations:

> *Therapy is a great time to work on your relationships; we can talk about what goes right or wrong.*

You and the patient can anticipate potential problems and how they might be handled, then discuss afterward how the contact actually went. Do not assign formal homework, as patients who do not comply with homework tend to feel like "bad" patients and may be more likely to drop out of treatment. Role play of difficult anticipated situations is often helpful and reassuring to patients. Indeed, patients in this category are likely to need considerable role play before risking encounters and developing social confidence.

If the patient contacted an old friend and arranged to see that person, you can ask:

> *Tell me how it went. How did you feel? What did you say? . . . Then what happened? Then how did you feel? What did you say?*

Each described encounter provides an opportunity for you to validate the patient's feelings, reinforce positive actions that she has taken, offer solace, encourage exploration of options, and then role play those alternatives for interactions that have not gone well. Each reconstruction of an interpersonal encounter also offers an opportunity to note differences between what the patient felt and what depression may have held the patient back from saying. The IPT therapist can frequently validate the patient's feelings and then encourage her to express them:

> *You felt angry when he said that. Was that a reasonable feeling? . . . If so, how might you express that? (Or: What would you think about just saying to him what you just said to me now?)*

If the patient arranged to enter a social situation, a party, a concert, a sporting event, or any type of situation, you can say:

> *Describe how it went. What did you do to meet people? How did you feel?*

Interpersonal difficulties are usually worsened by depression and—more to the point in IPT—may be a reflection of depression. Determine whether the deficits are chronic or acute, and just a consequence of the (possibly chronic) depression. Depressed patients lack the energy and confidence to pursue relationships. It is important *not* to assume that the patient has a personality disorder when seen in the midst of a depressive episode since apparent personality "traits" may wane or vanish with treatment of the depression. Moreover, depressed patients with and without personality disorders tend to blame something inherent in themselves for their difficulties—feeling defective and inadequate. Hence, whenever possible, the therapist should attribute such feelings and interpersonal cautiousness to the depressive disorder (or associated social anxiety disorder). The goal is to reduce social isolation and improve current relationships by improving skills in communicating and increasing the patient's social competence and confidence.

CASE EXAMPLE: "I CAN'T MAKE FRIENDS"

Diane, a 23-year-old single woman, had never been socially comfortable, but she had managed to fit in and make the best of it with friends she had known for years in high school, while living in a single-sex dormitory in college, and in planned school activities. She had avoided dating in school. Now she was on her own. In the year since she graduated from college she had found her first job and gotten her own apartment. Yet she felt at a loss.

Even though Diane had a good job that she had planned and studied for, she could not deal with her discomfort around men. She did not know how to talk to them, how to develop friendships, how to extricate herself from relationships that were uncomfortable, and how to avoid sexual involvement with men. She spent most of her time after work alone in her apartment. Her attempts to develop new friendships were disastrous. She went to a dance and became sexually involved with someone she hardly knew or liked. She described herself as bored and lonely. She had lost weight, was having trouble sleeping, and had missed several days at work. Her therapist defined her problem as major depression related to role deficits in social skills.

Therapy began with a detailed discussion of her daily activities: how Diane spent each day at work, her evenings, and the weekends. Therapist and patient also reviewed how her college relationships had developed since she graduated, finding a clear pattern of increasing withdrawal after her first, unsuccessful efforts to find friends when she had moved to town. She felt very shy, unattractive, and awkward, and did not know how to start a conversation or how to set boundaries in relationships.

On the positive side, Diane was a reasonably good athlete and had excelled in swimming in college, where she had one "best friend." The therapist encouraged her to act on her idea to invite the friend for a weekend visit, then to gradually increase her social activities with another trusted friend. Therapy included discussions of these opportunities and her anxieties and role play with the therapist: planning the weekend with her friend, approaching people at the swimming club she joined, and warding off premature or unwanted sexual advances from male acquaintances.

Diane made progress. By the end of therapy her depressive symptoms had decreased from the moderate to the mild range, she had bolstered her relationships with women friends, and she had successfully turned aside one unwanted man. She had yet, however, to begin dating comfortably or seriously. Patient and therapist agreed to a one-year maintenance course of monthly IPT (Chapter 9) in order to build upon and further the gains Diane had made acutely.

THERAPIST NOTE

Although Diane fit what could be termed interpersonal deficits, another formulation of this case might have been as a role transition—namely, the transition out of college and into adulthood. A key aspect of this shift would have been the need to adjust to social relationships. This might have been a more palatable formulation for a sensitive patient than the isolation/paucity of relationships rubric. The IPT formulation is intended to simplify problems and make them manageable so that the exploration of affect and interpersonal skill building can take place (Markowitz & Swartz, 2007).

CASE EXAMPLE: "RELATIONSHIPS NEVER LAST"

Bill was an attractive 41-year-old lawyer. He had been briefly married in his twenties, had a moderately successful career, and reported a series of relationships with women that never lasted more than four to six months. After the date—dinner, dancing, or a movie—he felt socially awkward and did not know how to get close to women. He described himself as sexually uninterested because he had not yet met the right woman, but further disclosure showed that he had low self-esteem and felt completely at a loss with regard to emotional intimacy. He felt unable to make a woman understand what kind of person he was, how to talk about himself, or how to encourage a woman to talk about herself.

In treatment with a female therapist, Bill clearly had great difficulty talking about his feelings. He confided in no one, even though he said he had several close friends. He wanted to marry and have children. He felt that he was getting older and more set in his ways and that this problem was becoming more difficult. In the last several months, following the breakup of his last relationship with Janet, who stopped answering his phone calls, he found himself increasingly depressed. His initial Hamilton Rating Scale for Depression score was 23.

The IPT therapist explored Bill's feelings about interpersonal encounters, helping him to voice these feelings in therapy, validating them (the therapist normalized much of what he felt and attributed some of his excessive anxiety to depression), and practicing interactions (role play). They role played Bill's being in a relationship with somebody he knew well, practicing what he might say and how he might reveal his feelings or get the woman to talk about herself. A clear pattern emerged from these practice sessions. Bill never let the other person finish a sentence, jumping in instead to lecture her, thus closing off further discussion. He came across as judgmental and controlling.

When the therapist pointed this out, Bill said that this was exactly how he would describe his own mother. In fact, last week they had had a major argument. When Bill told his mother about his relationship with Janet, his mother had responded with a lecture about his clothes, his manners, and his work schedule. He became infuriated, they argued, and he slammed down the phone. Communication ceased, and he could discuss neither his disappointment at the breakup of the relationship nor his anger at his mother. In IPT, as he discussed other relationships and how they had ended, he gradually became aware of his possible contribution to them. The therapeutic relationship provided a here-and-now laboratory for listening, gauging his feelings, speaking to another person, and gauging her feelings.

By the end of treatment he had not found a steady relationship but had become more aware of his feelings and his behaviors and was socializing somewhat more. He had confronted his mother about her lecturing, finished that conversation, and gotten her to back off. He was learning to listen to other people rather than interrupting out of anxiety. As he did so, his mood gradually improved, and his Ham-D score at termination was 10 (mildly depressed).

9

Termination and Maintenance Treatment

TERMINATION

IPT is a time-limited, not an open-ended, treatment. The time selected can vary: in IPT studies, the interval has been as brief as three to six weekly sessions and as long as thirty-six monthly sessions. Sessions usually run twelve or sixteen weeks for treatment of acute major depression. At the beginning of a course of treatment, the therapist and patient make an explicit contract about its frequency and length. By the end of the middle phase, the patient is usually improving, her symptoms diminishing. Several sessions before the end of the agreed-upon interval, the therapist begins the third, termination phase with an open discussion about the end of the treatment, and reviews what has been accomplished and what remains to be done. The patient is encouraged to discuss any feelings, positive or negative, about ending the therapy.

The therapist emphasizes that the goal of acute treatment has been to treat the depression and to help the patient deal successfully with life: work, love, and outside friendships. The patient–therapist relationship is a temporary one meant to enhance the patient's health, not to substitute for real-world relationships.

The goals of the termination phase are:

- To conclude acute treatment with the recognition that separations are role transitions, and hence may be bittersweet, but that the sadness of separation is not the same thing as depression
- To bolster the patient's sense of independence and competence, if treatment is to end, and to underscore new interpersonal skills the patient has developed
- To relieve guilt and self-blame if the treatment has not been successful, and to explore treatment options
- To discuss the options of continuation or maintenance treatment if IPT has been acutely successful but the patient faces a high risk for relapse or recurrence.

THERAPIST NOTE

If the patient is still symptomatic, it is also time to consider medication as an additional or solo treatment. If the patient has not received medication, a therapist who is not a physician may want to arrange a psychiatric consultation if the patient is still having sleep and appetite problems and low energy and/or expresses suicidal thoughts.

Feelings About Termination

Most patients have some discomfort with termination. A degree of sadness should be acknowledged as normal: you have been working on intimate matters together, it's been hard work, and it's hard to break up a good team. Indeed, the distinction between sadness and depression is a helpful one: *sadness is a normal signal of interpersonal separation or loss and does not mean the patient's depression is returning.* Depressed patients can feel uncomfortable with sadness, which can feel too close to depression, so this provides an opportunity to normalize sadness. Moreover, some patients, even if greatly improved, may have been feeling better for a matter of only weeks and may still feel somewhat shaky about handling matters on their own, without the therapist.

If a patient does not want to terminate, the therapist often suggests a waiting period of several months to see whether further treatment is really needed. Exceptions to this can be made if the patient has a significant burden of residual symptoms or has shown little or no improvement in the depression. In such cases, discussion should include consideration of alternative treatments: adding or changing medication or switching to a different type of psychotherapy; entering psychotherapy with a different therapist; or renegotiating the contract with the current therapist. If there have been additional changes in the patient's environment during the therapy (e.g., the unexpected death of a loved one during the treatment of a role transition), it may be appropriate to extend the therapy for a few additional sessions.

Competence and Interpersonal Skills

Depressed patients enter treatment feeling disorganized and incompetent. Many patients will improve during IPT, but even so they may feel anxious about stopping treatment because they recall that only a few weeks before they felt very depressed. You should help the patient terminate the IPT feeling organized and competent. One way to accomplish this is to review the patient's depressive symptoms (e.g., with the use of the Hamilton Rating Scale for Depression), note the great improvement (or achievement of remission [Ham-D < 8]), and then ask the patient: "*Why have you gotten better?*"

Patients tend to credit therapists for their gains, but in IPT the focus on the patient's activity outside the therapy office usually makes it clear that the patient has also done hard work and that the success is the result of their collabora-tive effort. You should emphasize the patient's agency in her own improvement. Termination is an opportunity to give patients credit for their own gains by reviewing their new strengths, noting how their use of new skills was associated with symptomatic improvement, and anticipating how they can use these skills to face upcoming situations. In short, the patient may not need you any longer at this point, although she is always encouraged to seek help again if symptoms return.

Some patients may require longer-term treatment or maintenance IPT to pre-vent relapse or recurrence. This includes patients with a history of recurrent depression: the more depressive episodes a patient has, the more episodes are likely to occur. Another high-risk group comprises patients who have responded to treatment but still have high levels of residual symptoms. For example, a patient whose Ham-D has decreased from 30 at intake to 13 after twelve sessions has certainly responded to IPT, but a score of 13 remains symptomatic and near the threshold for depressive relapse.

Some patients with recurrent depression that has resolved during twelve to six-teen weeks of acute IPT will do well and have a reduced risk of relapse or recur-rence with monthly maintenance IPT. If maintenance treatment seems indicated, a new treatment contract should be made. Monthly maintenance IPT is the best-tested interval, but some patients may want and benefit from more or less fre-quent sessions (Frank et al., 2007). The patient's preference for the frequency of sessions may be an important consideration. Some patients may want to meet every two weeks, whereas others may find such frequent meetings burdensome in their euthymic state.

Nonresponse

Patients who have not responded to IPT and who remain symptomatic should be evaluated for medication and/or a different type of psychotherapy (Markowitz & Milrod, 2015). Nearly all depressions eventually respond to some treatment, and the previous twelve to sixteen weeks have already been a long time to wait for treatment response. A risk of ineffective treatment is that depressed patients are likely to blame themselves ("This is supposed to be a great treatment, but of course I'm a failure") and may become too discouraged to persevere in treatment. If the patient has not improved, the IPT therapist invokes the medical model and—as the pharmacologist would do in a medication treatment—blames the treatment, not the patient, for nonresponse. The therapist can explain that only two-thirds of patients with major depression respond to their first course of pharmacological treatment, yet the majority of those nonresponders will likely respond to a subse-quent course of treatment. The goal of this discussion is to consider therapeutic options and to find a more effective treatment to alleviate the patient's pain. Some patients who have been initially unwilling to take medication may have built a sufficient alliance during an unsuccessful IPT treatment to now willingly consider a pharmacology trial. In that sense, even a failed IPT trial could lead to a success. The goal is always the patient's recovery, not an ideological belief in a particular therapy.

There is a good chance, however, that the patient will not be depressed after a brief IPT treatment (Cuijpers et al., 2011, 2016). You should acknowledge this improvement and congratulate the patient for having accomplished something that probably seemed very unlikely to her only weeks before. It may take a while for the patient to feel secure that the depression is truly gone and will not come back. Explain that the symptoms of depression and the kinds of interpersonal situations likely to be associated with the depression may recur. Encourage the patient by pointing out that she may be able to handle moods and situations differently when they occur and avoid a relapse or recurrence. If symptoms do return, the patient should know whom to contact and how to get help quickly, including contacting you again. Such a relapse or recurrence should not be seen as a failure on the patient's part but rather as a reappearance of a chronic vulnerability to illness, akin to hypertension or high cholesterol.

At the end of treatment, repeat the depression scale and other diagnostic assessments to concretely evaluate the patient's progress. To see how much progress has been made on the problem areas or whether new problems have developed, you could readminister the problem area questions on grief, disputes, transitions, or deficits that were asked at the beginning of treatment and discuss the results with the patient. See Appendix C for an Interpersonal Psychotherapy Outcome Scale, Therapist's Version, which might help guide the evaluation of progress in the problem areas (Markowitz, Bleiberg, Christos, & Levitan, 2006).

MAINTENANCE TREATMENT

IPT was designed as an acute, time-limited treatment. Resolving an episode of major depression using IPT takes twelve to sixteen weeks. It would be nice if the problem ended there, but unfortunately it often does not. Even patients who have remitted from a first episode of major depression face the likelihood of a relapse or recurrence at some point. Patients who have had multiple episodes are almost sure to have more unless given antidepressant prophylaxis (Judd et al., 1998; Judd & Akiskal, 2000; Kovacs et al., 2016).

The termination phase at the end of a successful course of IPT treatment should include discussion of the possibility that depression could recur; and that if it does, it is not the patient's fault but the return of a potentially recurrent and still treatable illness. Under such circumstances the patient should seek further treatment. If the patient has had a single episode of depression and has few residual symptoms, it may be appropriate to send her home with the following advice: although the patient is likely to experience another episode at some point in life, it may never happen or not occur for many years.

If, however, the patient has had multiple prior depressive episodes or has improved in IPT but still reports a high level of residual symptoms, then she faces a high risk of relapse, and prophylactic interventions should be discussed as part of the acute treatment termination. Medication has been the most carefully studied intervention and has yielded the most consistently efficacious prophylaxis of relapse of major depression, but it requires taking ongoing medication indefinitely. CBT and IPT have also shown preventive benefits for depressed patients. Thus, maintenance IPT should be considered as an option for continued treatment.

In addition to patients with recurrent depression, others deserving consideration for maintenance IPT include women during pregnancy and lactation, for whom taking medication may not be possible or optimal, but who can be maintained with a lower probability of relapse if they receive IPT. Elderly depressed patients who may not tolerate medication, as well as patients who have a history of recurrence but do not wish to take medication, are also candidates for maintenance treatment. The evidence for the efficacy of IPT weekly for six months (Klerman et al., 1974) as a continuation treatment, and weekly to monthly for up to three years of maintenance treatment, is quite strong (Cuijpers et al., 2016; Frank et al., 1990, 2007).

Repeated research trials have demonstrated not only that IPT can help patients to remit from major depression but also that maintenance IPT, even at the low dose of once monthly, can preserve euthymia for patients and forestall the return of depressive symptoms even for patients at very high risk for relapse (Carreira et al., 2008; Frank et al., 1990, 1991, 2007; Reynolds et al., 1999a, 1999b, 2006, 2010).

Adaptation

Maintenance IPT is in most respects like acute treatment. The focus remains on interpersonal functioning and mood in relation to life events.

TIME LIMIT AND FREQUENCY

Although maintenance IPT is a chronic treatment, the therapist and patient still arrange a time-limited contract for its duration. Maintenance IPT has been tested mainly as a weekly treatment for six months (Klerman, DiMascio, Weissman, Prusoff, & Paykel, 1974) or as a monthly treatment for three years. Its frequency can be varied in clinical practice depending upon what the patient and therapist deem appropriate and desirable. Maintenance IPT could conceivably continue the weekly schedule of acute IPT, or sessions might take place every two, three, or four weeks for a specified number of years. At the end of that period, you and the patient should again discuss a renegotiation of the therapy. The time limit is no longer intended to pressure the patient to action, as in acute IPT, but simply to define the duration of ongoing treatment.

FOCUS

Unlike acute IPT, maintenance IPT begins when the patient is not acutely ill. The goals of maintenance treatment are to minimize residual symptoms and to ward off the return of others, rather than to reduce the symptoms of an acute episode.

(The reduction of residual symptoms, however, is a worthwhile goal.) Sessions may include review of the emergence of symptoms or the appearance of problems that had been associated with their onset. Because the patient and therapist will have worked together in acute treatment, the themes of the acute treatment usually continue. It may be possible to complete work on role disputes, role transitions, and so on that began during the acute phase.

If maintenance treatment continues for several years, new life events may occur and new interpersonal foci arise. A patient who has previously worked on a role dispute may suffer bereavement when a loved one dies. Hence one aspect of maintenance IPT, is the flexibility to shift foci as circumstances dictate. Regardless of the focus, the general themes remain the same:

- Depression is a treatable illness that is not the patient's fault.
- Interpersonal situations influence mood, and vice versa.
- IPT works to help the patient recognize the connection between emotions and life circumstances and to develop skills to express those feelings in interpersonal circumstances in order to make life go better.

CONSOLIDATION
Patients who have responded well to antidepressant treatments often feel better but experience their euthymia as fragile (Markowitz, 1993, 1998). It may take weeks or months for self-confidence to really take hold in the aftermath of a depressive episode that had left the patient feeling helpless, hopeless, and worthless. Indeed, one function of ongoing treatment is to encourage patients to take appropriate social risks, to test their euthymia, rather than cautiously avoiding rocking the boat lest they become depressed again. Patients may require additional practice to feel comfortable using new social skills, as is reflected in research that shows that these skills grow during the year following acute treatment (Weissman, Klerman, Prusoff, Sholomskas, & Padian, 1981) and that seeming personality traits recede over time in maintenance IPT (Cyranowski et al., 2004). Hence maintenance treatment is a time to further initial growth in therapy and to encourage patients to test their abilities and take appropriate risks in social circumstances.

TECHNIQUES
Maintenance IPT uses the same techniques that are described in Chapter 10.

CASE EXAMPLE: SPEAKING UP TAKES TIME

Roger, a 34-year-old single male violinist in a prominent orchestra, presented with his third episode of major depression, which followed a panic attack at an important audition. He had hoped this audition would move him to the highest rung in his profession, but he had blanked, frozen, and forgotten his piece, then retreated in shame and horror to his room for two weeks. He presented with depressed and anxious mood; sleep and appetite disturbance; social withdrawal; extreme self-criticism;

feelings of helplessness, hopelessness, and worthlessness; and passive suicidal ideation. With a Ham-D score of 28, he met DSM-5 criteria for recurrent major depressive disorder, social anxiety disorder, and avoidant personality disorder. "My music
is my life," he said, and he had been too depressed to play in the past month.

Roger was a chronically shy, socially isolated man whose closest relationship had
always been with his single, artistically pretentious, domineering stage mother, with
whom he lived. He both resented her control of his life and depended on her. She had
interfered in the few romantic relationships he had dared to attempt. His two previous depressive episodes had occurred following his graduation from the conservatory
at age 21, and after his mother's humiliation of him in front of a would-be fiancée
when he was 25. Each episode had responded to a course of medication.

A twelve-week course of IPT focused on the role_transition in his career. With
the therapist's encouragement, Roger prepared for and sought another audition, in
which he played well and won a desired position. He and his therapist discussed
his problematic relationships, which included a fear of criticism by his famous and
famously stringent conductor, social discomfort in dealing with his colleagues, and
deferential ambivalence toward his mother. He increased his hobbies during acute
treatment but formed few new relationships. Nonetheless, his Ham-D score fell to 8.

Because of Roger's history of recurrent depression, his therapist congratulated him
on his gains in acute treatment and suggested that because he was at risk for recurrence, he might benefit from maintenance IPT to prevent a future depressive episode.
They contracted for two more years of monthly treatment, with the goals that he
use the additional therapy not only to further his career but also to work more on
interpersonal relationships. The first issue they dealt with was his social discomfort
in professional situations. Roger remained insecure about his status in the orchestra
because he believed that the conductor did not really like him. Roger and his therapist discussed this anxiety as a symptom of depression and social anxiety. After
considerable role play over several months, he made an appointment to speak to the
eminent and imperious maestro. To his surprise, when Roger expressed his worries
about his performance, the great man responded kindly and supportively. This successful experience enabled Roger to relax somewhat with his fellow musicians and
even to go out with them for drinks on occasion. This activity, however, aroused his
mother's ire.

In the second year of maintenance, Roger remained euthymic and less anxious.
He felt more comfortable at work, but now, at age 35, he wanted a romantic relationship, which meant setting limits with his mother. He had met Jeannie, a flautist
he liked, but was afraid to bring her home to Mom. Treatment shifted to a focus on
the smoldering role dispute between Roger and his mother. This was an unsettling
time for Roger, who asked for more frequent, fortnightly sessions for the subsequent
six weeks. The therapist agreed.

In these sessions Roger expressed anger about crossing his mother and fear that
she might either abandon him or have a heart attack and die if he disappointed her.
He had attempted few arguments with her and had never won one. The therapist
validated Roger's anger at his mother's selfishly oppressive behavior. They explored
his options for discussing the situation with her: he had never discussed relationships

with her directly. They role played his options in therapy. "Mom, it's time I had a girlfriend, and you shouldn't interfere. It doesn't mean I don't love you," he decided to say. He hesitated to confront her but finally did. His mother had a fit, but this had been anticipated in therapy, and Roger was able to stand his ground. His mother finally backed off, he continued his relationship with Jeannie, and he finally brought her home to meet his mother.

He had survived. Roger remained euthymic after the two years of maintenance IPT; his Ham-D score had hovered under 5 in the final six months. He re-contracted for an additional two years of bimonthly maintenance treatment, during which he got engaged, married, and moved out of his mother's apartment. He had developed some friendships and was prospering in his career. He no longer met criteria for either major depression or anxiety disorder.

10

IPT Techniques and the Therapist's Role

The strategies used in IPT, described in the preceding chapters, are distinctive. The techniques used to facilitate these strategies are neither unique nor new, however; most will be familiar to any experienced psychotherapist, particularly those familiar with affect-focused psychotherapies (Markowitz & Milrod, 2011). These aspects of the therapy constitute some of the "common factors" shared by many or all psychotherapies (Frank, 1971; Wampold, 2001). Our patient handbook (Weissman, 2005) explicitly states some of these methods from a patient's point of view. The time spent in IPT focuses on discussing feelings, normalizing them as responses to interpersonal interactions and as useful interpersonal information, and using them to take action to change the patient's interactions in order to resolve the identified problem area. You can use the following techniques to accomplish this.

NONDIRECTIVE EXPLORATION

Nondirective exploration uses open-ended questions to facilitate free discussion in order to gain information and identify problem areas. Some sample questions include *"Who are the important people in your life?"* and *"How have you been since we last met?"*

With a supportive acknowledgment, encourage the patient to continue: *"Please go on," "I understand,"* or, to deepen or extend the topic, *"Can you tell me more about the friend you mentioned earlier?"*

Nondirective exploration is useful with a verbal patient to focus the treatment, but it can make a less verbal patient anxious. As the therapeutic goal is to develop a comfortable alliance, more directed, active techniques are indicated for less verbal patients. The therapist must always weigh whether to intervene, providing structure and honing the direction of the therapy, or to wait, listening for the development and allowing the deepening of the patient's feeling state.

DIRECT ELICITATION

Use direct elicitation of material to obtain specific information, such as to develop the interpersonal inventory, to obtain symptoms in order to make a diagnosis, or where specific information is needed to demonstrate a point, such as defining a patient's role in a dispute or an unexpressed affect. For example: *"Can you tell me what you said before your wife accused you?"* or *"How did you feel when clearing out your husband's clothes after the funeral?"*

ENCOURAGEMENT OF AFFECT

Encouraging affect helps the patient to express, understand, and manage affect. The expression of affect may help her to decide what is important and make emotionally meaningful changes. Choosing options and making changes are more difficult if the patient does not recognize the range and intensity of her feelings about key interpersonal situations. Awareness of a sense of guilt, anger, or sadness, and reflecting on it, may help to clarify and point the patient in an interpersonal direction.

Further, tolerating strong affects, while not the primary goal of IPT, is an important byproduct of treatment. Many patients consider their strong negative emotions evidence of their defectiveness: many patients with depression view strong anger or hatred as indicating how "bad" they are; patients with posttraumatic stress disorder (PTSD) see anger as evidence of their dangerousness. For patients, learning that these feelings are normal—powerful, but not dangerous—and interpersonally informative (anger tells you someone is bothering you) can be transformative (Markowitz & Milrod, 2011). The IPT therapist encourages the patient to see strong emotions as human, as good rather than bad. Strong emotions can be converted into words that can lead to more adaptive interpersonal encounters, with benefits for overall mood and symptoms.

One way to help the patient deal with and accept painful affect, especially in grief reactions, is to elicit details of her interactions with others or to explore topics to which she has shown an emotional response. In the case example of Mitzi's grief in Chapter 5, she had idealized her husband but became able in therapy to express some of her disappointment and the burden she experienced following his sudden death. In the case of Phil in Chapter 7, direct exploration of his interactions at work allowed him to begin to make the transition into the retirement he had unexpectedly found so difficult. Patients who often feel guilty about expressing negative feelings may benefit from your direct reassurance, such as, *"Most people would feel like that,"* or *"Of course you're angry! It makes sense to feel angry."* This conveys your acceptance of the patient's feelings.

Although patients with many psychiatric disorders constrict their feelings and can be encouraged to express their emotions within the therapy, how they should act in close interpersonal relationships outside of the office varies by culture and situation (Markowitz et al., 2009; Verdeli et al., 2008). In some instances, strong expression of anger and resentment might damage already fragile relationships. The first steps are to elicit the feelings in the therapeutic situation, to normalize them where possible (but defining suicidal feelings, for example, as symptoms), and then to discuss the pros and cons of expressing them or how best to express them in existing relationships. When possible, the therapist can also encourage the patient to use social supports to express feelings. How best to do so, to whom, and what reactions can be anticipated are options to explore and to role play in IPT before the patient tries them out at home or work. Listen for emotionally important statements, and encourage their expansion by discussing them.

Yet constant repetition of angry, hostile, and sad outbursts can be counterproductive. When this occurs, you can help the patient to explore other options to break a maladaptive pattern of emotional expression. For example:

> *You seem to get into this pattern that doesn't really help you to feel better. Do you agree? . . . What other options might you have to express these feelings? How else might you communicate how you feel to your friend?*

Alternatively, an excessively affective display may be tempered by inquiring about the patient's thoughts about these strong feelings and exploring how she may delay acting on an impulse, allowing time to consider the consequences. If some behaviors or circumstances of the troubling problem change, this may reduce some of the patient's angry affect. Nor need the IPT therapist stop at encouraging angry and resentful feelings; many patients have difficulty expressing affection, gratitude, or caring, and can work on this in therapy sessions and in outside relationships.

CLARIFICATION

Clarifying a theme a patient has raised is a useful technique to increase the patient's awareness of how she is interacting or communicating. Patients can be asked to repeat or rephrase what they said. You may then rephrase this by saying, *"You were angry with her?"* You may call attention to the logical extension of a statement the patient has made: *"Do you mean to say that you would like your daughter to move out of the house?"*

The therapist can bring contradictions and contrasts to the patient's attention. For example:

- *You just described your husband's affair without showing any emotion. How do you feel about it?*
- *You were smiling when you told me about the angry exchange between you and your friend, but it hardly seems a happy matter.*
- *I noticed that you said X when you had previously said something else.*

- *Before, when you told me about this, you were sad, and now you seem to be calm.*

Such maneuvers help patients to reflect on their feelings and behaviors, a general benefit of psychotherapy that is a crucial element of IPT as a prelude to interpersonal action.

COMMUNICATION ANALYSIS

Communication analysis is a central IPT technique for examining and identifying problems in communication. It helps both therapist and patient to understand how the patient is interacting and to consider more adaptive alternatives when appropriate. The therapist elicits a detailed account of an important conversation or argument that the patient has had with a significant other in order to understand (1) the patient's feeling state and behavioral patterns, (2) the meaning of the transaction, and (3) the pair's methods of communication. The therapist listens to the communication in detail, stopping to understand the patient's feelings and intents at critical points:

Then what did (s)he say? . . . Then how did you feel? . . . Then what did you say?

Listen for a dissonance between what the patient feels and what she actually says, a discrepancy that may reflect how symptoms are interfering with interpersonal functioning. For example, a depressed patient may feel angered by an insult but say nothing, feeling that her reaction is inappropriate or might shatter the relationship if expressed. Ambiguous, indirect, nonverbal communication can be identified as less-than-satisfactory alternatives to verbal confrontation (e.g., the patient who sulks when angry). Patients are often not aware of how they communicate or how their depression may distort other people's messages and their own response to these.

Communication analysis provides a valuable interpersonal focus that may help patients detect these difficulties in communication, come up with alternatives ("*What other options do you have?*"), role play these, and ultimately improve the encounters. This interpersonal improvement leads to a greater sense of personal and environmental control, and an improvement in symptoms (Lipsitz & Markowitz, 2013).

At the same time, when treating patients from other cultures, it is important to take into account which forms of communication are accepted and which are proscribed in the patients' culture. Although therapists may be tempted to use their own culture as a referent, adopting the therapist's modes of communication might not always be in the patient's best interest (Chapter 24).

Another technique is to help the patient communicate directly her needs and feelings. Many patients assume that others will anticipate their wants or read their minds, the failure of which can result in anger, frustration, silence, and unexpressed affect that can destabilize a relationship.

Incorrect assumptions that one has been understood also need clarification. For example, was a friend's comment about the patient's hair meant as a criticism or a compliment? To identify faulty communication, listen for assumptions that patients make about others' thoughts or feelings. Rather than giving immediate feedback, encourage patients to draw their own conclusions. Follow through a particular conversation, again checking the patient's feelings as you progress. After she has offered her interpretation of events, you can elicit and suggest alternatives to poor communication and use role play (see below) to help improve communication.

DECISION ANALYSIS

Decision analysis helps the patient to consider alternative courses of action and their consequences in order to solve a given problem. Like most IPT techniques, the patient can learn to use it not only within the treatment but as a general interpersonal skill. Helpful questions may include:

- *What would you want to happen?*
- *What solution to this would make you happiest?*
- *What are the alternatives?*
- *What are the tradeoffs?*
- *Have you considered all the choices?*

ROLE PLAY

Role play has uses across the four IPT problem areas. You as the therapist can generally take the role of the other person, giving the patient needed practice in developing skills in self-assertion, confrontation, self-disclosure, and so on. For patients in the interpersonal deficits focus, it can sometimes be useful for them to take the role of someone in their life with whom they would like to develop a relationship. Role play can help prepare the patient to interact with others in different ways, particularly in acting more assertively or expressing anger. It clarifies for the patient and therapist how the patient reacts to others. In other cases (e.g., role disputes or role transitions), role play may helpfully rehearse the patient's handling of new situations or new ways to handle old situations. In instances of grief, it is often useful to role play an imaginary conversation between the patient and the deceased.

To avoid the role play feeling like artificial playacting, it is often helpful to just jump in, taking the role of the other person and implicitly inviting the patient to respond:

But Deborah, I wanted to go to this movie!

At the end of a role play, review with the patient:

- *Did you say what you wanted to say?* (That is, is the patient satisfied with the content of the message delivered?)
- *How did you feel about your tone of voice?* (Is the patient satisfied with the delivery of that content?)

Repeat the role play until the patient feels reasonably confident with the message and the medium. Consider contingencies: What might go wrong in the interchange, and how can the patient anticipate or respond to that?

THE THERAPEUTIC RELATIONSHIP

A large literature indicates the necessity of a therapeutic relationship as the basis for treatment outcome. A good relationship between therapist and patient does not guarantee the patient's improvement, but it is a *sine qua non* for that improvement. Without a good alliance, patients will not take medication (Krupnick et al., 1996); without a good alliance, the most elaborate psychotherapeutic approach will not matter. A good therapist helps a patient feel understood, listened to, and reasonably hopeful about prognosis, elicits affect, encourages success experiences, and so on. (Frank, 1971).

Common factors of psychotherapy are listed in Box 10-1, and implicit in that list are therapeutic authenticity, empathy, and warmth. IPT does not exploit or interpret the transference as in psychodynamic psychotherapy, where a transferential focus is an essential part of the treatment (Markowitz et al., 1998). However, IPT therapists do pay attention to the therapeutic relationship, recognizing that this may reflect how the patient thinks and acts in other close relationships. Although the focus of IPT treatment remains squarely outside

---

Box 10-1.

COMMON FACTORS OF PSYCHOTHERAPY

- Affective arousal (Response)
- Feeling understood by therapist (Relationship)
- Framework for understanding (Rationale)
- Expertise (Reassurance)
- Therapeutic procedure (Ritual)
- Optimism for improvement (Realistic)
- Success experiences (Remoralization)

Note: Adapted from Frank, 1971.

---

the office, rather than on the therapeutic dyad, the therapist can ask the patient to express negative feelings about both the therapy and the therapist, as well as to voice complaints, apprehensions, anger, and aversive feelings that may arise in the course of the treatment. (Psychiatric patients are notoriously averse to criticizing their therapists, even when the therapists make mistakes. IPT encourages patients to raise their interpersonal dislikes about therapist and therapy.)

These exchanges focus on the here-and-now interpersonal issues, not on childhood antecedents or other remote historical material. They allow the therapist to correct distortions or acknowledge genuine deficiencies or problems in the treatment. (IPT therapists need not hesitate to apologize for mistakes they may make. If you are late to a session or make a mistake, acknowledge it; apologize. If you sense the patient dislikes something in your style, ask about it in nonjudgmental fashion.) This approach helps patients to feel understood by the therapist (a "common factor" associated with better treatment outcome) and to see themselves as a partner in the treatment process.

The therapeutic relationship can be used in role disputes to give feedback on how the patient comes across to others and to help her understand maladaptive approaches to interactions. In interpersonal deficits, the patient's relationship with the therapist may provide a model for interacting in other relationships. Directive techniques include educating, advising, modeling, or directly helping the patient solve relatively simple, practical problems such as referrals for social services, housing, public assistance, medical insurance, or educational opportunities for family members. Advice, suggestions, limit setting, education, direct help, and modeling are elements of the therapeutic relationship but not necessarily major parts of it. They are best employed in early sessions to create an atmosphere in which the therapist is perceived as helpful. It is always preferable to encourage the patient's own sense of agency rather than to do something for her. Advice should ideally take the form of helping the patient to consider options not previously entertained (rather than direct suggestion).

THE THERAPIST'S ROLE

The therapist takes the stance of a friendly, helpful, hopeful, encouraging ally, evoking what would be expected of any physician, nurse, psychologist, social worker, or other health professional. This does not mean acting chipper and saccharine: it is important to sit with the patient's painful feelings rather than cutting them off, and before indicating that however difficult a situation may be, there is hope. As the therapist, you of course need to draw boundaries when necessary: being warm and friendly does not mean having a social friendship. Self-disclosure can be effective in rare circumstances but is generally discouraged. The focus should be on the patient, not on indulging the therapist's needs. IPT is an active therapy, and you should not allow long, painful silences. On the other hand, too much therapist activity can fragment patient affect, keeping sessions from building the depth of emotion that can make therapy effective. It takes practice to balance activity and reflective listening. Keeping interventions pithy—using a minimum of words—tends to maximize effectiveness. Patients with poor concentration can get lost in long speeches, which tend in any case to intellectualize the treatment.

In summary:

- The therapist is the patient's advocate and does not attempt a neutral stance. If the patient is self-deprecating, IPT therapists attribute such remarks to being depressed. Depressed patients are likely to take the therapist's silence after such self-criticism as agreement that the patient is worthless or as a withholding behavior on the therapist's part. Being the patient's advocate does not mean doing things for her. Rather, it means trying to understand things from the patient's point of view and validating her feelings (aside from the depressive outlook), siding with her against a sometimes hostile environment, and encouraging her to do things that she is capable of doing to change that environment.
- The therapist attempts to be nonjudgmental. Yet encouraging change in behaviors you believe are wrong, such as antisocial behavior, is a judgment that you should acknowledge as such.
- The IPT therapist does not view the therapeutic relationship through the lens of transference nor as the focus of treatment, but as an interpersonal relationship in which the patient may have feelings. The patient's expectations of assistance and understanding from the therapist are realistic and are not to be interpreted as a reenactment of the patient's previous relationships with others. The assistance that IPT therapists offer is limited to helping patients to learn and test new ways of thinking about their feelings, themselves, and their social roles and in solving interpersonal problems. When difficulties arise in the therapeutic relationship (e.g., the patient becomes angry at or feels criticized by the therapist), these are addressed in here-and-now, interpersonal fashion:

  Let's talk about what's going on between us. It's good that you're telling me you're upset—this is the sort of interpersonal communication we're working on, and with your feedback I can stop doing what's bothering you.

- Limits are set in the same way they would be in relationships with other medical clinicians.
- The therapist is active, not passive. As the therapist, you actively help to focus on improving the patient's current situation.
- The therapist encourages the patient to think of solutions to interpersonal problems. If the patient is unable to come up with new

approaches, despite your probing or leading questions, then you may suggest alternatives. The goal, however, is always to emphasize the patient's potential agency and autonomy, recognizing that the depressed patient has capacities she may not be recognizing or using while feeling hopeless and helpless.

11

Common Therapeutic Issues and Patient Questions

This chapter describes therapeutic issues that commonly arise when therapists begin practicing IPT. We also consider common patient concerns and ways to handle them. Psychotherapy is not a normal experience for most people, and these questions and answers can help with the educational component of IPT, especially in the initial phases. The chapter presents additional issues that arise when using IPT or interpersonal counseling (IPC; see Chapter 16) in primary care and other non-psychiatric medical settings.

THERAPEUTIC ISSUES

Personality

A frequent issue clinicians face is whether to focus on what DSM-IV called Axis I or Axis II: Is the main problem a psychiatric illness or a personality disorder? Syndromes on the two axes could coexist, but it was often unclear when to attribute symptoms to one axis or the other. (DSM-5 [2013] eliminated the multiaxial system, but the problem of comorbid psychiatric disorders and personality disorders persists.) A personality disorder may lead to dysfunctional behavior that yields poor outcomes in life and increases the risk of developing a depressive episode. Conversely, an episode of major depression or dysthymic disorder may heighten or mimic personality traits, creating the clinical impression of a personality disorder that may then remit if the mood disorder does (Markowitz, 1998; Markowitz et al., 2015).

IPT does not focus on the patient's personality, nor does it generally expect to change it. The exception to date is the effort to modify IPT to treat borderline personality disorder (Chapter 23). The focus on an Axis I disorder does not mean that the therapist should ignore manifestations of personality. The presence of a personality disorder may be illusory or may complicate treatment, but it should not dissuade you from IPT treatment.

The IPT stance on personality comprises the following:

- Patients who become depressed and who have other psychiatric disorders do not have unique personality traits.
- Symptoms of an Axis I disorder can mimic an Axis II diagnosis, and any definitive personality assessment should await resolution of the acute symptom state. For example, a major depressive episode may create the impression of a personality disorder that then remits if the mood disorder does (Markowitz, 1998). Depression instills social anxiety, dependency, passivity (which may sometimes be misinterpreted as passive-aggression), and avoidance of confrontation, which can easily be confused with Axis II Cluster C personality disorders. It can be almost impossible to accurately distinguish an illness state from a personality trait in the presence of an Axis I disorder. Treating the depression or other target disorder may clarify whether a personality disorder actually existed or just appeared to do so.
- A patient can have a mood disorder and personality disorder concurrently. In short-term psychotherapy, the outcome in such patients is expected to be less favorable than in those with mild or no personality pathology, just as other Axis I or Axis III (other medical) comorbidity may complicate treatment. Nonetheless, IPT may be used for acute symptom remission in the face of comorbid diagnoses.
- Personality problems may complicate treatment, altering the patient–therapist relationship and making it more difficult to manage (Foley, O'Malley, Rounsaville, Prusoff, & Weissman, 1987). Focusing on current interpersonal problems may be helpful even if the problems are largely due to the patient's behavior (as opposed to that of a significant other).

For example, you need to approach a patient with a paranoid stance with an understanding of the implications of that perspective. You can anticipate suspiciousness, disarm it with openness, and avoid threatening the patient by either acting too distant (and uninterested) or becoming too intimate (and hence threatening). A dependent patient is likely to defer to therapeutic authority, a behavior that may be linked to depression; with such a patient, you can gently encourage capability and independence, a sense of agency, rather than accept an authoritarian role. On the other hand, such patients may respond well to psychoeducation and clinical injunctions from the therapist ("*If you are feeling more suicidal, you must go to an emergency room!*").

A general clinical knowledge of personality disorders can be helpful in guiding the therapist's response to such characterological behaviors, whether these are artifacts of depression or not. As the IPT therapist, you attribute symptoms—including seeming character traits—to the depressive illness and do *not* blame the person's character (Markowitz, 1998). That is, the typical IPT use of the sick role (see Chapter 4) to excuse the patient for symptoms continues to apply. You can say:

You keep blaming yourself for these behaviors, but I see them as part of your depression. People who are depressed see themselves as defective, but that's a part of the disorder. Once we treat your depression and you're feeling better, we'll see what your "character" is like.

Personality may be a determinant of the patient's recurrent interpersonal problems. Although IPT therapists do not focus on exploring antecedents of personality functioning or changing personality, they may help patients to recognize maladaptive personality features. For instance, to a patient with mild paranoid tendencies, once having established an alliance, the therapist may point out a disposition to be touchy with certain people under certain conditions and then explore the interpersonal consequences. Personality has so far not been found to be an important determinant of short-term outcome in IPT (Markowitz et al., 1998, 2015; Zuckerman, Prusoff, Weissman, & Padian, 1980).

In the NIMH Treatment of Depression Collaborative Research Program, one analysis of patients who *completed* the study found that depressed patients with obsessive traits responded better to IPT than to CBT, whereas patients with avoidant traits (i.e., those isolated patients in the interpersonal deficits category) did better with CBT than IPT (Barber & Muenz, 1996). This finding did not apply to the treatment sample as a whole, however. In a study of depressed HIV-positive patients, the majority of whom met criteria for an Axis II personality disorder at the time of study entry, the presence of a personality disorder was associated with a slightly higher Hamilton Rating Scale for Depression score at both baseline and endpoint compared to depressed patients without personality disorders; however, the improvement in depressive symptoms was equal during the sixteen-week trial (Markowitz, Svartberg, & Swartz, 1998). In a study of IPT for chronic posttraumatic stress disorder (PTSD), personality disorder diagnosis did not predict PTSD outcome, and personality disorders often disappeared with treatment during the fourteen-week trial (Markowitz et al., 2015). These findings support the use of IPT for patients who have depression or PTSD with or without apparent personality disorders.

- Although IPT does not target personality disorder as a treatment (except for the adaptation for borderline personality disorder), it has been shown to build social skills. Without fundamentally altering personality structure, IPT can thus significantly improve overall functioning even in the presence of a personality disorder. Learning to be more assertive in disputes or to manage anger and to develop alternative ways of handling relationships may be as interpersonally useful as directly treating a personality disorder.
- By relieving depressive symptoms, IPT may improve maladaptive personality traits (Cyranowski et al., 2004; Shea et al., 2002; see case studies of interpersonal deficits [Luty], chronic depression [Markowitz], and maintenance IPT and personality pathology [Miller, Frank, Levenson] in Markowitz & Weissman, 2012).

Mobilizing the Passive Patient

Depressed patients tend to be passive, unassertive, and socially withdrawn. They fear the kinds of confrontations that often are necessary to many aspects of social interaction, particularly asserting their own needs and wishes, setting limits, and expressing anger. Therapists sometimes get patients to agree that they should be angry in a particular situation, but they are then reluctant or too guilty to express it, fearing that anger is a bad emotion, that it will destroy the relationship, and so on. A common clinical dilemma, then, is how to mobilize patients to take needed action.

One approach is to use the concept of a *transgression*. When a significant other breaks a social code, such as physically hurting the patient, having an affair, or behaving sadistically, the therapist may label this a transgression—the violation of a written or unwritten social rule, the kind of behavior that *everyone in society would agree is unacceptable*. This arms the patient with *the right to an apology*, at the very least. This conceptualization of interpersonal transgressions provides a helpful framework for some patients in thinking they have a moral right to redress.

Dealing with the transgression can then be explored in the usual IPT manner:

1. Exploring the patient's feelings (e.g., anger, sense of betrayal, disgust) about having been mistreated, which
2. the therapist can then validate. (*"Anyone would feel angry under such circumstances. Anger is a healthy interpersonal signal that someone is bothering you."*)
3. Investigating interpersonal options for expressing these feelings, and
4. having chosen an option, role playing the encounter so that patients can say what they want to say and in a tone of voice appropriate to the context.

Patients in role disputes who follow this route to seeking an apology or other redress often feel liberated and vindicated by the experience. "You owe me an apology" has been a rallying cry for many an IPT patient.

Another approach to mobilizing a passive patient involves using the treatment time limit, which exerts pressure on both the therapist and patient to accomplish something in a limited treatment interval. Although IPT assigns no formal homework, the agreement to resolve a focal interpersonal problem area (e.g., complicated grief, role dispute), followed by exploration of patient options and role playing of those options, puts the patient in a position of having a new approach to a problematic situation and only so much time to try it out.

The Intellectualizing Patient

Some patients avoid dealing with frightening affects by distancing therapy on an abstract, intellectualized plane. They may do unassigned background reading about psychotherapy, employ psychotherapeutic jargon, and speak in generalities. None of this is conducive to effective psychotherapy.

It is important to keep IPT grounded in affect. Therapy feels meaningful when it teems with emotion related to important issues in the patient's life. The structure of IPT sessions facilitates this approach by focusing each meeting on a recent, affectively charged event in the patient's life. *("How have things been since we last met? . . . I'm sorry to hear that; did something happen in the past week that contributed to your feeling so bad?")* As an IPT therapist, focus on specific events and the patient's reactions to them as a way of keeping the therapy affectively alive. One guide to the emotional vitality of the session is therapeutic boredom, which may indicate that the treatment is becoming affectless. If the patient becomes vague or discursive, you can ask, *"For example?"* and then elicit the patient's emotional responses to that example.

When emotion wells up during a session, linger and savor it. As a therapist, you want the patient to come to understand that strong emotions need not be avoided. (*"Feelings are powerful, but they're not dangerous. They can even help you understand what's happening with another person."*) Such shared emotional epiphanies are likely to stay with the patient and add impact to the therapeutic process. Even if the patient's emotional response makes you a little uncomfortable, do not intervene until she has had some time to recognize, live with, reflect on, and develop some comfort with and control over the feelings. Patients should learn in IPT that feelings, depressive and otherwise, are powerful but, at the same time, are only feelings. In IPT, patients should recognize that they can use these emotions to understand interpersonal events. They should grasp that they can come to express themselves effectively and develop some control over their feelings.

For the patient who keeps a distance by giving evaluative and intellectualizing interpretations of events (e.g., "My wife is narcissistic," "My boss is paranoid," or "Work has been hectic"), it is useful to get the details of the conversation or situation that leads the patient to these conclusions:

> *What does that ["narcissistic"] mean? Can you tell me what she did or said that gave you that sense? . . . How did you feel about that behavior?*

Details of what the patient said, how others responded, how the patient then felt, and what he said, etc., may helpfully break the barriers to feelings and help the patient to begin working on the problem.

Keeping the Focus

Holding the patient to the agreed-upon focus can be a challenge. Particularly at the start of treatment, patients may not know what to expect and may digress to a variety of topics. Once you have determined the focal problem area, described it to the patient in a formulation, and obtained the patient's agreement to work on this focus, you can and should invoke it as the therapy progresses. Bringing up the focus reminds the patient of the central theme of the depressive episode and provides a sense of thematic continuity.

If you have chosen the interpersonal problem area well, the incident elicited at the start of most sessions (*"How have things been since we last met?"*) will fit within the treatment framework. For example, sadness and loneliness during the week may be tied to complicated bereavement; anger or marital strife may be connected with a role dispute. Sometimes the patient will raise an interpersonal situation that resonates with the current theme (e.g., an office disagreement parallel to a marital role dispute). If so, help the patient solve it, and then point out the parallel. With your encouragement, the patient will soon learn to stay on track until the problem area is resolved.

Short digressions can be tolerated, but you do not want the treatment to meander so far as to lose its direction and shape. If the patient deviates, listen carefully—you do not want to disparage information that the patient feels is important—but try to resolve the extraneous issue quickly and remind the patient of the focus you had both decided would be central to the treatment. (*"What you're bringing up is interesting, but we only have X sessions in this treatment to resolve the role transition you're going through."*) Returning to the focus should not be a mechanical and artificial process but rather an organizing motif for the treatment. If (rarely) the problem area clearly needs to shift because of new material that arises (e.g., the sudden death of a significant other during the course of treatment), make this move explicit.

Sticking to the Time Limit

Psychotherapists unused to time limits may need practice to adjust to the pressure induced by a predetermined eight- or twelve-week cutoff point. Such a constraint indeed pressures both therapist and patient to work hard and quickly. It also provides the patient with a clear structure for the treatment. Hence, you should resist the temptation to dilute this pressure by failing to fully define the treatment length or granting extra sessions without an imperative rationale. *"We'll work for twelve to sixteen sessions"* is unnecessarily vague; make the limit precisely twelve, fourteen, or sixteen. *The exact number is less meaningful than that there be an exact number.*

Sessions generally should occur weekly, allowing time between sessions for things to happen in the patient's life yet maintaining momentum. Plan for vacations at the start of treatment. Try to make up sessions if you or the patient has to cancel one (therapist flexibility is a virtue patients appreciate), while keeping to the overall threshold. If you take the time limit seriously, so will the patient.

THERAPIST NOTE

Patients with many obligations—such as those caring for small children or who live far away—need flexibility. If need be, holding a session by telephone or secure

Skype may be preferable to breaking the momentum of therapy by missing a session altogether.

If a patient comes late to or misses sessions, attribute this lateness to the patient's depressive illness rather than personality pathology or "resistance." Such an attribution fits the IPT medical model, facilitates the therapeutic alliance, and is likely to be accurate for depressed patients. If you have the time to tag on a few minutes at the end of a late-starting session, it is worth doing so. On the other hand, if a patient repeatedly cancels or misses sessions without plausible rationale, continue to count down the sessions, sticking to the time limit and increasing pressure to attend.

Silence

Silence occurs in any therapy and is a normal part of the treatment. It may indicate the patient's discomfort with treatment and avoidance of emotionally charged material. In IPT, the patient and the therapist share responsibility for raising topics to discuss and explore. When emotionally laden material has been discussed, a period of silence may follow. If a situation is very charged, there may be a few moments during which the patient cannot talk about it. In such situations, you probably will not probe, as it might be more helpful to wait for the material to come up spontaneously. You might explain:

> *Silence does not necessarily mean that no work is going on. The therapy involves sharing the experiences of the time, which may include silence as well as active discussion.*

On the other hand, don't make this comment if you are simply anxious that there has been a silence.

If silence becomes a persistent problem, it will require discussion. You might say:

> *It's possible that you have done so well and are feeling so good that there's nothing more to talk about. In this case, we should talk about terminating treatment. . . . If you don't feel that the problems are solved, then you might try to figure out what is making it hard to discuss how you're feeling. Are you feeling guilty about something? Ashamed? Fearful of what I might think about what's on your mind? Do you feel that something is inappropriate? That I'll disapprove?*

Some patients use silence as an interpersonal style: they pout or sulk rather than voice legitimate complaints. If your patient does this, you may address the issue directly without framing it as a criticism:

> *When you're feeling depressed, is it hard to let someone know when you're feeling upset with him? . . . If this is the case, it might be helpful to look at the effects*

your silence has on others and whether it is an effective form of communication for you.

You may also gently make the point that:

There are no "bad" feelings. Your feelings tell us something about what's going on in your life, and they can be helpful guideposts to understanding your situation. Even if it feels awkward, I encourage you to let me know as much as you can about how you're feeling. Often it feels better to bring uncomfortable feelings up rather than bottling them inside.

TECHNICAL ISSUES

Some therapists may view psychotherapy purely as two people talking in a room and may consider rating scales and recording devices uncomfortable intrusions at first. Yet both can be important aspects of IPT.

Choose a rating instrument for depression (or the appropriate target syndrome) and get to know it. The American Psychiatric Association's *Handbook of Psychiatric Measures* (2008) lists various scales that either you (e.g., the Hamilton Rating Scale for Depression—see Appendix A at the end of this book) or the patient (e.g., the Beck Depression Inventory or Patient Health Questionnaire—see Appendix B) can complete to assess symptom severity. Get used to administering the scale both at intake and at regular intervals during the treatment. Measuring symptoms facilitates psychoeducation—the patient will leave having memorized the symptoms of depression—and keeps both you and the patient attuned to progress. As symptoms diminish, you can congratulate patients on their progress:

- *You've cut your score in half already!*
- *Your Hamilton Depression score is now 7—a big improvement from the 22 you started with. You're officially in clinical remission! Good work!*

Many clinicians who get into the habit of using rating scales in IPT subsequently use them in all of their treatments.

You may also want to audio- or video-record your treatment sessions for supervisory purposes. An actual tape of the session is the best way to evaluate the therapeutic process: it is far more accurate and less intrusive than process notes. Like a therapist in an IPT session, your supervisor will want to know what each of you said and how it felt. If you do record sessions, first obtain the patient's written consent for taping and explain the purpose of doing so, your concern for protecting the patient's confidentiality, and what will happen to the tapes:

I will be using this only for supervisory purposes; only my supervisor, an IPT expert, will be reviewing the tape, which I will keep in a locked drawer and erase at the end of the treatment [or in two years, or whatever you stated in the consent form].

Therapists tend to be more worried about the taping process than patients are. You may at first feel self-conscious with a tape or video recorder running, but you are likely to learn a lot from the experience and to adjust to the process after a few sessions. Later you may be pleased to have recorded your finest therapeutic moments on tape—rather than your worst, as you may initially fear!

COMPARISON WITH OTHER TREATMENTS

The literature of the past century lists hundreds of kinds of psychotherapy. Most of these represent the personal approaches of charismatic psychotherapists, and the overwhelming majority of these approaches have never been tested for efficacy. IPT inevitably overlaps with some of these approaches in using particular techniques. It is the coherence of its interpersonal strategies and its targeting of psychiatric disorders as medical illnesses, rather than the particular techniques involved, that define IPT as a treatment. Nonetheless, there are techniques that IPT does not use (which also helps to define it as a treatment).

The two psychotherapies to which IPT is most often compared are psychodynamic psychotherapy and CBT. Many IPT therapists have received training in one or both of these backgrounds. IPT and psychodynamic psychotherapy are both affect-focused treatments. However, compared to psychodynamic psychotherapy, IPT focuses more on the here and now, rather than on childhood antecedents; it focuses on the patient's life outside the office rather than on the therapeutic relationship within it; and it does not interpret dreams or transference. Compared at least to psychodynamic therapies that are not diagnosis-focused and time-limited, IPT takes a more organized, outcome-focused approach to changing interpersonal patterns as a method of relieving symptoms of a depressive or other psychiatric syndrome (Markowitz et al., 1998).

THERAPIST NOTE

If an IPT patient raises a dream, you might comment on its manifest interpersonal content and underlying affect, such as, *"What was your mood in the dream?"*, and then steer the treatment back to the agreed-upon focus.

Like IPT, CBT is an often time-limited treatment that has been applied to a range of psychiatric diagnoses. Whereas IPT focuses on affect and behavior in interpersonal relationships, CBT focuses on the irrational thoughts (cognitions) that arise in such contexts. If IPT is more structured than psychodynamic psychotherapy, CBT is still more structured than IPT, frequently beginning each session by developing an agenda for the meeting. CBT therapists assign homework, including undertaking specific activities and making lists of cognitions. In contrast, IPT has no formal agenda and assigns no homework—unless the resolution of the interpersonal problem areas (e.g., role dispute) within the framework of the treatment time limit is considered a kind of grand therapeutic assignment.

Thus, IPT differs from both psychodynamic psychotherapy and CBT, eschewing many of their key techniques. IPT has been called a "supportive psychotherapy." This often amorphous and originally pejorative term once referred to diluted psychodynamic psychotherapy for patients too ill to tolerate transferential interpretations. As IPT does not employ interpretations, it is in that sense a supportive psychotherapy. More modern definitions of supportive psychotherapy (e.g., Novalis, Rojcewicz, & Peele, 1993; Pinsker, 1997) emphasize the so-called common factors of psychotherapy (Frank, 1971): release of affect, helping the patient feel understood, building a strong therapeutic alliance, and so on (refer to Box 10.1). In this sense, IPT contains elements of supportive psychotherapy but also emphasizes specific interpersonal interventions and strategies that supportive therapists use far less often and less systematically (Amole et al., in press; Markowitz et al., 2000). No other psychotherapies explicitly focus on the IPT problem areas.

PATIENT QUESTIONS

How Does IPT Work?

Most patients, especially if they have never been in psychotherapy, have legitimate questions about how talking to a stranger can help them with their problems. You can explain:

> *Psychotherapy is not a mystery. Psychotherapy involves a relationship with someone you can trust, who is here to try to help you, who will hold what you say in strict confidence, and who will not take a judgmental approach or decide what is right or wrong for you. In interpersonal psychotherapy, we work on the connection between your feelings and your life situation. In the next X weeks, we will work on unfulfilled wishes and problematic relationships that are contributing to your depression. You should begin to become more comfortable with your feelings in problematic close relationships and decide how to use them to change the relationship/situation you're in.*
>
> *We're not sure exactly how IPT works, but some of its benefits come from learning to understand your own feelings, using them to fix difficult interpersonal situations, and finding people in your environment who can give you emotional support.*

What Credentials Should My Therapist Have?

IPT is designed for use by psychiatrists, psychologists, primary care physicians, psychiatric social workers, psychiatric nurses, and other health professionals who have had at least several years of clinical experience in psychotherapy with depressed patients. There is increasing interest and experience in training health workers good at focusing on relationships through didactic training and supervision (see Chapter 24).

If patients ask, tell them your credentials. Usually, questions about credentials reflect discomfort with the therapeutic situation. In the beginning, patients without prior treatment experience may find that the therapeutic situation feels unnatural. Encourage patients to discuss their discomfort directly and determine with you whether the problem is not just discomfort in seeking help. You can reassure the patient that, beyond knowing your credentials, she needs to feel comfortable with you. Encourage the patient to raise any criticisms or complaints that may arise (this parallels the encouragement of raising feelings and confronting others in the patient's outside life). Apologize if you're late or mix up an appointment. Make it clear that you will not be insulted if the patient wants to consider a different treatment or therapist. At the same time, it is important not to present such nonchalance in offering an alternative referral that the patient finds you uncaring or rejecting.

I Thought It Didn't Matter If I Came Late

Patients new to psychotherapy who are used to attending crowded clinics with long waits, where appointment times are relatively meaningless, may fail to show up on time. In such cases, help the patient acculturate to psychotherapy. This means explaining that the sessions will begin and end on time, and that you have set aside this time for the patient. The IPT time limit can be used to emphasize the importance of the therapy session: *"We have only nine sessions left."*

Sometimes patients may arrive late because of practical problems such as transportation or babysitters. This should be discussed. However, it is also useful when appropriate to relate the lateness to patients' feeling of hopelessness about their condition and the value of treatment, and moreover the fact that being depressed may make it difficult for them to get to sessions. Depressed individuals are in fact often late to many things, not just therapy, and it's helpful to model blaming the disorder rather than the patient. You can offer a supportive statement such as:

> *It's hard to get to treatment when you are feeling so bad and when you haven't slept and don't have much energy.*

This avoids blaming the patient for depressive symptoms that may underlie not coming to treatment.

Of course, the patient's attendance may waver in the face of sessions on top-ics that are anxiety-provoking and stressful. The patient may also feel that treat-ment is not helping her or that her life perhaps is getting better, and thus she may not want to spend the time in discussions. It is useful to talk about these issues directly, distinguishing between true lack of progress and subjective depressive perceptions of hopelessness. (This is another juncture where rating scales have benefits.)

Can My Family Come to the Treatment?

IPT was designed as a treatment for individual patients and has been adapted for couples and groups (Chapter 25). Most IPT therapists have been individual psy-chotherapists who have had less expertise in other treatment formats. Depressed patients may ask about involving family members because they feel inadequate to the task of therapy themselves. Yet their prognosis is good, and if they do partici-pate in individual IPT, they can leave with full credit for their gains.

Bringing in family members is likely to shift the role of the therapist, who may be pushed into a more coordinating, mediating role. Family members and patients may appeal to therapists for approval. Thus, whereas individual IPT focusing on a role dispute is, in essence, unilateral "couples therapy" (Chapter 6) that the patient actively solves on his own—an agency the IPT therapist wants to encourage—bringing in family is likely to shift credit to the therapist.

It is occasionally helpful to have significant family members (spouse, parents) participate in one or more therapy sessions if there are marital or parent–child problems and if both the patient and the significant other are willing to do so. These joint sessions may be used to acquire additional information, obtain the cooperation of the significant other, or facilitate some interpersonal problem solving and communication. For couples who have marital disputes, a conjoint marital IPT has been developed for use when both parties want to participate (Chapter 25).

The patient should feel free to ask you whether a family member can attend, and you may also request the person's attendance, especially in initial sessions. In treating minors, parents should be involved to provide consent and often attend the initial sessions (Chapter 14).

Family member participation, however, must not violate confidentiality. Clarify beforehand with the patient what will and will not be discussed in con-joint sessions: that you will not discuss the content of patient sessions with the other person, and that you will discuss and report any additional contact you have with the other person. Your allegiance should remain to the patient's improvement.

The increasing use of IPT cross-nationally may require local modification of the extent of including families (Chapter 24). In countries where family mem-bers almost always accompany the patient for treatment, the therapist must make accommodation to include the family. Beyond custom or curiosity, family members may have legitimate reasons for attending the patient's treatment, and these must be understood and respected.

Do I Need a Different Treatment?

No one treatment benefits all patients. In some cases, IPT patients will need different or additional treatment, including referral to a different kind of psychotherapy (e.g., CBT) or for psychotropic medication (with or without IPT). That multiple options exist to treat the disorder merits open discussion at the beginning of therapy so that the patient feels permitted to inquire about alternatives during the course of therapy. A consultation with a psychiatrist may be useful for patients not in therapy with a psychiatrist. This exploration of therapeutic options is consonant with the IPT medical model and with the pragmatic IPT emphasis on the exploration of options.

On the other hand, some depressed patients ask the question because they are skeptical about *all* treatment. You may reassure them that their chances of improving are good even if they won't fully believe that until they're better. If a patient has not had at least a 50 percent reduction in symptoms or a complete remission at the end of twelve sessions or twelve weeks, consider a different psychotherapy or the addition of medication (or a switch of medication) (Markowitz & Milrod, 2015).

Will I Get Along on My Own at the End of the Treatment?

Patients are apt to have this concern during time-limited psychotherapy. Even if they have achieved remission by the end of the brief treatment, they will not have been feeling well for very long and may lack confidence that their improvement will last. Yet depressed patients (and sometimes their therapists) often underestimate their capabilities. The patient may expect to miss the therapist's guidance, especially if it has been useful. Yet a goal of IPT is to inculcate a method: a patient should leave treatment with knowledge that depression can potentially recur, and with an understanding of the link between mood and life events and new skills for handling interpersonal situations. That is, the patient should leave treatment having learned the IPT method—something to reinforce during the IPT termination phase. (Providing a clear approach for the patient to take from therapy is a reason to adhere strictly to IPT rather than venturing into eclectic therapy.) You can tell the patient that dependency on the therapist is focused and limited. The therapist helps the patient recognize her own personal strengths and capabilities. As a patient begins to feel better and to deal better with interpersonal problems, some reliance on the therapist will disappear. However, the option for additional (or different) therapy always remains at the end of a course of treatment.

What If I Want to End Treatment Early?

The patient may wish to terminate early because the patient and therapist disagree about the therapy contract; because the patient feels the continuation of therapy is threatening; or because she believes the problem has been satisfactorily addressed and feels better. A frank discussion here is useful. Ask questions such as:

- *Why do you want to stop at this point? If you want to end the treatment early, it's your choice, but we should consider why you do.*
- *Are you no longer depressed?* [Perhaps repeat the rating scale.]
- *Do these issues feel too painful or frightening to confront?*
- *Is there some problem between the two of us that we haven't discussed?*
- *Do you feel that IPT is not the right treatment for you, and that alternatives should be considered?*

Make it clear that the goal of therapy is to help the patient feel better, not to tie the person to the IPT treatment.

Is My Depression Biological?

As information about the biological bases of depression reaches the popular press, patients increasingly ask questions about a cause: "Is my depression due to a chemical imbalance or to my stressful marriage?" Debates about whether depressions are biological or psychological miss the point. You can say:

All depressions have a biological component. They are associated with changes in sleep, appetite, energy levels, and concentration. The feelings of depression reflect brain chemistry. These biological changes, and increasing information about genetic vulnerability to depression, do not change the fact that all depressions also occur in a psychosocial context. A person's mood can be markedly altered by upsetting changes in relationships with others— in your case, by the marital dispute we've been talking about. Research has shown that stressful life events can trigger episodes of depression in genetically vulnerable people.

We can't do much to change genes, but psychotherapy can do a lot to identify and handle your stressful life situation. Depression usually responds to medication, or psychotherapy, or a combination of the two. Biology and psychosocial context are intimately related and difficult to separate from each other. That may explain why both psychotherapy and medication work on symptoms that appear very biological (e.g., loss of appetite), as well as those that appear more psychological (e.g., feelings of guilt, low self-esteem). Neuroimaging studies have shown that psychotherapy changes your brain chemistry [Brody et al., 2001; Martin et al., 2001]: it's a biological treatment.

Can I Give Depression to My Children?

There is little question that depression runs in families. The children of depressed parents carry a two to three times greater risk for becoming depressed than the children of parents who have never been depressed (Weissman, Berry, Warner, et al., 2016; Weissman, Wickramaratne, Gameroff, et al., 2016). Put another way, if the overall average rate of depression is 3 percent, the risk for children of depressed parents is 6 to 9 percent. The good news is that most of the children will *not* develop depression. We do not know the mechanisms by which depression is transmitted in families—whether it is through genes, learning, stress, or some combination. You can tell the patient:

> *If you are depressed and your children seem to be having similar problems, pay attention, take it seriously, talk to them about it, and get them help. There is good evidence that improving your symptoms will have a positive effect on your children. It's harder to be a parent when you're feeling depressed. Relief from stressful events and figuring out better ways to handle them may help to reduce or eliminate triggers of depression both for you and for any vulnerable family members.*

Remission of parental depression has beneficial effects on their children's symptoms (Swartz et al., 2016 Weissman, Berry, Warner, et al., 2016; Weissman, Wickramaratne, Gameroff, et al., 2016; Weissman, Wickramaratne, Pilowsky, et al., 2015). Consonant with the IPT model, emphasize that the depressive risk to children, like the patient's depression itself, is not the patient's fault: depression is a medical illness, comparable to high blood pressure or arthritis, that tends to run in families.

What About Alcohol and Drugs?

There is high comorbidity between depression and alcohol abuse, particularly in depressed men. Depressed patients may try in various ways to relieve their symptoms before coming for treatment, and alcohol can seem an enticing solution. In the short run, alcohol may relieve anxiety, improve mood, help the depressed individual sleep, and dull painful memories and anxiety. On the other hand, you can tell the patient:

> *Alcohol feels good in the short run, but it's bad for depression in the long run. While it may help your mood and sleep at first, over time it disturbs sleep and depresses your mood. It can diminish your ability to cope, it creates additional problems with family and at work, it interferes with treatment, and it may increase suicide risk. There's also the danger of ending up with two problems, depression and alcoholism.*

Part of taking a good initial history involves exploring substance use. Ask patients about their use of alcohol, recreational drugs, and prescription medications. Antidepressants and other medications may potentiate the effects of drugs or alcohol. Patients with heavy or chronic substance use may require detoxification prior to or concomitant with antidepressant treatment. Your goal as an IPT therapist is to help the patient substitute healthy interpersonal responses, using improved communication to reach outward, for the tendency to reach for the bottle and retreat inward.

Is My Depression Incurable?

Patients with acute depressive symptoms feel hopeless. You can say:

> When you're depressed, it often feels like the symptoms will last forever. However, with an evidence-based treatment, more than half of the time depression responds in four to six weeks. As your sleep and appetite problems begin to resolve, you will find that your mood improves. There are many different types of effective treatments for depression. IPT is just one of them. I can't promise you that this treatment will help you, but there's a very good chance it will. If it doesn't, there are other types of psychotherapies and a range of medications that can help. So if one treatment does not work, there are plenty of alternatives to try. Give the treatment time to work. Don't let the hopelessness of depression discourage you from continuing: that hopelessness is a very misleading symptom of depression, and your prognosis, in fact, is good.

What If I Have Thoughts of Suicide?

Because depressed patients suffer, and most feel hopeless about the future being any less painful, thoughts of suicide are common. Suicide is the greatest risk that depression brings. Inquiries about suicidal thoughts, plans, and attempts are a necessary part of the initial evaluation and should continue during treatment as needed:

> Have you been feeling so bad that life hasn't felt worth living?
> [If yes:] How far have those thoughts gone? . . . Do you have a plan for how you might kill yourself?

A person who has a plan to end her life in the near future needs urgent care and referral to keep safe. You must ask such patients direct questions about suicide throughout the assessment and intervention. Too many clinicians avoid asking direct questions about suicide even if they suspect a patient has these troubling thoughts. This is often because they fear that talking about suicide will put ideas in the patient's head. One unfortunate consequence of therapist silence about suicide is that the suffering patient will remain alone and unsupported in addressing this painful, potentially lethal symptom. It is important to encourage the patient to feel comfortable in talking openly about suicide (like any topic) and to show her that you are not shocked by anything she might say. Because suicide can be such a sensitive topic, you must put aside personal beliefs about suicide.

> *The symptoms of depression can be overwhelming and invade every part of your life. You feel your life is out of control. If you feel great pain and distress and are hopeless that things will ever improve, you may feel life is not worth living, wish you were dead, or perhaps think about killing yourself. If you feel this way, please let me know! The pain, hopelessness, and suicidal thoughts are all symptoms of the depression; they're treatable, and they're not your fault. Suicide is the worst outcome of depression. It's important that you stay alive long enough to treat the depression and get better—after which, you'll very probably want to live. People who are no longer depressed don't want to kill themselves, and you have in fact a great chance of getting better in treatment. If the feelings get stronger, we can have more frequent contacts either in person or by phone.*

Will Depression Return When IPT Ends?

Most patients who recover from a depressive episode are understandably concerned about having a relapse or a recurrence. About 30 percent of people who have a single depressive episode will never have another one (Judd et al., 1998). Over a lifetime, then, most patients will have recurrences, usually in the face of a life event. Patient education during IPT can help them to understand and anticipate situations that could provoke recurrence and either find ways to handle them or seek early treatment. Understanding of prevention of recurrences is increasing. You could tell the patient that vulnerability to depression is the same kind of chronic medical vulnerability that puts people at risk for high blood pressure, asthma, high cholesterol, or heart disease:

> *We will talk about situations that might put you at risk for another episode, and hopefully you'll be able to deal with those situations before they get to you and result in symptoms. You should leave here expert in recognizing early symptoms of depression. Depression is a medical vulnerability, sort of like having an ulcer. If you should get depressed in the future, the important thing to remember is that it's a treatable illness, it's not your fault, and you just need to return for treatment, the way you would for any other medical problem.*

Patients who have had multiple episodes of major depression carry high risk for further episodes. IPT has shown efficacy as a maintenance treatment for depression (Chapter 9). Thus, ongoing maintenance IPT is an option for patients who have benefited from acute IPT but remain at high risk for relapse or recurrence.

PROBLEMS MORE OFTEN SEEN IN PRIMARY CARE SETTINGS

Depression Presenting as Physical Symptoms

As the use of IPT and its briefer forms like IPC (Chapter 16) increases in primary care clinics, more clinicians will see patients with problems related to the ambiguity and overlap between physical and mental symptoms. Many patients going through life crises present with physical symptoms (headaches, pain, indigestion, fatigue, sleep problems) unrelated to a (non-depressive) medical condition. Review physical examination and laboratory tests, if available, with the patient and ensure that tests are negative.

The possible relationship between symptoms and concerns and stress in the patient's life deserves explicit discussion. Ask about recent changes in life circumstances, mood, and social functioning to determine how life circumstances may relate to the onset of symptoms, and reassure the patient that you will explore current problems that may be contributing to the physical symptoms. If you are not a physician, consult with the patient's primary care physician as appropriate.

Patient reactions to this type of exploration can take at least three directions:

1. The patient may insist that he has an undetected physical illness.
2. The patient may remain focused on the somatic distress—sleep disturbance, fatigue—and deny any possible connection to life stress.
3. The patient may acknowledge to varying degrees some current life stress.

The first response is the least frequent and most difficult one to address. If the patient responds in either the first or second way (i.e., with denial), do not push or lecture her. If this stance persists, it may be necessary to consult with the treating physician, delay further contacts, and offer to review the physical examination. As in usual clinical practice, it may reassure the patient to provide information about why her worries about medical illness are improbable. Consider whether he is alexithymic, and is not registering emotional symptoms of depression, and may need affective attunement in psychotherapy; or whether the problem is a somatic delusion that might require antipsychotic medication.

Proceed gently with such patients. Don't argue with or try to convince the patient, and never deny the reality of the depressive symptoms and the real discomfort they produce. Always leave the door open and attempt to arrange another visit, gently stating that you'd like to give the patient another chance to explore what is going on in her life and to see how she is doing.

Recognize, too, that depressed patients with a comorbid medical illness may unavoidably have to repeatedly cancel appointments, causing disputes with their health-care providers. If so, IPT can address this situation as a role dispute or role transition.

Poor Adherence to Medication or Medical Regimens

Nonadherence to medical treatment can be a persistent problem leading to treatment failure or suboptimal benefit, poor outcomes, and poor quality of life. This nonadherence may become a topic in IPT. The *sick role* excuses patients from what their illness precludes them from doing, but it carries the responsibility to work as a patient to get better.

Nonadherence includes the patient's not taking medications for medical or psychiatric conditions, not following medical recommendations such as diet or exercise, and missing medical or therapy appointments. Following the no-fault IPT approach, you should attempt to blame the patient's depressive symptoms where appropriate rather than making her feel bad for noncompliance: diminished energy and lack of concentration do make exercise and remembering to take pills more difficult, and depressed patients tend to be late to many events, not just medical or therapy appointments.

> *People who are depressed have a harder time taking care of their medical health.*

You can remark upon the benefits of adherence and the health threats of nonadherence. Elicit the patient's perception of the problem and her understanding of why adherence problems exist. Find ways, where possible, to simplify the regimen tailored to the patient: for example, one higher-dosage pill rather than two; simplifying diet; and understanding practical obstacles to attendance, such as transportation, cost, and family disappointment.

Your understanding, concern, and interest in the patient's viewpoint are essential. Often the solutions need reinforcement over time.

Adaptations of IPT for Mood Disorders

12

Overview of Adaptations of IPT

The success of IPT as a treatment for acute major depressive episodes (Cuijpers et al., 2011) has led to its adaptation and testing for patients diagnosed with other mood and non-mood disorders and in different formats (Cuijpers et al., 2016). All of these modified treatments follow the general IPT principles already described. Some have been detailed in separate manuals, which contain usually minor changes relevant to the specific disorder, age group, or treatment format they address (see Chapter 26). We summarize here some of the numerous adaptations researchers have made; there is simply no room to include them all. Parameters to consider are time requirements (treatment duration), clinical experience, and empirical support. We recommend that you review the DSM-5 diagnostic criteria for the disorder of interest (American Psychiatric Association, 2013) and have some clinical experience in treating patients with that diagnosis before attempting to use IPT to treat them.

TIME

Studies of IPT for acute major depressive disorder have typically used a preset time limit of twelve or sixteen sessions in as many weeks. Some of the following adaptations have altered this time, or "dosage" interval. Swartz and colleagues have tested IPT in as few as eight sessions (Swartz et al., 2008, 2014), and interpersonal counseling (Chapter 16) may use even fewer weekly sessions. As is true for most psychotherapies, the optimal number of sessions in IPT has received relatively little testing. In clinical practice, some flexibility may be reasonable to adjust for vacations, upsetting events occurring late in therapy, and so on. Yet it is important in IPT to set and hold to a time limit of some kind. The time limit provides structure so that the patient knows what to expect, and the pressure of time helps propel the acute therapy forward.

EXPERIENCE

This book will not equip you as a clinician to treat all patients with all diagnoses or to use IPT in a group format if you have never done group therapy. To effectively treat patients who carry a particular diagnosis, you must not only learn IPT but also have experience in working with patients to whom that adaptation applies. To treat depressed adolescents, patients with eating disorders, or those with borderline personality disorder, you should know the clinical terrain as well as the psychotherapeutic approach. To work with patients in conjoint (couples) or group IPT, you should have familiarity with those treatment modalities.

EMPIRICAL SUPPORT

The level of empirical support for each of these adaptations varies and will shift as new studies are conducted. To guide you, we have developed the following shorthand scale to rate the strength of empirical foundation for each adaptation that follows:

> **** (four stars):** Treatment has been validated by at least two randomized controlled trials demonstrating the superiority of IPT to a control condition. This generally qualifies treatments for inclusion in treatment guidelines, as is the case for IPT for major depressive disorder.
> *** (three stars):** Validation by at least one randomized controlled trial or equivalent to a reference treatment of established efficacy
> ** (two stars):** Encouraging findings in one or more open trials or in pilot studies with small samples (less than twelve subjects)
> * (one star):** Undergoing testing or not tested
> **(no stars):** Negative findings (IPT has been found to be no better than a control condition)

Thus, IPT for acute major depression has a four-star rating based on multiple positive comparisons to control conditions (Cuijpers et al., 2011, 2016).

13

Peripartum Depression

Pregnancy, Miscarriage, Postpartum, Infertility

OVERVIEW

IPT is based on the hypothesis that patients who experience social disruptions face an increased risk for depression. This in itself has made IPT an interesting potential treatment for addressing symptoms that develop during the perinatal period.

The idea of pregnancy as a time of unconditional well-being is a myth (Cohen et al., 2006). Ten percent of pregnant women experience major depression, and for many, the depressive episode continues into the postpartum period. Rates are even higher in low- and middle-income countries (Fisher et al., 2012). Complications of pregnancy and miscarriage can lead to chronic depression. "New baby blues" (i.e., mild depressive symptoms in the six months following childbirth) are so common as to be considered normal. Yet these blues may be prolonged, impair functioning, and require treatment. Risk factors for depression during this period include a personal or family history of depression; chronic marital, family, or financial problems; a history of child abuse; young age; medical complications during pregnancy; or unwanted pregnancy.

Adequate treatment of depression is important for the health not only of the mother but of the infant and other children in the family. There is good evidence that maternal depression impairs mother–infant bonding and may harm the child's later cognitive and emotional development. Infants of mothers depressed during pregnancy display poorer motor performance, dysregulated behavior, low birth weight, and altered amygdala functional connectivity (Grote, Bledsoe, Swartz, & Frank, 2004; Rifkin-Graboi et al., 2013). Pregnancy is a good time for health interventions, as pregnant women have already entered the health-care system if they are receiving prenatal care, and almost certainly have during delivery and the postnatal period.

The U.S. Preventive Services Task Force in 2016 recommended screening for depression during pregnancy and the postpartum period, implemented with adequate services in place to ensure accurate diagnosis, effective treatment, and follow-up (Siu et al., 2016). Thus we can expect better identification and treatment of more depressed pregnant women. The choice of treatment is complex, as the full effects of maternal medication treatment (compared to untreated maternal depression) on the developing fetus remain unclear. The topic is difficult to study because pregnancy precludes randomized clinical trials, researchers must disentangle the effects on the fetus of maternal depression from the effects of maternal medication, and potential sequelae require long-term follow-up. Recent studies of the use of serotonin reuptake inhibitors (SSRIs) during pregnancy urge caution because of short-term effects on infant motor scores and arousal (Salisbury et al., 2016), infant speech perception, and later motor and language difficulties (Brown et al., 2016; Weikum et al., 2012). There may also be a delayed effect of increasing depression risk when the child reaches adolescence (Malm et al., 2016). Mouse model studies of in utero exposure to SSRIs found these latter depression effects in early adolescence, and the findings have been supported by human birth cohort studies, even after controlling for maternal depression (Malm et al., 2016). Psychotherapies, in contrast, present minimal fetal risk but need to demonstrate efficacy for peripartum women.

The U.S. Preventive Services Task Force noted only a small risk of harm from in utero exposure to SSRIs on fetal health and lack of evidence of harm in postpartum women (O'Connor et al., 2016). Oddly, the task force found only three clinical trials of psychotherapy in pregnant depressed women, all involving CBT. Fourteen additional clinical trials included postpartum depressed women, seven of which studied CBT and the rest nondirective psychotherapy (N = 3), psychodynamic psychotherapy (N = 1), and other (N = 3). Only three trials did not support the favored intervention.

In fact, IPT ranks among the best-studied treatments for depressed peripartum women. Contrary to the selective findings of the task force (Siu et al., 2016), which located no IPT studies, we found five clinical trials of IPT in pregnancy, six in the postpartum period, and others addressing depression in the context of infertility treatment or following miscarriage. The unknown effects on the fetus of in utero medication exposure and the effects of untreated maternal depression on mother and fetus make psychotherapy an important treatment during pregnancy and breastfeeding.

Levels of evidence for IPT are as follows:

IPT during pregnancy: **** (four stars; validation by five randomized controlled trial or equivalent to a reference treatment of established efficacy)

IPT for miscarriage: ** (two stars; encouraging findings in one or more open trials or in pilot studies with small samples)

IPT for infertility: * (one star; one clinical trial with a small sample)

IPT during the postpartum period: **** (four stars; six randomized controlled trials and one open trial)

ADAPTATIONS

The adaptations of IPT needed to treat depression during pregnancy, miscarriage, the postpartum period, and infertility have been minimal (Grote et al., 2009; Klier et al., 2001; Koszycki et al., 2012; Mulcahy et al., 2010; Neugebauer, Kline, Bleiberg, et al., 2006; Neugebauer, Kline, Markowitz, et al., 2006; O'Hara et al., 2000; O'Hara, Stuart, Gorman, & Wenzel, 2000; Reay et al., 2012; Spinelli & Endicott, 2003; Spinelli et al., 2013; Zlotnick et al., 2006, 2011). The usual IPT problem areas neatly suit the issues that arise for women at these times. The birth of a child is a major role transition and may cause family disputes. Miscarriage and infertility are times of grieving and role transitions. The adaptations involve:

1. *Differentiating between depressive symptoms and symptoms of normal pregnancy*: Symptoms associated with pregnancy and the postpartum period can overlap with those of depression, particularly fatigue, appetite change, low energy, and sleep problems. It is useful to try to differentiate those that result from normal pregnancy from those that may be depressive. In reviewing symptoms, find out whether they began before or during pregnancy or postpartum. For mild symptoms following childbirth, determine their impact on the mother's functioning and the duration and history of major depression.

2. *Interpersonal inventory and pregnancy history*: To determine the triggers of a depressive episode, explore the woman's feelings about the pregnancy, the delivery, the baby, the father's role, whether it was a wanted pregnancy, the types of social support available, who is living in the house, and the ages of other children. A sexual and reproductive history, including previous miscarriages, pregnancy difficulties, and use of in vitro fertilization, is indicated. The interpersonal inventory remains unaltered, except that the concept of family may need expansion to include a parental surrogate and the anticipated newborn.

3. *Time flexibility*: Some modification of the timing and duration of treatment may be necessary depending on the stage of the pregnancy. A flexible therapist should take into account the pregnancy stage at which the woman presents for treatment, the expected time of delivery, and other family obligations. A break in therapy may be needed around delivery, with continuation into the postpartum period. Less frequent visits following childbirth or telephone sessions should sometimes be considered so that attending treatment sessions does not add to the new mother's burden. On the other hand, some women find therapy sessions a welcome break from the seemingly overwhelming responsibilities of childcare; in fact, if the woman remains seriously depressed and it is possible to telephone or meet with her during the obstetrical admission for delivery, such contact may cement the therapeutic alliance and provide relief during a potential crisis. There is substantial support

for using the telephone to provide psychotherapy, including IPT (see Chapter 25).

If the woman would find it helpful and agrees, it may sometimes be appropriate to involve other family members who may have substantial roles in caring for both the child and the mother during the pregnancy and postpartum.

IPT for Depression During Pregnancy

The potentially positive impact on both mother and child of preventing or reducing depressive symptoms in pregnant and new mothers has led to several adaptations of IPT. A pilot study comparing four-session group IPT to treatment as usual found IPT beneficial in reducing postpartum depression in pregnant women at high risk for major depression because of a history of depression and/or poor social supports (Zlotnick et al., 2001). The four IPT sessions provided psychoeducation about new baby blues, discussed the role transition associated with the birth and ways to manage it, and, in the final session, focused on identifying and handling disputes.

Zlotnick et al. (2011) later offered four-session individual IPT plus a booster session within two weeks of delivery to pregnant women with domestic partner interpersonal violence. They found effects for reducing posttraumatic stress disorder (PTSD) and depression symptoms during pregnancy and a large effect up to three months postpartum. Standard IPT was used, with the initial sessions including description of the abusive relationship and a safety plan.

Grote et al. (2009) conducted eight-session IPT before birth and up to six months postpartum in a difficult-to-engage, impoverished, non-treatment-seeking population. The treatment added a motivational interviewing engagement session at its start designed to understand obstacles to treatment. To increase the cultural relevance of treatment, therapists used the term "stressed" instead of "depressed." IPT showed significant benefits versus usual care after three months of treatment during pregnancy and six months postpartum. Grote et al. (2015) studied brief IPT in a collaborative care setting, offering low-income depressed pregnant women "MOMCare," a choice of brief (nine-session) IPT, pharmacotherapy, or the combination versus intensive maternity support services. The IPT condition had superior outcomes for depression (Grote et al., 2015), and particularly when the pregnant women had comorbid PTSD (Grote et al. 2016). Moreover, they found that MOMCare lowered perinatal maternal depression scores whether or not there was an adverse neonatal birth event, whereas the comparison condition did not protect against depression in the setting of an adverse event (Bhat et al., 2017).

Replicating the Grote et al. approach, Lenze and Potts (2016) conducted a small randomized trial comparing nine sessions of prenatal IPT to enhanced treatment as usual in depressed, pregnant, low-income women. IPT proved feasible, depression scores declined, and social satisfaction was higher in the IPT group.

Spinelli et al. (2003) compared sixteen weeks of individual IPT to parenting education for depressed pregnant mothers, finding significant effects for IPT and a significant positive relationship between maternal mood and mother–infant interaction. Repeating this study in three New York City sites using twelve weeks of IPT (Spinelli et al., 2013), they found high recovery rates and equal benefit across conditions. A reanalysis, however, found that among women with moderate depressive symptom severity, IPT was markedly effective compared to parent education and that parent education produced no change during the last four weeks of the study (Spinelli et al., 2016). While using standard IPT, Spinelli wrote a useful unpublished manual with detailed clinical illustrations.

IPT for Postpartum Depression

The first study of IPT for depression in the postpartum period offered twelve weeks of individual treatment (O'Hara et al., 2000; Stuart & O'Hara, 1995). O'Hara et al. (2000) showed that IPT reduced Ham-D depressive symptoms in postpartum mothers from a mean score of 19 to 8, significantly greater improvement than a waiting list had. Klier et al. (2001), Reay et al. (2006), and Clark et al. (2003) later independently produced group adaptations. The group format was used to reduce social isolation and ranged from eight to twelve sessions, with the group format drawing from the work of Wilfley et al. (2000).

Individual IPT treatment for postpartum depression in Chinese first-time mothers included a one-hour education session and a telephone follow-up two weeks later after discharge using the principles of IPT; the researchers reported positive effects as compared to standard treatments (Gao et al., 2015).

Although no studies have directly compared treatment formats, a meta-analysis (Sockol et al., 2011) reported that individual psychotherapy was superior to group psychotherapy in reducing perinatal depressive symptoms from pre- and post-treatment. This same review found that IPT had a greater effect size than a variety of comparators, including CBT. A Cochrane database review of psychosocial intervention for postpartum depression (Dennis & Hodnett, 2007) comprising nine more trials and 956 women found IPT, peer support, nondirective counseling, and CBT effective in reducing the symptoms of postpartum depression.

IPT for Depressive Symptoms After Miscarriage

Neugebauer et al. (2006, 2007) successfully adapted a brief telephone version of IPT in a small study of women with subsyndromal depression after miscarriage. By extension, IPT appears a reasonable intervention for women with full major depression after miscarriage. The same issues apply: Was the pregnancy wanted? What is the woman's relationship with the father and other social supports? What was her experience of the miscarriage? Does she feel guilty? What were her expectations of life with the baby? The woman's sense of loss may relate to whether the miscarriage occurred early in pregnancy (before the quickening around week 20) or whether she had felt fetal kicking, had marked changes in her body, had begun furnishing a nursery, and so on. It is therefore helpful to learn about the timing of the miscarriage. Moreover, depression and a history of miscarriage may co-occur without necessary relation: some patients in this study had both, but the miscarriage was not necessarily the trigger of the depressive episode. The patients tended to respond to IPT either way.

Koszycki et al. (2012) compared twelve sessions of unmodified IPT to brief supportive psychotherapy in a pilot study for depressed women in an infertility clinic. The completion rate was high, and two-thirds of women in the IPT arm responded (73 percent for IPT vs. 38 percent for supportive therapy, $p = .04$). There was a suggestion that women in the IPT condition might be more likely to achieve parenthood as well, either through pregnancy or adoption. This is a promising use requiring a full clinical trial. The variety of available approaches to addressing infertility, including in vitro fertilization and gamete donation, and the expanding concept of family, including same-sex marriages (Weissman, 2016), suggest many opportunities for adapting IPT for depression associated with infertility.

PROBLEM AREAS

The problem areas of IPT aptly apply to pregnancy, miscarriage, postpartum depression, and depression associated with infertility.

Grief

Women may have grief reactions due to a miscarriage or the mourning of a deceased child. A woman who has had a miscarriage, a stillborn child, or a child who died soon after birth must be helped through the grieving process as she would for any death. Grief in such cases often entails mourning not only the past but also the future the mother had imagined—the life she had hoped to have with her child.

Role Disputes

The postpartum period may bring numerous role disputes as the woman undertakes the care of the new infant, especially if she feels tired or overwhelmed. This is especially likely if the pregnancy was unwanted or the partner is absent or unsupportive. Disputes about autonomy and income might also arise for a woman who has had to give up work in order to care for a child. If disputes do not arise in connection with giving up work, many women may still find the change a difficult role transition. Disputes may arise with other children, or the partner, who feel jealous of the new baby and angry at the loss of the mother's attention.

In infertility, the partners seeking to get pregnant may blame or feel unsupported by one another.

The use of surrogates, in vitro fertilization, and same-sex parenting may raise not fully described disputes. These forms of parenting are not necessarily more prone to disputes than more conventional relationships, but they deserve consideration in taking the interpersonal inventory and in discussion in therapy.

Role Transitions

Pregnancy and the postpartum period are role transitions, especially in the instance of a first child. Transitions may include giving up an outside work role or the loss of time, sleep, income, and intimate time with the partner or other children.

Deficits

As at other times, patients with a paucity of relationships or attachments can have difficulty during this period and may require additional help in obtaining support from other family members, friends, or social service agencies in managing the burdens of childcare. Yet pregnancy and delivery also inherently provide a role transition and a new relationship for the patient to deal with. The interpersonal deficits category is only used in the absence of a life event, which pregnancy, miscarriage, and infertility invariably provide. Hence one of the other, preferable interpersonal problem areas should be invoked as a focus of treatment.

Complicated Pregnancy

Spinelli (1999) identified a fifth area, "complicated pregnancy," in the case of rape, concurrent illness such as HIV, unplanned or untimely pregnancy, or a child born with anomalies. The clinician should be sensitive to the impact of these situations and become knowledgeable about them. The usual IPT problem areas apply to these pregnancy-related events.

14

Depression in Adolescents and Children

ADOLESCENT DEPRESSION

Background

Cross-national epidemiological studies of the last two decades have found that major depression has an early onset, often in adolescence, and especially in girls. Untreated adolescent depression is associated with substantial morbidity, including school dropout, teenage pregnancy, suicide attempts, and substance abuse, in addition to considerable health expenditures. Depression that begins in adolescence frequently continues into or recurs in adulthood (Weissman et al., 1999, 2016).

Although early intervention is ideal for what is often a chronic or recurrent disorder, adolescent depression is vastly undertreated: less than a third of adolescents with mental health problems in the United States receive any mental health services. In recent years, school-based health clinics have emerged as an important treatment setting for adolescents with mental and general health problems, and some treatment studies have been conducted in these settings. Mufson et al. (1999) developed an adaptation of IPT for depressed adolescents (IPT-A; manual: Mufson, Pollack Dorta, Moreau, & Weissman, 2004, 2011) and have shown its efficacy in a study (Mufson et al., 1999) and in a school-based clinic, modified to address the constraints of this setting (Mufson, Dorta, Wickramaratne, Nomura, Olfson, & Weissman, 2004). Psychotherapy is an important treatment for depressed youth because of the controversy surrounding the use of psychotropic medications in this age group.

Depressed adolescents experience the range of DSM-5 depressive disorders, including major depression, persistent depressive disorder, bipolar disorder, and unspecified depressive disorder. Persistent depressive disorder requires only a one-year duration in adolescents. The only other diagnostic difference is perhaps a predominance of irritability over depressed mood. Adolescents are also much more reactive than adults to external situations or stressors and may experience transient but acute episodes of depression, resolving in a few days. Yet the morbidity of even these transient episodes should not be underestimated. They often fluctuate with current life and interpersonal situations but can be impairing. Depressed adolescents carry a much higher risk for suicide attempts than adults or elderly people, and although these attempts may at times reflect a wish for attention rather than death, they can be serious or even lethal.

Depression in adolescents is further significant because of its tendency to recur over the life span and to significantly impair psychosocial functioning, particularly if the patient is left untreated when important developmental educational or relationship tasks arise.

The role of being a patient undergoing treatment is uncomfortable for many people, particularly for adolescents. The therapist, while still establishing a time limit—the adolescent may be relieved to hear that the treatment is relatively brief, not lasting forever—should take a flexible approach to working with youths, staying available and rescheduling as needed.

Multiple studies have demonstrated the efficacy of IPT for depressed adolescents, among them Mufson et al. (Mufson, Dorta, Wickramarante, Nomura, Olfson, & Weissman, 2004; Mufson, Weissman, Moreau, & Garfinkel, 1999) and Rossello and Bernal (1999, 2012).

Mufson et al. (1999) found that adolescents receiving twelve weeks of IPT-A, compared to clinical monitoring (a brief supportive therapy) significantly more often met recovery criteria, had decreased depressive symptoms, and displayed improved social functioning. Rossello and Bernal (1999) reported similar results comparing IPT-A to CBT or a waitlist control condition. Both IPT-A and CBT were better than the waitlist control, and IPT had a larger effect size and was superior to the control condition in improving self-esteem and social adaptation. Both studies had relatively small samples and lacked follow-up. The Rossello IPT manual maintained the IPT theoretical framework but was an adaptation.

Mufson et al. (Mufson, Dorta, Wickramaratne, Nomura, Olfson, & Weissman, 2004) later conducted a randomized clinical effectiveness trial of IPT versus treatment as usual in a school-based clinic using community clinicians. The study showed the feasibility of training community workers in IPT-A, its acceptability as a treatment in an impoverished urban Latino sample, and its effectiveness relative to standard school clinic treatment.

Mufson, Gallagher, Pollack Dorta, and Young (2004) have also adapted IPT-A as a group intervention and carried out a pilot study in which adolescents received IPT as group or individual treatment. Both treatment formats showed comparable rates of recovery. A larger study found considerable obstacles to implementing a school-based treatment in an impoverished, inner-city community (Mufson, 2010).

The level of evidence for IPT for depressed adolescents (IPT-A) is **** (four stars; validation by at least two randomized controlled trials or equivalent to a reference treatment of established efficacy).

Adaptations

Therapists treating depressed adolescents using IPT must have experience in working with depressed adolescents and in practicing IPT (Mufson, Pollack Dorta, Moreau, & Weissman, 2011; Mufson, Pollack Dorta, Wickramaratne, et al., 2004). IPT therapists generally take a relaxed and informal stance in conducting psychotherapy, but therapists working with this population must be comfortable in collaborating with teenagers. The adaptations that have been made for this age group are limited and concern the content of the IPT sessions, not the structure or techniques of the treatment. The content issue relates entirely to the developmental concerns of youth, not to any uniqueness of adolescent depression. Following are the adaptations important for treating depressed adolescents with IPT.

FLEXIBILITY

The treatment should mesh with the adolescent's school schedule and other educational needs. Sessions, particularly if conducted in a school-based clinic, may need to be shortened to accommodate an academic schedule. Therapists can use telephone sessions to make up appointments missed due to scheduling conflicts. For a remitting youngster, attending basketball practice may be a sign of recovery rather than resistance to psychotherapy. This should be discussed and accepted.

THE SICK ROLE

The sick role in the initial phases of IPT exempts the depressed patient from overly onerous responsibilities. The sick role is a state that, if chronic, would be socially undesirable and so should be resolved as quickly as possible. It labels the need for help. Except in rare, extreme cases, the sick role should not exempt the adolescent from attending school. It can accommodate lower grade performance or excusal from extracurricular activities, but school attendance must be maintained.

INVOLVEMENT OF PARENTS OR GUARDIANS

Parents should be involved in at least the initial phase of treatment. The therapist makes seeing the parent a requirement of the adolescent's treatment. Clarify to the patient that you will not convey what is discussed in individual sessions to parents unless there is a risk of suicide or harm to the adolescent or to a parent by the adolescent. Explain your contact with the parent to the adolescent as adding another perspective on the adolescent's problems. During the initial phase, meet with both the adolescent and a family member. Ideally everyone should meet together so that you can explain the conduct of the initial evaluation and discuss the goals of treatment. Explain to the parent the structure and overall content of the therapy sessions, the outline of IPT, the duration of treatment, and expectations of what will be discussed.

To the extent possible (and this is not always possible), enlist parents as facilitators rather than antagonists of the treatment, for their child's and their family's sake. In rare cases in which the parent refuses involvement or the child refuses to have the parent involved, treatment should not be denied, but parental involvement should again be raised later in the treatment.

OUTSIDE INFORMATION
Relative to standard IPT, treatment with adolescents expands the sources of clinical information, including not only the adolescent but also parents, other family members, teachers, school personnel, and other health professionals or caretakers, such as pediatricians and clergy. The therapist does not routinely seek clinical information from all of these sources but chooses among them as seems appropriate and relevant, guided by the content of the treatment sessions. For example, it might be appropriate to contact the teacher of an adolescent who is having school problems. This requires the adolescent's permission.

CONFIDENTIALITY
It is essential to discuss confidentiality with adolescents, as with all patients. As the therapist, you guarantee that you will not discuss the content of the sessions with the parents or with anyone else, unless the patient and you jointly decide that such communication would facilitate the treatment. The exception is if the adolescent is in danger: you would then discuss breaching confidentiality with the patient before acting to make contact for the patient's safety. If possible, update the parent in a general sense about the adolescent's progress (e.g., symptomatic improvement, therapy attendance, recommendation to see a psychiatrist to consider medications). You should first review this contact with the adolescent for her approval. If she refuses to allow you to speak to a parent, encourage her to discuss such information with her parents directly.

Defining the Interpersonal Context

Obtaining information about the interpersonal context of depression and using the interpersonal inventory are similar in adolescents and adults. Mufson, Pollack Dorta, Moreau, and Weissman (2004, 2011) graphically modified the interpersonal inventory for adolescents by using a visual "closeness circle" with an X in the middle, representing the patient. The patient is asked to place markers for significant relationships at appropriate distances from the central X to illustrate their relative intimacy. This technique may benefit adolescents who are having difficulty differentiating among relationships.

The events associated with depression in adolescents are age-appropriate: typically, role transitions or disputes such as changes at school or in the family structure, the onset of sexuality, and sexual relations. These issues readily fit the four problem areas used with adults. An earlier version of IPT for adolescents (IPT-A) added a fifth problem area, single-parent family, but subsequent experience has indicated that the issues this category captures fit within role disputes or transitions.

Depression Is a Family Affair

Depression runs in families. Quite commonly one or both of the adolescent's parents also suffer from depression or related psychiatric disorders (e.g., alcohol or drug abuse). Many parents refuse interventions for themselves but encourage or allow the adolescent to accept treatment. On the other hand, parents may view the child's treatment in a negative light, perhaps because they have previously had unsuccessful treatment themselves. The more that you can involve parents in a successful course of an adolescent's treatment, the more likely the parents may be to enter treatment themselves. There is evidence that successfully treating a parent's depression to remission can reduce the child's symptoms as well (Weissman, Pilowsky, Wickramaratne, et al., 2006; Weissman, Wickramaratne, Pilowsky, et al., 2015), including IPT for depressed mothers (Swartz, Cyranowski, Cheng, et al., 2016; Swartz, Frank, Zuckoff, et al., 2008).

THERAPIST NOTE

Although the purpose of meeting with parents is not primarily to assess their clinical state, the therapist should be attuned to cues that may open up the topic. Caution is required in discussing parental psychopathology with the adolescent present.

Adolescents with a strong family history of depression, particularly if crossing multiple generations, may have a more difficult course, more recurrences, and may require maintenance treatment (Weissman, Wickramaratne, Gameroff, et al., 2016).

Special Issues with Adolescents

Issues that arise in treating adolescents reflect their developmental phase. Some of special importance, which usually fall into the standard IPT problem areas, include nonnuclear or single-parent families, sexual identity, school refusal, sexual abuse, substance abuse, learning disabilities, sexual activity, birth control, and pregnancy. The manual by Mufson et al. (2004, 2011) outlines the specific handling of these situations.

Suicide Risk

Because suicidal thoughts and attempts are common among depressed adolescents, you should ask the adolescent directly:

- *Do you ever feel life is not worth living?*
- *Do you think about death?*

- *Do you wish you were dead?*
- *Do you think about killing yourself?*

Positive answers require a follow-up:

Have you ever made a suicide attempt? When? How? What happened? Did you think you would die? Who was around when you did this? Did you receive medical treatment? Did you tell anyone about it? Did your parents know? What are you thinking about doing to hurt yourself? How close are you? Will you be able to stop yourself? Will you be able to tell someone before you hurt yourself?

You must evaluate the degree of suicide risk, including lethality of plan, the adolescent's history, and the availability of a stable family and other social supports. Seek a second opinion if you feel uncertain in determining the need for hospitalization. A possibly suicidal patient must be capable of establishing an alliance with the therapist. You should feel confident that no suicidal plan will be carried out and that the adolescent will notify you or go to the emergency room if the suicidal urges become compelling. Parents should be notified if the adolescent has a clear suicidal plan, will not form an alliance with the therapist, or cannot guarantee that the plan will not be carried out.

Depression Prevention for Adolescents

Adolescent Skills Training (IPT-AST) is a depression prevention program based on IPT-A. IPT-AST targets interpersonal disputes and poor social support, interpersonal vulnerabilities that have been linked prospectively to adolescent depression (e.g., Allen et al., 2006; Brendgen, Wanner, Morin, & Vitaro, 2005; Sheeber, Davis, Leve, Hopes, & Tildesley, 2007; Stice et al., 2004). IPT-AST comprises two individual pre-group sessions, eight group sessions, and an individual mid-group session that parents are invited to attend. Groups consist of three to seven at-risk adolescents with at least subthreshold depression, and two group leaders.

During pre-group sessions, the group leaders provide a framework for the group and conduct an abbreviated interpersonal inventory to identify interpersonal goals for group. During the initial phase of group (group sessions 1, 2, and 3), adolescents learn about the symptoms of depression, discuss the relationship between feelings and interpersonal interactions, participate in activities that help them understand the impact of their communication on others, and are introduced to communication strategies that can be helpful in improving their relationships. In the middle phase (group sessions 4, 5, and 6) and the mid-group sessions, the leaders encourage the adolescents to apply communication strategies in interpersonal problem solving to their own relationships. Communication analysis, decision analysis, and role playing are used to facilitate this work. Finally, in the termination phase (group sessions 7 and 8), the adolescents review the strategies learned and discuss ways to continue using the skills in their lives once group ends (see Young, Mufson, & Schueler [2016] for treatment manual).

IPT-AST was initially developed as an indicated preventive intervention for adolescents with subthreshold depression. Three school-based randomized clinical trials have compared IPT-AST to usual school counseling or group counseling for youth with elevated depressive symptoms (Young, Benas, Schueler, Gallop, Gillham, & Mufson, 2016; Young, Mufson, & Davies, 2006; Young, Mufson, & Gallop, 2010). In the first two studies, which compared IPT-AST to usual school counseling, IPT-AST yielded significantly greater improvements in depressive symptoms and overall functioning and significant reductions in depression diagnoses. Supplemental analyses demonstrated that IPT-AST youth also experienced significant reductions in anxiety symptoms relative to youth in usual school counseling (Young, Makover, Cohen, Mufson, Gallop, & Benas, 2012). In the most recent clinical trial, which compared IPT-AST to groups matched on frequency and duration of sessions, the data have only been analyzed through the six-month follow-up. As in the earlier studies, adolescents participating in IPT-AST experienced significantly greater improvements in depressive symptoms and overall functioning than adolescents in group counseling. There were no significant differences between the two conditions in onset of depression diagnoses in the short-term follow-up, however (Young et al., 2016). Additional analyses are underway to examine the longer-term data.

IPT-AST has also been studied as a universal depression prevention program. Horowitz et al. (2007) compared eight weekly sessions of ninety-minute IPT-AST, a cognitive-behavioral (CB) prevention program, and a no intervention control condition for ninth graders enrolled in health class. After the intervention, students in both the CB and IPT-AST groups reported significantly lower levels of depressive symptoms than did those in the no intervention group; the two intervention conditions did not significantly differ from each other.

Overall, the research to date supports the efficacy of IPT-AST as a prevention program for adolescent depression, particularly when targeting adolescents with subthreshold depression.

Tang et al. (2009) in Taiwan tested IPT-A in 73 high school students who reported suicidal risk among a screening of 347 classmates. These 73 students were assigned to receive IPT-A versus treatment as usual two sessions per week for six weeks. Results showed that school-based IPT-A reduced depressive severity, suicidal ideation, and anxiety significantly more than usual treatment. The adaptation did not require parent involvement because of the reluctance of students and, at times, parents.

Jacobson and Mufson (2012) described the rationale for and a detailed case summary of using IPT-A for adolescents with non-suicidal self-injury. The emphasis is on increasing communication and problem solving in behavior triggered by interpersonal stressors or disputes. In theory, interpersonal disputes or loss from death or transition leads to an overwhelming negative effect that, when combined with deficits in emotional regulation, distress intolerance, and a predisposition to experience affect intensively, may lead to non-suicidal self-injury as a temporary, maladaptive coping mechanism.

The level of evidence for IPT-A for depression prevention is **** (four stars; validation by at least two randomized controlled trials or equivalent to a reference treatment of established efficacy).

PREPUBERTAL DEPRESSION

In contrast to adolescence, depression in school-aged prepubertal children (ages approximately six to eleven years) is uncommon. The precise symptoms and clinical course are unclear at present. Few antidepressant treatments have been developed and tested for this age group.

The level of evidence for IPT in preadolescents is *** (three stars; validated in one controlled trial demonstrating superiority to a control condition). Dietz et al. (2008) carried out a small open trial of sixteen nine- to twelve-year-olds using the standard IPT-A manual (Mufson, Pollack Dorta, Moreau, & Weissman, 2004, 2011) developed for adolescents, with the adaptation of having parents systematically involved in weekly sessions (an average of fourteen). Individual and conjoint meetings called family-based IPT were held. Family-based IPT includes several developmental modifications for eight- to twelve-year-olds:

1. Increased parental involvement and structured dyadic sessions, with individual meetings with parents, and parent–child sessions for teaching and role playing communication and problem solving skills
2. A limited sick role, to shape parental expectations for depressed preadolescents' performance across contexts and to provide parenting strategies for decreasing conflict
3. An increased focus on comorbid social anxiety, to decrease depressed preadolescents' interpersonal avoidance and to enhance their communication and interpersonal problem-solving skills with peers.

During the initial phase, therapists conducted individual parent meetings to gather information about parental concerns and family stressors and to establish a contract and goal. Dyadic sessions with a parent provided the opportunity to practice new communication skills and for the clinician to coach in these skills. A plan for monitoring symptoms and initiating treatment was covered in termination.

The study compared ten patients treated with family-based IPT alone to six who received family-based IPT plus a serotonin reuptake inhibitor. Results showed good outcomes in both groups, demonstrating the feasibility and acceptability of the treatment. Children attended treatment and had fewer symptoms and less impaired functioning.

A second clinical trial comparing child-centered therapy, a supportive nondirective treatment for preadolescents (ages eight to twelve) to family-based IPT found higher rates of remission and of symptomatic decrease in IPT (Dietz et al., 2015). Decreases in interpersonal impairment with peers mediated the association between family-based IPT and preadolescents' post-treatment outcomes, providing support for improving peer relationships as a mechanism of action for family-based IPT.

To date, family-based IPT is one of the few psychosocial interventions for depression in preadolescents that has demonstrated superior outcomes when compared to an active comparison treatment condition. As such, family-based IPT has promise as an efficacious intervention with readily measurable targets and mechanisms of action. Future directions include implementation and effectiveness trials in community settings to expedite the dissemination of this promising intervention for depressed preadolescents.

The two major adaptations are that most sessions involve the mother or caretaker along with the therapist and child and use play as part of the treatment. The assessment process may take longer for young children because of the child's limited insight and the need to gather information from multiple sources. Many of the problems that children face reflect their parents' interpersonal problems. Therefore, determination of the parents' clinical status and the emergence of current problems (grief, disputes, or transitions) in the parents' lives often explain why the child's symptoms have emerged and can be used to help both the child and the parent. Recent data showing that successful treatment of a mother's depression can reduce the child's symptoms need to be considered in working with the parent (Weissman, Pilowsky, Wickramaratne, et al., 2006; Swartz, Cyranowski, Cheng, et al., 2016; Swartz, Frank, Zuckoff, et al., 2008). While these studies focused on the depressed mother, it is likely, albeit not tested, that the impact on the child of successfully treating the depressed father may also be helpful. In any case, when treating the child, awareness of the parents' current clinical state is important. This study makes clear that the absence of a father predicts a more difficult course for the depressed mother and her child in some circumstances (Talati et al., 2007).

COMPARATIVE EFFICACY IN CHILDREN AND ADOLESCENTS

A meta-analysis integrating direct and indirect evidence from randomized controlled studies investigated the comparative efficacy and acceptability of psychotherapies for depression in children and adolescents (Zhang et al., 2015). Systematic searches located fifty-two studies of nine psychotherapies and four control conditions. After treatment, only IPT and CBT were significantly more effective than most control conditions and more beneficial than play therapy. Only psychodynamic therapy and play therapy were not significantly superior to waitlist. IPT and CBT were more beneficial than problem-solving therapy. At follow-up, IPT and CBT were significantly more effective than most control conditions, and only IPT retained this superiority at both short-term and long-term follow-up. With regard to acceptability, IPT and problem-solving therapy had significantly fewer all-cause discontinuations than cognitive therapy and CBT. These data suggest that IPT and CBT should be considered the best available psychotherapies for depression in children and adolescents. However, several alternative psychotherapies are understudied in this age group.

CONCLUSION

The work of Mufson, her protégés, and other investigators in this area has been impressive in this crucial area of early life intervention. IPT-A has demonstrated efficacy and effectiveness as a treatment for adolescent depression and has shown the best outcomes in this understudied area. There are suggestions that variants of IPT-A may help prevent depression in at-risk adolescents and treat depression in preadolescents.

15

Depression in Older Adults

OVERVIEW

Depression ranks among the most common psychiatric diagnoses in older adults, but the first episode rarely occurs at this age. When it does, it may reflect an overwhelming stressor, perhaps the loss of a spouse of many years, important social changes associated with retirement, or changes in health. The IPT therapist should also consider medical problems, including neurovascular disease, as the source of the patient's depressive symptoms. Most older patients with depression, however, are experiencing a recurrence of previous episodes. The symptoms of depression remain similar across the life cycle, but older patients may focus more on physical symptoms, including somatic preoccupations, pain, and sleep disturbance.

The fact that older adults have more medical problems may complicate not only the diagnosis but also the treatment of depression. The onset of a disabling medical illness is a major life event and a risk factor for depression. Conversely, depression itself is associated with poor self-care (e.g., Gonzalez et al., 2007) and may contribute to different illnesses, such as ischemic heart disease and stroke (Evans et al., 2005). Patients with both depression and cardiovascular disease or diabetes face an increased mortality risk (Gallo et al., 2005). Psychotherapy is an important modality for depressed older patients because they may have greater sensitivity to medication side effects and more difficulty tolerating antidepressants. Because they are often taking several other medications, they carry greater risk for drug interactions. However, Reynolds et al. (2006) showed that depressed persons over age 70, many of whom may have had neurovascular disease, did better taking antidepressant medication than in IPT.

Often the biggest barrier to the use of IPT in depressed elderly people is the belief of some therapists (contrary to the scientific evidence) that older patients do not fare well in psychotherapy or are inflexible and cannot change. Ample evidence from controlled clinical trials now demonstrates that psychotherapy, particularly IPT, is a useful, efficacious, and accepted treatment in depressed elderly adults (Hinrichsen & Clougherty, 2006; Reynolds, Frank, Dew, et al., 1999). Case reports suggest that IPT can be used as an augmenting treatment in depressed elderly people who are responding poorly to an antidepressant medication (Scocco & Frank, 2002).

Reynolds and colleagues in Pittsburgh have conducted a series of maintenance IPT studies with older depressed patients. In each trial, they treated patients with both IPT and a medication until their depression remitted and stabilized, then randomly assigned them to continued combined treatment, monotherapy with IPT or medication, or pill placebo. Patients aged 60 to 69 did best on the combination of IPT and medication, did well on monotherapy with either treatment alone, and relapsed quickly on placebo (Reynolds, Frank, Perel, et al., 1999).

Yet results have not always been uniform. Depressed patients aged 70 and older were more likely to relapse than patients aged 60 to 69 on monthly maintenance IPT alone compared to medication alone or in combination with IPT (Reynolds et al., 2006). The oldest patients had late-onset major depressive disorder, and some may have suffered from early stage Alzheimer's disease or vascular dementia. These findings suggest that elderly patients with their first onset of depression in this age period may have a comorbid medical problem that compromises the effectiveness of psychotherapy and may require greater caregiver involvement. On the other hand, a further analysis of patients from the Reynolds et al. (2006) two-year study found that monthly maintenance IPT was associated with a longer time to recurrence than clinical management in patients with cognitive impairment and a history of remitted depression (Carreira et al., 2008).

Another trial of 124 patients with major depression aged 60 or older of combined treatment, comparing escitalopram plus IPT to escitalopram plus a control condition titled depression clinical management, found benefits for both treatments but no significant advantage for IPT in inducing remission: 58 percent versus 45 percent (Reynolds et al., 2010).

Van Schaik et al. (2007) compared IPT to treatment as usual in treating major depression among 143 older (more than 55 years old) patients in a primary care practice in the Netherlands. IPT was more effective than general practitioners' usual treatment for patients with moderate to severe major depression. Patient compliance with treatment was considered high (77 percent).

Miller (2009), long a member of the Pittsburgh IPT research team, developed a variant of IPT for late-life patients with depression and comorbid mild cognitive impairment. Cognitive difficulties complicate the patient's independence and agency, which are typical goals of an IPT treatment. This adaptation, which attempts to integrate a caregiver as surrogate to provide some of that agency (Miller & Reynolds, 2007), has yet to undergo rigorous testing.

Elderly depressed patients who were offered case management that included IPT, compared to patients receiving routine care, showed a decrease in suicidal ideation over a one-year period and a more favorable course in both severity and speed of depressive symptom reduction, changes that were significant by four months (Bruce et al., 2004). These results covered several primary care clinics and a range of ethnic groups in the United States. Patients who declined medication received acute, continuation, and maintenance IPT treatment delivered by master's-level clinicians. The dosing of IPT was twelve weekly sessions during the first three months of acute treatment, and monthly thereafter during the six-month continuation phase for patients showing some remission. Then, during a fifteen-month maintenance phase, IPT sessions were held bimonthly. If a patient relapsed, weekly sessions could resume. Interestingly, serotonin reuptake inhibitors (SSRIs) were considered the first-line treatment, and IPT was administered only if patients refused medication. Eleven percent of the patients initially requested IPT, but over a twelve-month period, the use of IPT as either monotherapy or augmentation of medication increased (Schulberg et al., 2007).

The level of evidence for IPT in older depressed persons is **** (four stars; treatment has been validated by at least two randomized controlled trials demonstrating the superiority of IPT to a control condition).

ADAPTATIONS

When dealing with any age or ethnic group, the clinician should understand the generational experiences that shape the values and worldview of the population under treatment: in this instance, the difficulties of later life, particularly retirement, aging, medical problems, and bereavement.

Because depressive symptoms such as sleep and appetite disturbance, fatigue, and aches and pains overlap with many chronic medical illnesses, an older patient presenting for treatment of major depression should have a complete medical evaluation to rule out comorbid general medical illness that may account for the symptoms. *The presence of comorbid general medical illness does not mean that depression should not be treated*: it is not normal or expected to develop major depression in the context of medical illness. Yet it is imperative, particularly for patients seeing nonmedical therapists, also to address other medical problems. This follows from the medical model of IPT and from clinical common sense. Patients with pain or sleep disturbances—which can often coexist—take longer to remit in treatment (Karp et al., 2005). By contrast, there is no evidence that older patients, even those hospitalized for a medical illness (Mossey, Knott, Higgins, & Talerico, 1996), cannot tolerate fifty-minute therapy sessions, a finding that contradicts impressions in earlier writings.

PROBLEM AREAS

The IPT problem areas generally apply to the common difficulties of aging. However, it is useful to understand how they nest within the IPT problem areas.

Grief

Elderly people face more experiences of bereavement: the death of a spouse, partner, close friend, or relative. With the loss of a spouse, the patient must face not only the loss of a partner but also disruptions in the practical aspects of living. For the surviving spouse, bill payment, financial burdens, leisure activities, and relationships with children may change dramatically. These disturbances can lead to role disputes or transitions.

Resolving grief reactions may be more complex than with younger patients, as older patients have more extended histories with the deceased person to discuss and resolve. The possibilities of meeting a new partner and interest in doing so may be more limited. Insecurities about how to reenter the dating scene after many years in a stable relationship may contribute another element of distress. The compounding effect of additional deaths of friends, other relatives, or acquaintances around the same period of time, which is not unusual in this age group, may increase the patient's sense of vulnerability and exacerbate the symptoms of depression. For an older patient, the death of a significant other may frequently evoke the patient's own approaching mortality.

Role Dispute

Some older adults have longstanding disputes with a spouse, partner, or adult children that are exacerbated by life changes such as retirement, financial problems, or the assumption of care for a family member. Issues and disputes with adult children often include disagreement over the frequency of visits or assistance; an adult child's financial, mental health, or substance use problems; unhappiness over the child's choice of spouse or partner; financial disagreements; or issues related to grandchildren.

Role Transition

Role transitions are common for older adults. Modal issues are the transition into the role of providing care to an infirm spouse or partner; transition to the role of an aging person with health problems and accompanying disability; retirement; or change of residence or community.

Interpersonal Deficits

This problem area is rarely identified in IPT with older adults. One explanation is that older adults often seek mental health services at the behest of a significant other, and individuals in the interpersonal deficits category typically lack such close relationships. Older depressed individuals may come to the attention of staff when they enter assisted-living residency or long-term care facilities. Some older adults may find that the loss of a critical relationship such as a spouse or sibling confronts them with the reality that they have very limited social resources or experience in obtaining new ones. The IPT therapist formulates this as complicated bereavement if the significant other has died, or as a role transition if the partner providing social support has moved away.

OTHER FEATURES

The basic IPT approach remains unchanged in treating older individuals, but as with any population, there are variations on the theme.

Medical Model

Older adults find the medical model of depression appealing because their other health problems often render it familiar. They may be less acquainted with the view of depression as a medical illness and may need psychoeducation about depression and its treatment.

Interpersonal Inventory

Because older adults have accumulated many relationships, the interpersonal inventory may take longer to complete. While reviewing key past relationships and relationship patterns, the therapist should focus on the present insofar as possible, where the list of current relationships may be all too short.

Maintaining the IPT Focus

Cognitive researchers have described a phenomenon of "off-target verbosity" in older people and suggest this may be related to changes in the aging brain (Arbuckle, Nohara-LeClair, & Pushkar, 2000). IPT researchers have observed that older depressed patients are more likely to reminisce about the past (Reynolds, Frank, Dew, et al., 1999). You can address this by initially clarifying to patients the framework of IPT and subsequently redirecting them to the relevant, agreed-upon focal problem area.

Therapist's View

Therapists who have limited clinical experience working with older adults may be pessimistic about the likelihood of substantive change, daunted by patients' multiple medical problems, and discouraged by the sense that elderly individuals have limited options or abilities. Efficacy studies have found, however, that older, depressed adults are resilient, adaptive, and capable of change, and outcomes have been very positive overall in IPT (APA Working Group on the Older Adult, 1998; Reynolds et al., 1999; Scogin & McElreath 1994). Psychotherapists who are treating geriatric patients thus need to fight ageism—negative therapeutic prejudices that depressed elderly patients themselves may well echo. You can teach an old dog new tricks!

Physical Accommodations and Liaison with Medical and Social Service Agencies

Older adults may need more concrete social services and are usually in medical treatment. Therefore it may be particularly important, with the patient's permission, to contact the patient's physician to clarify medical problems. Older patients may need help in obtaining transportation to IPT sessions, temporary housing, and long-term care. Focusing on psychological issues can be a hollow pursuit if basic activities of daily living are in disarray (Grote et al., 2008). The integration of these interventions may become more common when people age and are confronted with major role transitions that they cannot personally master.

Depression with Cognitive Impairment

Miller et al. (2006; Miller, 2009) have modified IPT for elderly patients with cognitive impairment. This adaptation engages both patient and caregiver in treatment by giving psychoeducation to both, offering practice in solving problems for both parties individually, and providing a forum to resolve role disputes through joint meetings. Caregivers have regular input into the therapy and are encouraged to extend the work between meetings to help the patient maintain progress despite memory loss or impairment.

Primary Care Treatment of Depression and Suicidal Ideation

Because older depressed patients frequently present to a primary care physician, efforts have been made to treat depression and suicidal ideation in depressed, older primary care patients (Alexopoulos et al., 2005). Treatment of suicidal ideation is important because suicide rates are highest in late life, and the majority of older adults who die by suicide have seen a primary care physician in the preceding six months. Depression is a strong risk factor for late-life suicide and its precursor, suicidal ideation.

CASE EXAMPLE: I LOST MY WIFE AND MY LIFE

David, a 66-year-old widower and retired lawyer, was brought to treatment by his family. He acknowledged being quite depressed in the aftermath of the death of his wife, Margaret, from breast cancer five months earlier. On questioning, he stated that his depression had really begun a year and a half earlier, when he retired from his job in order to care for his wife's declining health. Margaret had been fighting breast cancer on and off for eight years, an onslaught that he described as having gradually taken over their lives. He was distracted from his work, and what he described as a previously warm and close relationship had suffered.

"But why shouldn't I be depressed?" he asked. "My life is ruined, over."

He reported agitation, rumination, decreased sleep and appetite, a fifteen-pound weight loss, and passive suicidal ideation, with a sense that he might be reunited with his wife in death. His Hamilton Rating Scale for Depression score was 27.

David reported one prior episode of depression in his early twenties; he had also abused alcohol many years before but denied current use. He reported mild prostatic hypertrophy but was otherwise in good medical condition. He was adamant that he would not take an antidepressant medication.

Given a choice between a role transition based on retirement and complicated bereavement, both therapist and patient agreed to focus for twelve sessions on the latter. David felt guilty that he had let his wife down, believed that he should have cared for her better, and considered her the love of his life—an irreplaceable loss after some forty years of marriage.

The therapist encouraged him to reminisce about what he missed about Margaret and their marriage. She also noted that David had barely discussed his feelings with his friends and had not really used available social supports. David said that many friends and family members had either moved away or died in recent years, and that he was not in any case one to talk about his feelings. He had withdrawn and kept to himself from the time of his wife's funeral. The therapist encouraged him to consider building new skills in this area, inasmuch as social supports could provide him with some comfort in his difficult situation.

As therapy continued, David reported having begun to attend synagogue for the first time in years, and that his rabbi had provided some solace. At the same time, David began to discuss his ambivalent feelings about his wife: how her illness had distracted him from and ultimately ended his career and how she had annoyed him at times despite his wanting to care for her. Although they had had a wonderful marriage, there had (inevitably, his therapist noted) been some problems. He began to discuss these issues with a new level of affect, initially apologizing for his tears but gradually relaxing and accepting his feelings. His Ham-D score decreased to 13, and he began to become more socially active.

In the latter part of the twelve-week therapy, David returned to practicing law, conducting pro bono work for senior citizens. He also became active as a volunteer for a local cancer society, raising funds and—somewhat to his surprise—developing new friends. He saw this cancer work as a tribute to his wife. He also reengaged with his children and other family members. By the end of treatment, his Ham-D score had fallen to 7, signaling remission. He was still sad about his wife's death but not depressed, and proud to have improved "by myself" without medication. Given his history, David and his therapist agreed to monthly maintenance IPT to help him preserve his gains.

16

Depression in Medical Patients: Interpersonal Counseling and Brief IPT

OVERVIEW

There has been a marked increase of interest in the psychological impact of having a medical illness. This interest is high in medical specialty clinics for patients undergoing treatment for serious illnesses and in primary care clinics for distressed patients in routine care.

In many parts of the world, including resource-poor countries, ambulatory mental health care is part of primary care. In the United States, increasing recognition that far more patients with psychiatric problems receive care in medical settings than in mental health settings (Katon et al., 2010) has led to a focus on integrating mental health care into primary care settings. The U.S. system is transitioning, beginning with the simple addition of mental health professionals to primary care offices; the full extent of changes in U.S. health-care delivery is currently unclear. Models have developed for training primary care clinicians (not necessarily physicians) to provide basic problem-focused psychotherapy, with psychiatrists and other mental health professionals consulting in collaborative care models. This approach has become standard in some large integrated health systems (Gerrity, 2016; Goodrich et al., 2013). Each step has improved mental health outcomes and associated cost savings. These integrated models have also demonstrated some early success in improving the care for chronic medical diseases, such as hypertension and diabetes, which are prevalent among patients with mental illnesses (Katon et al., 2011).

This systematic transition is reflected in numerous studies of IPT, adapted in a new, briefer version in medical practice and primary care to accommodate time constraints and different levels of training of mental health care providers. Interest in depression and other psychiatric problems in medical patients and in primary care stems from their high co-occurrence with medical conditions such as cardiac disease, HIV infection, cancer, stroke, and diabetes (Evans et al., 2005).

Depression has been associated with cardiac events such as myocardial infarction, increased risk of hospitalization, and increased morbidity and death after bypass surgery or heart attack. Depression has been linked to accelerated immune system decline in HIV-positive women and poorer adherence to antiviral medications. Depression may lead patients to neglect treatment of other medical conditions. Conversely, some medical syndromes (e.g., hypothyroidism, pancreatic cancer) may predispose to depression.

Across a wide range of comorbid medical conditions, depression is a risk factor for nonadherence with medical treatment and poor self-care (Swenson et al., 2008). Depression can diminish expectations of treatment benefits, reduce the level of support from family members, and interfere with patient–physician communication. In one report on patients with diabetes, the presence of comorbid depression was associated with poor communication between patients and physicians, including diminished elicitation of patient problems and concerns, decreased explanations about the patient's condition, and reduced patient involvement in decision making. Depression treatment that is coordinated with care for comorbid chronic conditions improves control of both the depression and the chronic medical diseases (Katon et al., 2010).

The time allotted to primary care physicians to manage patients with major depressive disorder (MDD) is greatly limited by competing priorities to treat comorbid medical conditions. Doctors in the United States average only seven to eight minutes of patient contact (Dugdale et al., 1999). Such time constraints limit adequate assessment, diagnosis, and treatment of depression. As a result, depression often escapes clinical detection, and even when appropriately diagnosed, treatment is often limited (Gonzales et al., 2010). Deficiencies in the quality of depression care may be especially glaring among low-income and minority patients (Miranda & Cooper, 2004).

Medical staff and many patients long tended to consider depression an expected consequence of medical illness: "Who wouldn't be depressed with cancer?" Yet most medically ill individuals are not depressed, and those who are often have histories of depression predating their medical illness, which a medical episode re-evokes. Most importantly, depression in the context of medical illness is usually treatable. Antidepressant medication is probably the most common treatment approach, due to ease of administration and continuing lack of trained psychotherapists in most medical settings. Clinical interest in psychotherapy has been increasing, however. Medical patients often have illness-associated social and interpersonal distress, and some hesitate to take additional medication or face the risks of interactions and side effects from adding psychotropic medication to their current medication regimens.

Interpersonal problem areas are relevant to the experience of medical illness. Receiving the diagnosis of a serious illness constitutes a role transition, one that can involve changes in physical appearance, loss of work or productivity, change in familial responsibility, or the loss of an expected future and anticipatory mourning of one's own approaching death. The role transition of medical illness and its treatment may isolate the patient from social supports. Medical illnesses can produce interpersonal disputes with medical staff and family members. These are problems therapists can approach with IPT.

Schulberg et al. (1996) conducted the first IPT study of medical patients, treating MDD in 276 patients in a primary care practice, and showed that sixteen weeks of pharmacotherapy with nortriptyline and IPT each treated major depression more effectively at eight months than usual care with the primary care physician. The study transplanted psychiatrists and Ph.D. psychologists into the medical clinic setting. How medically ill the study sample was is unclear. This model did not spread because importing these mental health professionals was not considered cost-effective for primary care. Subsequent studies have typically employed trained master's-level therapists. Van Schaik et al. (2006), using psychologists and nurse therapists, found that ten sessions of IPT were more effective than usual general practitioner care in treating 143 elderly patients with a diagnosis of moderate to severe major depression.

Markowitz et al. (1998) found IPT to have equal efficacy to pharmacotherapy plus supportive therapy, and greater efficacy than CBT or supportive therapy alone, for 101 depressed HIV-positive patients. Ransom et al. (2008) observed that six-session, telephone-delivered IPT for HIV-infected rural individuals (N = 79) with depression lowered depressive symptoms and overall levels of psychiatric distress more than usual care. The same group replicated these findings in a subsequent study of 132 depressed rural HIV-positive patients who received either nine sessions of tele-IPT or treatment as usual (Heckman et al., 2016).

A negative study by Lesperance et al. (2007) documented the efficacy of citalopram administered in conjunction with weekly clinical management for twelve weeks for MDD among 284 patients with coronary artery disease, but they found no evidence of added value for IPT over clinical management. Attrition was significantly higher in the medication group, primarily due to side effects, whereas 86 percent of the IPT patients finished all twelve weeks.

Gois et al. (2014) in Portugal treated thirty-four patients with type 2 diabetes and depression, comparing psychiatrist-delivered IPT to sertraline for twelve weekly sessions with a three-month continuation phase. Both groups improved, with no significant differences in response rate between treatments. Response may have been slower on IPT, but the sample was too small for definitive determination. The authors concluded that IPT may benefit this treatment population.

Powers et al. (2012) in Scotland tested CBT, IPT, and treatment as usual by general practitioners for depression in 125 primary care patients, providing twelve to sixteen weekly sessions and a five-month follow-up. Therapists included psychiatrists, psychologists, and nurses. All groups improved, with IPT having the largest symptom reduction, followed by CBT and then treatment as usual. Attrition was 52 percent in the treatment-as-usual group, 30 percent in CBT, and less than 4 percent for IPT. At five months the outcomes were equivalent. The authors concluded that response to focused psychotherapy, especially IPT, may provide faster relief.

ADAPTATION

The need for flexibility in scheduling medical patients is critical so as not to conflict with treatment of the medical condition. If possible, schedule sessions in the hospital if the patient is admitted, or on the telephone if the patient is incapacitated by illness or just prefers telephone contact (see Chapter 25). Accommodating to the patient's suffering and needs frequently consolidates the therapeutic alliance with patients, who may fear abandonment. Therapists and patients face confusion about whether somatic symptoms derive from depression or the medical comorbidity. In the case of HIV and depression, treating the depression often alleviated fatigue, insomnia, and poor concentration that both therapist and patient had attributed to HIV infection (Markowitz et al., 1998). The interpersonal inventory should explore family histories of illness and medical treatment, as well as the patient's own experience with doctors, hospitals, and medicine. Aside from scheduling and a focus on medical issues, the basic IPT approach remains unchanged.

Patients with serious or incapacitating medical regimens (e.g., cancer patients undergoing chemotherapy) appear to appreciate the use of telephone sessions (Donnelly et al., 2000). When families are involved, it may be helpful in the initial phase (with the patient's consent) to educate both the family and the patient about the medical regimen the patient is undergoing. This has been useful in patients receiving cancer chemotherapy, where both the family and the patient had many questions about the course of illness and disability, and needed social services to help maintain family functioning and arrange transportation.

Some research groups have suggested sending the IPT patient guide and monitoring forms to patients before treatment begins in order to maximize the therapeutic effect and educate patients who are seeking psychiatric treatment on what to expect in psychotherapy (Weissman, 2005).

PRIMARY CARE AND ELDERLY PATIENTS

Because older people have elevated rates of depression and frequently attend primary care clinics, this setting provides an opportunity to detect and treat it (Alexopoulos et al., 2005; Schulberg et al., 1996; Bruce et al., 2004) (see Chapter 15).

CASE EXAMPLE: DIABETES WAS NOT
THE ONLY PROBLEM

Len, a 21-year-old college student, was admitted to the hospital with his fourth episode of diabetic ketoacidosis. His chief complaint was: "I've had it."

Since Len's diagnosis with diabetes mellitus 3 years before, near the start of his freshman year of college, both his sugar and his emotions had been out of control. Despite the pleas of his doctors, parents, and friends, he had refused to follow a diet, test his blood sugar, or take insulin regularly. His glycosylated hemoglobin (A1c) level was 9 percent.; the normal range is 4 to 5.9 percent.

On evaluation, Len appeared both angry and despairing. He reported neurovegetative symptoms of depression, including changes in sleep, appetite, weight, and energy level. It was difficult, however, to determine how much of this was attributable to a mood disorder and how much to his endocrine status. He reported feeling hopeless, helpless, and worthless. He believed that he was defective and that his life was over. "College is supposed to be, like, partying, girls, and beer," he said. "The doctors tell me I'm not allowed to drink like I want to. And who's going to go out with a damaged freak like me?" He felt diabetes had ruined his college experience, his body, and his life. He had alienated most of his few friends on campus and was failing courses. He wanted to die and seemed to have invited his diabetic crises on occasion with sporadic drinking binges. His Hamilton Rating Scale for Depression score was 22.

Len refused to take antidepressant medication because he was against medications altogether. He did, however, vent his feelings to the consultation-liaison psychiatrist, who validated Len's anger and frustration about his condition.

"No wonder you're depressed," said the therapist. They began to discuss the social and career expectations Len had brought to college and how "this sugar bit" had shattered them. In the second session, the therapist reinforced the diagnosis of major depression, showed Len a pocket DSM-5, and linked the depression to the role transition of a major medical illness—diabetes mellitus.

"You have two related medical problems, and either one can kill you if you don't take care of them. On the other hand, we can work on treating these problems, both of which can get in your way but neither of which is untreatable or your fault. If you can get them under control, you can live more of the life you've wanted."

Once Len's blood sugar was acutely controlled in the hospital with diet and insulin, he was discharged to outpatient follow-up in continuing IPT with the same psychiatrist. They agreed to a twelve-week course of IPT focusing on resurrecting Len's college life. In the sessions, Len mourned his loss of health, the imposition of a strict schedule on what had been a pleasantly slovenly life, and his sense that diabetes made him unattractive to women. He felt that the illness was "forcing me to grow up" prematurely: college was supposed to be the end of youth, not the beginning of adulthood.

The therapist agreed that Len had put his finger on the role transition he faced: he had lost an innocent, "party animal" role and had to grow up faster than he wanted to. That was sad, frustrating, enraging. He had definitely lost something, and it was appropriate to be upset. But was there anything good about the new role he had to adapt to?

Len mentioned that, despite his hostility toward doctors and hospitals, he had started to feel some interest in his illness and had thought about shifting his academic concentration from prelaw to premed. However, with his sugar out of control, he had trouble concentrating in class and studying, so the idea seemed unrealistic. The therapist encouraged this interest and urged Len to become expert both about diabetes and depression. Len got his roommate to remind him to check his blood *sugar and to snack more regularly. His concentration and study habits began to improve.*

Yet Len's overriding concern was his social life. He felt that diabetes was taking from him the drinking and partying that had been the focus of his college fantasies and the only comfortable venue in which to meet women. He and his therapist began to talk about his feelings of inadequacy around women—which predated his diagnosis of diabetes—and to role play interactions in nondrinking situations. Encouraged by the therapist, Len began to make overtures to women in his classes and in other activities, such as pick-up Ultimate Frisbee games. Not all of these encounters went smoothly, but enough did that he began to feel more confident and to date.

As this occurred, Len became less depressed and more willing to take care of his diabetes. At the end of twelve weeks, he was doing better on medical, academic, and social fronts. He drank only rarely and in moderation, and his Ham-D score had fallen to 7 and his hemoglobin A1c to 4 percent, both in the normal range. He now described himself as a more adult diabetes "survivor."

For another clinical example of IPT with medical patients, see Hoffer et al. (2012).

INTERPERSONAL COUNSELING (IPC) AND BRIEF IPT

National health reform in the United States has increased interest in cost-effective care models that expand access to mental health services for diverse populations. In the traditional model of primary care treatment of depression, primary care physicians often struggle without support to manage the mental health problems of their patients. Their well-intentioned efforts are too often undermined by competing clinical imperatives to treat acute and chronic medical conditions and deliver preventive care. Primary care physicians in the United States lack both training in psychotherapy and the time to deliver it.

Although depressed primary care patients usually receive medication, if given the choice they often prefer to talk about their problems (McHugh et al., 2013; Vidair et al., 2011). Less than 40 percent of adults entering psychotherapy receive more than three to five sessions. Whether the brevity of treatment episodes is primarily driven by patient preference or economic considerations is unclear, but short treatment is the norm and constrains the feasibility of traditional psychotherapy approaches in primary care.

Interpersonal Counseling

Interpersonal counseling (IPC), which (confusingly) has sometimes been called "brief IPT," derives directly from IPT. IPC originally was designed to have fewer and briefer sessions, up to eight sessions of fifteen to thirty minutes each, with the patient determining the number as treatment progresses. IPC addresses current stressors, and patients may decide to end treatment after fewer than eight sessions if they have made adequate progress. IPC delivered by non-mental health professionals of varying training can lower the burden on the primary care doctor. This model is used around the world, especially in resource-poor countries. IPC was designed to treat patients with subsyndromal depressive symptoms or distress. To aid non-mental health practitioners in its use, Weissman (2005) outlined IPC scripts for each session and added homework to facilitate treatment.

IPC has been used as a ten-session treatment administered by psychiatric clinical nurse specialists for medically ill, hospitalized elderly patients (Mossey et al., 1996), and by Australian general practitioners in combination with pharmacotherapy in a primary care setting (Judd et al., 2001, 2004). The management of stress, distress, and depression in medical patients is important but requires an easy-to-learn format that is sufficiently simple and scripted for medical personnel without psychotherapy experience to provide, and sufficiently flexible to combine with primary medical treatment and to accommodate patients with compromised energy. For patients with comorbid medical conditions, it is important to rule out the medical illness as the explanation for the symptoms. For patients who deny distress or psychopathological symptoms associated with the medical condition, therapists may suggest that some of their symptoms extend beyond and compound the medical condition, and may be helped by psychotherapy.

IPC is best used with patients who have low levels of depressive symptoms, or distress, and where more highly trained therapists are not available but health personnel are interested in providing counseling. Only one small study (Kontunen et al., 2016) has directly compared IPT to IPC. IPC has been used in varying ways across a range of patients and contexts. A 2014 review found thirteen clinical trials of IPC (Weissman et al., 2014), and another trial has been published since. The studies reviewed included the original Klerman and Weissman Harvard Community Health Plan study (Klerman et al., 1987), which employed medical nurses to treat medical patients with depressive symptoms. They found significantly higher remission rates in the IPC group (83 percent) than in treatment as usual (37 percent) three months later. Up to six IPC sessions were provided (average 3.4).

Mossey et al. (1996) assessed IPC as a treatment for medically hospitalized patients age 60 or older (N = 76) who had elevated depressive symptoms. Several adaptations were made to accommodate the needs of the medically ill elderly. The number of IPC sessions was increased to ten, session length was extended from thirty minutes to sixty minutes, and IPC sessions were flexibly scheduled from once weekly to a schedule reflecting the individual's medical status. At three months, the IPC treatment group showed greater improvement than the usual treatment group. This difference was not statistically significant at three months but reached significance at six months.

Holmes (2007) examined the effectiveness of IPC in decreasing psychological distress following severe physical trauma, recruiting 117 patients with major physical trauma and psychological distress at two trauma centers for a randomized clinical trial comparing IPC delivered by clinical psychologists to usual treatment. Three- and six-month follow-up showed no significant differences between the two treatment conditions for symptom level or psychiatric diagnosis. The dropout rate was high, and patients with a history of major depression randomized to IPC showed significantly increased levels of depressive symptoms at six months. Thus, this was a negative study.

Badger et al. (2004, 2005a, 2005b) compared IPC versus usual treatment for forty-eight breast cancer patients receiving adjuvant treatment who reported depressive symptoms and fatigue. The therapists were master's-level clinical nurse specialists. IPC was associated with significant reduction in depressive symptoms, fatigue, and stress; an increase in positive affect; as well as better outcomes among women in a long-term marriage who had no prior history of depression or cancer.

In a second randomized controlled trial, Badger et al. (2007) evaluated both ninety-six breast cancer patients undergoing adjuvant treatment and their supportive partners. Depressive symptoms were not required as inclusion criteria. Patients were randomized to either telephone IPC for both patients and partners, self-managed exercise, and three telephone calls with partners, or an attention control group that included six weekly telephone calls and six biweekly calls to partners. At six weeks and ten weeks after the intervention, the women's depressive symptoms decreased across all groups. Their anxiety symptoms decreased significantly in the IPC and exercise groups, but not the attention control group. Assessment of partners' depressive and anxiety symptoms yielded similar findings: partners reported significantly decreased depressive symptoms overall, and anxiety symptoms decreased in the IPC and exercise groups but not in the attention control group.

In a third study, Badger et al. (2011, 2013a) randomized seventy-one men with prostate cancer and their intimate or family supportive partners to IPC or health education attention condition. No distress or depression symptoms were required as entrance criteria. IPC-trained counselors/research assistants held eight weekly thirty-minute sessions and found the health education attention condition superior to IPC.

Finally, Badger et al. (2013b) examined seventy Latina women with breast cancer receiving adjuvant treatment and their supportive partners. Again, no distress or depression symptoms were required for entry. This randomized controlled trial divided patients between IPC and telephone health education interventions, assessing their progress at eight and sixteen weeks after the intervention. Both interventions, which were provided by master's-level social workers, yielded significant improvements in psychological, physical, social, and spiritual quality of life for both breast cancer patients and their partners over sixteen weeks, with no significant between-treatment differences.

Oranta et al. (2010, 2011, 2012) implemented IPC for 103 inpatients with recent myocardial infarctions in Finland. Patients received up to six IPC sessions, with at least the first session occurring in the hospital. Post-discharge sessions took place over the telephone. A psychiatric nurse with one day of IPC training delivered treatment. Depressive symptoms decreased significantly in the IPC group compared with the usual-treatment control group across age groups. IPC did not improve overall health-related quality of life at follow-up.

Preliminary research tested IPC for women experiencing elevated depressive symptoms after miscarriages (Neugebauer et al., 2007; see Chapter 13).

A pilot study in Israel compared telephone-administered IPC and supportive counseling, assessing depression, anxiety, and somatization symptoms and quality of life of frequent attenders in primary care (Sinai & Lipsitz, 2012). Frequent attenders are believed to have elevated rates of depression, anxiety, and psychological distress; lower social functioning and limited social networks; and increased primary care usage. Treatment provided six thirty-minute sessions over twelve weeks of IPC focusing on an interpersonal problem that was identified in the initial session, or an equal dosage of supportive counseling without a specific focus. Patients receiving no treatment were assessed at baseline and after twelve weeks with the PHQ questionnaire. Overall results found IPC significantly superior in decreasing symptoms compared to supportive counseling and controls. Only IPC showed marginal significance in decreasing somatization symptoms and reducing anxiety and depression symptoms. Quality-of-life measurements and health care utilization and costs did not significantly differ between before and after the intervention in any of the conditions. Doctor, hospitalization, and clinic costs each showed nonsignificant trends for greater cost reduction in IPC only. A marginally significant time × group interaction for number of primary care visits decreased only for IPC, at a trend level.

The first published study combining IPC with antidepressant medication took place in an Australian general practice setting (Judd et al., 2001). Thirty-one patients with major depression received venlafaxine-XR and were randomly allocated to IPC or to usual psychosocial interventions. Doctors in the intervention group received IPC training with video and written material. Twelve IPC patients and nineteen patients in the standard treatment group were included in the intention-to-treat analysis of efficacy at twelve weeks. Both treatments yielded statistically significant reductions in Beck Depression Inventory (BDI) scores from baseline, with IPC showing greater improvement.

The largest IPC study (Menchetti et al., 2010, 2014), a multicenter randomized controlled trial in Italian primary care centers, compared the effectiveness of IPC to selective serotonin reuptake inhibitors (SSRIs). Patients referred by primary care physicians were eligible for the study if they met criteria for major depression and were in their first or second depressive episode. They were randomly assigned to IPC or to antidepressant medication. IPC was adapted to accommodate the patients' needs; the recommended number of sessions was six thirty-minute weekly sessions. Therapists determined whether one or two additional sessions were needed. Therapists were residents in psychiatry or in clinical psychology with at least two years of clinical experience.

Menchetti et al. (2014) reported that the proportion of patients with mild depression who achieved remission at two months was significantly higher for IPC than SSRIs (58.7 percent vs. 45.1 percent, $p = .02$). IPC and SSRI appeared equally effective in treating moderate to severe depression. Mild depression, low functional impairment, first depressive episode, and absence of comorbid anxiety disorders predicted better outcome with IPC. IPC was feasible, easily learned, and well suited to the primary care setting. These results encouraged investigators working with Menchetti et al. to use IPC elsewhere in Italy.

Since the 2014 review, Kontunen et al. (2016) in Finland randomized forty patients with MDD to either seven sessions of IPC or sixteen sessions of IPT delivered by psychiatric nurses in primary care. Both treatments were well tolerated (90 percent completion), and within-group effect sizes were large (>1.4). Outcomes were similar at one year, with 59 percent in IPC and 63 percent in IPT recovered. The authors concluded that IPC was a sufficient first-phase intervention for mild to moderate depression in primary care. This study, although underpowered to find differences, is the first to compare IPT and IPC.

Researchers are currently adapting and testing IPC in lower-resource settings and with less skilled health workers. Feijò de Mello (personal communications, 2013, 2016) is currently evaluating IPC in a Brazilian family health program. Verdeli (personal communication, 2013) is testing IPC in a stepped-care model within a primary care network of Partners in Health in Haiti; and Ravitz et al. (personal communications, 2013, 2016) are disseminating it in a nationwide training program in Ethiopia. The therapists in these settings include psychiatric and general medical nurses and community health care workers (Weissman, 2013). IPC is also being adapted in Edinburgh as an acute intervention for patients presenting at a crisis service with high levels of self-harm and suicidality (Graham & Lamaigre, personal communication, 2013). It is being adapted under the sponsorship of WHO for primary care in Muslim countries by Weissman and Verdeli and in Lebanon for refugees.

Summary of IPC

Fourteen studies have tested IPC. Aside from the 2010 study by Menchetti et al. (N = 300), sample sizes have been small. The studies generally found that IPC improves depressive symptoms and functioning, excepting the Badger et al. study (2011, 2013a) of men with prostate cancer comparing IPC to health education attention, and the Holmes et al. study (2007) of psychological distress after major physical trauma. The studies not requiring depressive symptoms or distress as entrance criteria showed weaker findings for IPC (Badger 2007, 2011, 2013a), perhaps because of a floor effect with milder symptoms or a weakening of the medical model in the absence of a psychiatric target diagnosis. In the trial for Latina women with breast cancer comparing IPC to treatment as usual, both groups improved (Badger et al., 2013b). The largest, most important study (Menchetti et al., 2014), which took place in primary care sites, found that IPC yielded greater remission than an SSRI regimen.

Clearly more research is needed, including more details about the adaptations and training provided. Studies comparing IPC to collaborative care are needed.

Although IPC was developed for non-psychiatric health workers to treat patients with subsyndromal symptoms, its use has spread more widely.

Brief IPT

Whereas IPC was designed as a shorter, simplified, more structured offshoot of IPT, brief IPT (IPT-B) had a different origin. Little research has been done to evaluate the optimal dosage—length and frequency—of any psychotherapy, IPT included. Swartz and other researchers (Swartz et al., 2014) have experimented with concentrating IPT within a tighter time limit and fewer sessions for specific treatment populations, thereby creating a shorter form of IPT that to some degree converges in length and principle with IPC. This has led to some confusion about terminology.

The first test of IPT-B was a matched, case-control study comparing eight weeks of IPT-B to sertraline for thirty-two women who met DSM-IV criteria for MDD. Patients completed a mean 7.1 (± 2.0) sessions. Both groups improved, but response was quicker with IPT-B than with sertraline (Swartz, Frank, Shear, Thase, Fleming, & Scott, 2004).

Depressed mothers of children with psychiatric illness were identified as a group likely to benefit from brief psychotherapy. Open pilot testing of IPT-B (N = 13), combined with a single initial engagement session (Swartz et al., 2004), demonstrated the feasibility of treating depressed mothers of psychiatrically ill children ages 12 to 18 years for MDD. A larger study then compared IPT-B (N = 26) to usual treatment (N = 21) for MDD in mothers of children ages 6 to 18 years who were receiving treatment for a psychiatric disorder. Children were treated openly in the community. Controlling for baseline values, analyses of covariance comparing mean maternal symptom and functioning scores at three- and nine-month follow-ups found significantly better outcomes among mothers receiving IPT-B than usual treatment on Ham-D scores at three months. At the nine-month follow-up, children of IPT-B–treated mothers had significantly better child self-report depression and functioning scores than children whose mothers received usual treatment (Swartz, Frank, Zuckoff, Cyranowski, Houck, Cheng, et al., 2008).

To minimize barriers to care, ameliorate antenatal depression, and prevent postpartum depression, Grote et al. (2004) conducted an open trial of acute IPT-B during pregnancy and before childbirth (N = 12), initiated with a pretreatment engagement session (Swartz et al., 2004) and followed by monthly IPT maintenance sessions up to six months postpartum. Findings demonstrated the feasibility of treating depressed, pregnant women on low incomes who were receiving prenatal services in a large, urban obstetrics and gynecology clinic and who were not receiving pharmacotherapy or other psychosocial treatments. Intent-to-treat analyses showed that patients reported significantly reduced depressive symptoms on the Edinburgh Postnatal Depression Scale (EPDS; Cox et al., 1987) after acute IPT-B and six months postpartum, with high treatment satisfaction (Grote, Bledsoe, Swartz, & Frank, 2004b).

A larger study subsequently assessed IPT-B in treating antenatal depression in socioeconomically disadvantaged women. Once again, IPT-B involved a multi-component care model comprising a pretreatment engagement session (Grote et al., 2007), acute IPT-B before childbirth, and monthly maintenance IPT up to six months postpartum. Fifty-three non-treatment-seeking pregnant women not receiving depression care were randomly assigned to receive either IPT-B (N = 25) or enhanced usual care (N = 28), involving referral for mental health services in a clinic located in the same hospital as the obstetrics clinic. Intent-to-treat analyses found patients in IPT-B, relative to those in usual care, had significantly reduced depression diagnoses both before childbirth and at six months postpartum, and reported fewer depressive symptoms (Grote et al., 2009).

Poleshuck et al. (2010b) adapted IPT-B for women with co-occurring depression and chronic pain (Poleshuck et al., 2010a). Interpersonal psychotherapy for depression and pain (IPT-P) uses IPT-B as its core structure but incorporates components of pain management, including an evaluation of pain intensity and interference. In an open study of IPT-P (N = 17), women with MDD experiencing at least three months of self-reported pelvic pain were treated with IPT-P and had statistically significant declines in scores on the Ham-D and Social Adjustment Scale (SAS; Weissman & Bothwell, 1976) but no significant change in Multidimensional Pain Inventory scores (Poleshuck et al., 2010b).

Consistent with the aims of IPT-B for perinatal depression, Brandon et al. developed a conjoint form of treatment, partner-assisted IPT (PA-IPT), for pregnant or immediately postpartum depressed women. Retaining the eight-session brief treatment framework, PA-IPT includes a partner as an active participant throughout. The intervention incorporates elements of Emotionally Focused Couples Therapy (Johnson et al., 1999) to strengthen the couple's interpersonal bond and address attachment needs within the context of the transition to parenthood. In an open study (N = 10) of PA-IPT, consisting of eight sessions delivered over twelve weeks, 90 percent of women had Ham-D scores of 9 or less following acute treatment, but no statistically significant changes in relationship satisfaction were reported.

In parallel to the version of IPT-B used in the United States, clinical investigators in Scotland developed an eight-session IPT. Although independently developed, the two treatments are very similar. Pilot testing of IPT-B (Scotland) was conducted in primary care settings (Graham, 2006). Individuals clinically diagnosed with MDD were randomly assigned to either IPT-B (N = 26) or a waitlist control group (N = 23). IPT-B yielded a significantly greater reduction in depressive symptoms as measured by the Ham-D and Beck Depression Inventory (BDI-II), though no greater improvement in quality of interpersonal relationships. Seventy-three percent of IPT-B patients experienced significant change at the two-month follow-up.

Finally, Mufson et al. (2015) developed and pilot tested brief IPT for adolescents in primary care, treating ten low-income, depressed adolescents. Ninety percent completed and reported satisfaction with treatment. Symptom reduction suggested the feasibility of the approach.

IPC and Brief IPT

Back in the 1970s when IPT began, a twelve-session psychotherapy treatment was considered almost radically brief. Now a clear need exists for even briefer psychotherapeutic approaches. Their development has been uneven. In 1983, Klerman and Weissman developed IPC directly from IPT. IPC was briefer than IPT, had scripts to follow, and was intended for training professionals with no mental health background in the treatment of primary care patients with depressive symptoms (Klerman et al., 1987) (Table 16.1).

The IPC manual was updated in the mid-2000s in response to an increasing emphasis in the United States on efficient, accessible, cost-effective mental health service models and a growing demand for psychosocial approaches to care in developing countries devastated by war and natural disaster. The IPC manual was shortened from six to three sessions, and the section on termination, which was renamed triage, was made more explicit. The three-session version was determined based in part on observations that patients in IPC efficacy studies used only about three sessions on average; in keeping with broader mental health service utilization patterns in the United States; and in planning for use in developing countries lacking resources for extended psychotherapy. This updated IPC version was renamed Interpersonal Psychotherapy, Evaluation, Support, Triage (IPT-EST; Weissman & Verdeli, 2012). The name change caused confusion, as it seemed unconnected to IPC and thus appeared to be a new treatment—which was not true. It also appeared to separate these procedures from existing efficacy data. We have hence rescinded the name IPT-EST; the revised manual is again titled IPC.

The content and structure of IPC have not changed over the years. While the latest version emphasizes three sessions, it allows flexibility in the context of the setting and resources.

While IPC was originally designed for subsyndromal symptoms for non-mental health workers and in primary care, IPT-B targeted major depression and delivery by mental health workers. IPT-B, by further compressing an already short treatment, may require the therapist to work harder, under greater pressure. In practice, IPC has been used for major depression and by mental health workers and

Table 16.1 IPC AND IPT-B

	IPC	IPT-B
Length (sessions)	1–6	8 (+1)
Scripted	Heavily	Far less
Therapists	Often non-mental health professionals lacking psychotherapy experience (but this varies by study)	Mental health professionals
Target	(Usually) subsyndromal depressive symptoms	Major depressive disorder

in testing medical settings. The development of parallel brief versions of IPT and their considerable overlap reflect the interest and need for brief psychotherapy. Further adaptations of both brief IPT and IPC are underway. At this point we can't say which should be used under which circumstances. With few exceptions the samples have been small. There is high interest in developing briefer approaches, a wealth of evidence-based choices, and much work to be done.

The level of evidence for IPT/IPC in medical patients and brief IPT is **** (four stars; treatment has been validated by at least two randomized controlled trials each demonstrating their superiority to a control condition).

17

Persistent Depressive Disorder/Dysthymia

DIAGNOSIS

Dysthymia is a syndrome similar to acute major depression, generally of slightly lower symptomatic intensity but of longer duration. The severity of symptoms may not reach the threshold for major depressive disorder (MDD; when it does, it is called "double depression"), but symptoms typically begin early in life and continue for decades. The DSM-5 (2013) has combined what had been called dysthymic disorder with chronic major depression as a single chronic mood diagnosis, termed persistent depressive disorder. Its criteria for duration require a minimum of two years (one year in adolescents) with no more than two months of relief, but patients frequently report having felt miserable for their entire lives, with no more than a day or two of improvement here or there.

This chronic debility takes a toll not only in constant dysphoria but also in impaired psychosocial functioning. Individuals who became depressed in childhood or adolescence may never have learned appropriate interpersonal skills, and those who did may have seen them erode in subsequent years of suffering. They tend to have limited social supports and few confidants. They often believe that their depressed mood is part of their personality, rather than a symptom that can be successfully treated. Chronically depressed patients do not necessarily have as severe neurovegetative symptoms of depression as patients with acute MDD, but they have greater cognitive symptoms such as pessimism, guilt, helplessness, hopelessness, and worthlessness (Riso et al., 2003).

All of the interpersonal issues typically seen in MDD tend to be exaggerated for patients with dysthymia/persistent depressive disorder: social withdrawal, passivity, difficulty with self-assertion and confrontation, and the sense that expressing needs is selfish and that anger is a "bad" emotion. Having recognized that other people do not want to hear about their chronic suffering, they typically put on as bright a front as they can, shunning the spotlight and trying to pass as "normal." If they then succeed in some aspect of life, they tend to feel that they are frauds.

Similarly, feeling undeserving and unlovable, they put the needs of others ahead of their own, but feel increasingly resentful of this over time. They then see their anger as evidence of their selfishness and toxic defectiveness: Who would want to be around someone who feels so angry over such slight matters? In consequence, these patients tend to withdraw socially, or at least to limit and distance their social interactions, in which they constantly feel like second-class citizens. Thus, individuals with dysthymia often avoid intimate relationships or feel unable to form such attachments, fearing that closeness will reveal to the other person how defective, fraudulent, or unlovable they are.

Because dysthymic symptoms are chronic and indolent, people with dysthymia can often use all of their limited energy to eke out adequate work functioning. If an episode of major depression does not occur, these people may avoid treatment, believing that the problem is simply their personality. Alternatively, individuals with dysthymia may have sought long-term psychotherapy for character change—a setting in which they have been reputed to have a poor prognosis—and have achieved little change in mood or social functioning.

Although treatment works to reduce symptoms, the chronicity of chronic depression tends to make it less responsive to standard treatments than acute depression. None of the proven treatments for acute depression works as well as for chronic depression: that includes pharmacotherapy, CBT, and IPT.

IPT for patients with dysthymia has been tested in two clinical trials. In one, ninety-four patients with pure dysthymic disorder (i.e., no history of major depression) were randomly assigned to IPT adapted for dysthymic disorder (IPT-D), brief supportive psychotherapy, sertraline, or sertraline and IPT-D for sixteen weeks (Markowitz et al., 2005). Patients improved in all conditions. The study was underpowered, but medication was superior to the other treatments in achieving response and remission. IPT-D and brief supportive therapy had equivalent outcomes. The degree of change that IPT-D patients made in their focal interpersonal problem areas correlated with the degree of symptomatic improvement (Markowitz, Bleiberg, Christos, & Levitan, 2006).

A large Canadian trial randomly assigned 707 patients with dysthymic disorder or double depression (now called persistent depressive disorder) to receive unmodified IPT, sertraline, or a combination of both (Browne et al., 2002). Unfortunately, the IPT treatment comprised twelve weekly sessions, whereas medication was continued for more than two years, a somewhat unbalanced comparison. The investigators reported a 47 percent response rate for IPT alone, significantly less than the 60 percent rate for sertraline alone and 57.5 percent for combined treatment. Yet IPT was found to be associated with lower health and social service costs, rendering combined treatment most cost-effective (Browne et al., 2002.). IPT actually performed well in this study, considering the dosage disparity between IPT and sertraline. Nonetheless, this trial did not technically demonstrate efficacy for IPT.

Schramm and colleagues (2011) compared IPT to the cognitive behavioral analysis system of psychotherapy (CBASP) in a randomized pilot trial of twenty-two sessions in sixteen weeks. Treating thirty patients with early onset chronic depression, they found no statistically significant difference between treatments on the primary outcome measure, the Hamilton Rating Scale for Depression, although CBASP had higher remission rates (57 percent vs. 20 percent) on the Beck Depression Inventory.

Two other studies provide some support for IPT as an augmentation of medication for dysthymic patients. In one small trial, chronically depressed patients who received the antidepressant medication moclobemide plus IPT had somewhat better outcomes than those who received moclobemide alone (Feijò de Mello, Myczowisk, & Menezes, 2001). In the other, patients responding to fluoxetine showed suggestions of greater benefits when given a group therapy combining interpersonal and cognitive interventions for depression than those who received fluoxetine alone (Hellerstein et al., 2001).

In the past decade there have been no further IPT trials for persistent depression. Other psychotherapies have also generally struggled in treating chronic depression (e.g., Kocsis et al., 2009). It is not that they are entirely ineffective, but that their effects are more modest than for acute depression (Markowitz et al., 2006). The psychiatric treatment literature indicates that medication is the first-line treatment for chronic persistent depression. Psychotherapy, including IPT, may be a useful adjunct and would seem to target important interpersonal difficulties endemic to the disorder, but strong evidence for the specific efficacy of IPT is lacking.

Yet some chronically depressed patients do not want to take or do not respond to medication, and for them IPT may provide an alternative treatment. Further modification of the IPT manual for dysthymic disorder may be helpful. IPT remains to be systematically tested in patients with both dysthymic disorder and MDD. Since IPT-D did not fare badly in the trials described and various methodological problems (e.g., changes in therapist personnel during the trial) may have hurt its chances, IPT still should not be dismissed as a potential sole treatment for patients with chronic depression. Further, based on clinical experience and preliminary data (Feijó de Mello et al., 2001; Markowitz, 1993), IPT may be helpful as a kind of social rehabilitation treatment for chronically depressed patients who respond to medication and feel better but find themselves risk-averse, socially avoidant, and lacking in the interpersonal skills needed to conduct a euthymic life, skills that have either atrophied or never developed in the setting of chronic depression.

For these reasons, this chapter describes the adaptations of IPT for the treatment of patients with dysthymic disorder (Markowitz, 1998; see manual list, Chapter 26). Some of these adaptations may also apply to other chronic psychiatric syndromes such as social anxiety disorder (Chapter 21).

The level of evidence for IPT alone is no stars (IPT has been found to be no better than an active control psychotherapy as monotherapy). However, the level of evidence for IPT as a combined treatment with medication is ** (two stars; encouraging findings in one or more open trials or in pilot studies with small samples).

ADAPTATION

Although the IPT approach to chronic depression generally resembles the treatment of acute major depression, there are several important changes.

The usual IPT model connects a recent temporal event in the patient's interpersonal life with current mood and symptoms. For patients who have been depressed for many years or for as long as they can remember, this model makes less sense. Even if there has been a recent, upsetting life event, this does not explain past years or decades of suffering. For such patients we developed the concept of an *iatrogenic role transition* (a transition initiated by the doctor), in which the patient moves from recognition of illness to health and from psychosocial functioning impaired by persistent depressive disorder to better functioning and mood. This transition focuses on patients' confusion of who they are and their longstanding mood disorder, which after so many years they may naturally confuse with their subjectively "defective" personality. The IPT therapist thus makes treatment itself a role transition in which the patient learns to recognize depressive symptoms of long duration and how they have affected her social functioning. In addition, the patient learns to handle interpersonal situations in a euthymic, nondepressed fashion. Learning such new ways of managing interpersonal interactions in a healthy way should not only ameliorate the life circumstances and give a greater sense of environmental mastery but improve mood and self-esteem.

The therapist takes a careful history and interpersonal inventory, looking for patterns in relationships and for good relationships and strengths the patient may have shown. Patterns to expect in chronic depression include shyness (avoidant personality traits), passivity (particularly in social situations; less so in situations defined by a job description), and discomfort with self-assertion, anger, confrontation, and social risk taking.

The therapist then offers a formulation that shifts the blame for the patient's situation from the patient (who he is) to the illness (chronic depression):

> As we've discussed, you are suffering from persistent depressive disorder, a chronic form of depression. It's a treatable illness, and it's not your fault. You have been depressed for so long that you very naturally have trouble distinguishing depression from who you are: you think it's your personality, but it isn't. You've just been depressed for so long that you can't tell the difference. Persistent depressive disorder has to make it harder to handle social situations: social discomfort is a hallmark of the condition.
>
> I suggest that we spend the next fourteen weeks helping you to figure out what depression is and what you might be like when not depressed. If you can learn to handle situations in your life in a nondepressed way, not only should that make life go better, but you're also likely to feel better and more in control. And then maybe you'll begin to see that what you're suffering from is a treatable depression, not your personality.

With the patient's acceptance of this formulation, treatment proceeds. Therapists work hard with such patients to identify emotions—and particularly negative affect and feelings of competitiveness, anger, and sadness—that arise in everyday situations. The therapist and patient discuss whether such feelings are understandable and warranted. The idea of a *transgression*—that there are some behaviors that break expected social conduct, warrant anger, and deserve at the least an apology—may be helpful in normalizing such feelings for patients (see Chapter 11):

> *If you're selfish all of the time, that's a problem. But if you're selfless all of the time, you're a martyr, and you're going to have trouble getting what you want and need. Everyone does better if they are a little selfish; if you don't speak up on your own behalf, who will?*

Once feelings are identified and normalized, a lot of role play is often needed to help patients become comfortable with self-assertion or confrontation. They may never have expressed a wish and almost never have said "no" to anyone. Yet if a patient has a successful experience in one of these situations (e.g., asking for and receiving a raise, confronting a spouse), the patient will have learned a new skill, discover some sense of control over the local environment, and likely feel better.

The adaptation of IPT-D includes sixteen weekly sessions to drive these points home. Patients who improve are still likely to feel shaky: after what may be decades of depression, a few weeks of feeling better is unlikely to instill a feeling of security. For this reason we have routinely offered monthly continuation sessions and sometimes maintenance therapy (Chapter 9). In our experience, it takes several months for patients' euthymic self-image and new track record of healthy interpersonal functioning to sink in and for them to believe they are really better.

CASE EXAMPLE: TAKING ALL OF THE BLAME

Elaine, a 53-year-old woman, sought treatment because "My husband is disgusted with me." She reported having always felt sad, shy, and inferior. She completed college and had worked briefly before marrying a high-powered executive who expected her to run the house and care for their three children, one of whom, Kayla, had major developmental problems. She saw Kayla's problems as her own failure.

Elaine presented for treatment with double depression when her two other children were leaving home, leaving her with her increasingly handicapped daughter and her angry, unsupportive spouse. She felt quietly indignant about the way her family treated her but felt that anger was a "bad" emotion that confirmed what a damaged person she was. She tended to comply and suffer silently, seeing other people's needs and meeting them at the sacrifice of her own. Indeed, she was hard pressed to state what her own needs were. Never one to risk confiding in others, Elaine had few social supports outside of or even within her immediate family. She had had numerous prior trials of antidepressant medication with little benefit. She similarly felt that a two-year supportive psychodynamic psychotherapy, which had focused on understanding her childhood more than her current problems, had been a waste of time and money. She had never told her therapist this, not wanting to complain.

In the initial session, Elaine's IPT therapist diagnosed dysthymic disorder that had worsened into major depression. He noted her Hamilton Rating Scale for Depression score of 23 as evidence of this and reviewed the DSM criteria to try to reify the disorder. The therapist then suggested that they spend the next fifteen weeks (for a total of sixteen sessions) looking at how chronic depression was affecting her life and her interactions with important people in her life. He explained persistent depressive disorder as a condition from which she had suffered for so long that she seemed to consider it part of herself. He also stated, however, that she could learn in therapy to distinguish herself from the depression. IPT itself was defined as a role transition to health.

Elaine was skeptical but compliant. Early sessions focused on identifying and validating emotions such as her resentment of her husband and recasting them as useful and appropriate signals of frustrating situations. This took longer than it would have in treating acute depression, but after a couple of sessions she was able to tentatively role play expressing such feelings. She and the therapist tried to anticipate how her husband might respond: with anger, interruptions, and denials. Then, with trepidation she began to try to set protective limits ("as self-defense") with her husband and handicapped daughter, practicing saying no and carving out a little private time for herself. They also explored Elaine's needs and discussed whether she needed to feel "selfish" in pursuing them:

E: So, I guess I should talk to Jack about his helping with Kayla, but it's not going to work.
Therapist: What would you want him to do? What would be helpful to you?
E: I'd like him to really understand how hard it can be to live with her. He's never home, and when he is, the kids are my responsibility. . . . It's my fault for not bringing her up better; that's why she's having these problems. I know we've discussed that I blame myself because I'm depressed, but he blames me, too.
Therapist: Do you agree? Is that fair?
E: Sometimes I get confused. But no, I guess I more and more don't think it's fair. The psychologists say that we didn't do anything wrong to Kayla.
Therapist: So how do you feel when Jack blames you?
E: Angry? I don't like that feeling. But yes, it feels unfair. I resent it.
Therapist: And do you think that's a reasonable feeling?
E: I don't like the feeling. But yes, it's called for.
Therapist: So what options do you have in dealing with Jack?
E: It hasn't felt like there were any options. . . . I guess—I guess I could say what I just said. That Kayla's problems aren't my fault and that I resent it when he blames me. We should work together to try to help her. That would be best for all of us.

Therapist: How did that sound?

E: Pretty good, I guess.

Therapist: Is there something you would say differently? Did you say what you wanted to say? . . . Were you happy with your tone of voice?

E: Yes, but he'll probably not even let me finish. On the rare occasion when I start to say something, he cuts me off.

Therapist: Let's talk about what you would specifically like Jack to do to help you out and also about how you can handle it if he should interrupt.

To Elaine's surprise, her husband listened to her feelings without interrupting. He told her for the first time how much he respected her handling of Kayla's difficult behaviors and offered to provide more help around the house. Although he briefly became irritated, Elaine was able to tolerate this, and overall their encounter went far better than she had expected. Her mood improved, and her Ham-D score fell to 13. She was then willing to make further efforts to confront her family members and to gratify her own wishes in small ways. By the end of treatment, Elaine was shakily euthymic, with a Ham-D score of 8. She eagerly consented to monthly follow-up sessions for the ensuing six months, during which period she maintained her euthymia (Ham-D = 5 after six months) and began to consolidate her nondepressed track record and identity. She developed new friendships and independent interests outside of her home. She remained improved at a two-year follow-up.

CONCLUSION

This patient was not treated with medication, but many chronically depressed patients will respond best to the combination of medication and psychotherapy. In such instances, an antidepressant medication can relieve many of the symptoms of persistent depressive disorder, freeing the patient to work on interpersonal issues in IPT-D.

18

Bipolar Disorder

DIAGNOSIS

Bipolar disorder has long been recognized as a serious psychiatric disorder. The treating clinician should be familiar with the symptoms of mania as well as depression. Most bipolar patients present for treatment during the depressive phase of the disorder, but the clinician should obtain a history of manic symptoms from currently depressed patients to clarify the diagnosis. Because bipolar patients require special attention, nonmedical clinicians should always consult with a psychiatrist if a manic history is suspected to confirm the diagnosis and to introduce or monitor medication. The risks of suicide and social disruption in family and work situations are high for individuals with bipolar disorder. When patients are manic, they are reluctant to stay on medication or remain in any treatment.

For much of the late twentieth century, treatment research on bipolar disorder had focused almost exclusively on pharmacotherapy. There is no question that pharmacotherapy is essential to the treatment of bipolar I disorder; less is known about bipolar II disorder, in which symptoms range from depression to hypomania. In the last decade, research has explored the utility of psychotherapies as adjuncts to pharmacotherapy for bipolar I patients and is beginning to explore its utility as a primary treatment for bipolar II disorder.

There are clinical reasons to expect that psychotherapy might benefit these patients. Bipolar disorder is a profoundly dislocating condition, disrupting relationships through its depressive, manic, and psychotic symptoms. Patients often emerge from episodes with their sense of self shattered and their life situation in upheaval. Moreover, life events can trigger new episodes of depression or mania.

There is evidence that Interpersonal and Social Rhythm Therapy (IPSRT), an amalgam of IPT with behavioral therapy developed by Frank and colleagues, is an efficacious adjunct to medication for patients with bipolar I disorder. The behavioral component addresses coordination and stabilization of daily behaviors, especially the preservation of sleep, which is a critical factor in avoiding manic episodes, and modulation of environmental stimulation, whereas IPT targets the depressive aspects of the disorder. This combination represents an important extension of IPT into novel treatment territory.

Bipolar I Disorder

In a randomized clinical trial of 175 patients with bipolar I, Frank et al. (2005) found that mood-stabilizing medication was more efficacious in combination with IPSRT than when administered in an intensive clinical management (ICM) control condition. The study was complex, with a design involving dual random-ization to IPSRT or ICM at both the acute and maintenance phases of treatment. Initial time to stabilization did not differ between IPSRT and ICM, although IPSRT patients regularized their social rhythms more in the acute phase (Frank et al., 2005).

Patients treated with acute IPSRT remained euthymic longer in the mainte-nance phase before developing a recurrent episode, regardless of whether they received IPT or ICM in the maintenance phase. Ability to stabilize social rhythms using IPSRT during the acute phase was also associated with reduced likelihood of recurrence during the maintenance phase. This suggested that early introduc-tion of IPT and social rhythm therapy for bipolar I disorder in the acute phase has a prophylactic benefit. However, bipolar patients with multiple medical prob-lems took longer to reach remission and fared better in ICM (which focused on the patient's somatic symptoms) than in IPSRT (which focused on increasing the social stability of the patient's life) (Frank et al., 2005). Finally, patients with comorbid panic disorder had poorer outcomes.

A subsequent trial, a segment of the STEP-BD study, compared psychothera-pies as adjunctive treatments for 152 depressed outpatients receiving pharmaco-therapy for bipolar I or bipolar II disorder (Miklowitz et al., 2007). Eighty-four patients were randomized to thirty sessions over nine months of either IPSRT, CBT, or family-focused therapy, whereas sixty-eight received three-session psy-choeducational collaborative care. All three active therapies were associated with better patient functioning, relationship functioning, and life satisfaction than the collaborative care condition, although work and recreational scores did not improve. There were no meaningful between-therapy differences.

Data for adolescents are limited. In a small open trial, Hlastala et al. (2010) found that treatment comprising sixteen to eighteen sessions of adjunctive IPSRT over twenty weeks was well tolerated and was associated with significant improve-ment in a sample of twelve adolescents with bipolar disorder. A pilot study attempted to test IPSRT for thirteen at-risk adolescent children of patients with bipolar disorder (Goldstein et al., 2014). Attrition was a problem, but preliminary results suggested sleep stabilization for participants.

Bipolar II Disorder

Bipolar II disorder has received too little study, and its definitive treatment remains unclear. Patients with this diagnosis become hypomanic rather than manic but spend lengthy stretches of their lives depressed. They have difficulty distinguishing between euthymia and hypomania: what occasionally occurs and feels "normal" may actually be an elevated state, and what is objectively euthymic may feel substandard and depressive. Mood instability and chronic depression hurt relationships and self-esteem. The mood-stabilizing medications efficacious for bipolar I disorder have some but less clear benefit for bipolar II disorder, and psychotherapies have been little researched (Swartz, Levenson, & Frank, 2012).

Swartz, Rucci, Thase, Wallace, Carretta, Celedonia, and Frank (in press) recently completed a randomized, twenty-week trial comparing IPSRT alone to IPSRT plus quetiapine for ninety-two otherwise unmedicated patients with bipolar II disorder presenting with a major depression. Both treatments yielded significant improvement, with comparable response rates (≥50 percent reduction in Ham-D-25 item scores), with a 67.4 percent response rate overall. A significant time × group interaction favored the combined condition on the Ham-D-17 ($p = .048$) and Yale Mania Rating Scale ($p = .044$). Patients receiving IPSRT + quetiapine developed significantly higher body mass index over time ($p = .012$).

Quetiapine benefits patients with bipolar II disorder but has weight gain as a well-known side effect. IPSRT combined with quetiapine produced greater symptomatic improvement but also more weight gain than IPSRT alone. Swartz et al. concluded that IPSRT monotherapy may be an appropriate treatment for patients with bipolar II depression who wish to avoid weight gain. These promising initial findings bear attempts at replication.

The level of evidence for IPSRT for bipolar I disorder is **** (four stars; treatment has been validated by at least two randomized controlled trials demonstrating the superiority of IPT to a control condition). The level of evidence for IPSRT for bipolar II disorder is *** (three stars; validation by at least one randomized controlled trial or equivalent to a reference treatment of established efficacy).

ADAPTATION

IPSRT is the first IPT adaptation to be designed as an adjunct to medication, rather than as a standalone, primary treatment; it is also the first attempt to integrate IPT with a behavioral approach.

The problem in adapting IPT to bipolar disorder lay not with the depressive phase of the disorder, for which IPT approaches were already well developed, but with the mania. Frank and colleagues recognized that a crucial aspect of mania was the disruption of the diurnal life schedule, particularly the loss of sleep, which commonly triggers mania. Accordingly, they developed a behavioral approach to regularize daily social activities (especially sleep). Patients fill out a weekly grid of activities, the Social Rhythm Metric (Table 18.1), starting each morning and running throughout the day, to mark social anchors of daily routines. They review the SRM with therapists to see how regular their schedule is, how stimulating their activities are (how many people they encounter at breakfast, etc.), and what sorts of things may be interfering with a predictable, organized day and night. Focusing on such daily behavioral patterns can enable patients to regularize their schedules, thus decreasing the likelihood

Table 18.1 Social Rhythm Metric II, Five-Item Version (SRM-II-5)

Week of _____

Directions:
1. Write the *ideal target time* you would *like* to do these daily activities.
2. Record the *time* you actually did the activity each day.
3. Record the *people* involved in the activity: 0 = alone; 1 = others present; 2 = others actively involved; 3 = others very stimulating

Activity	Target Time	Sunday Time/P*	Monday Time/P	Tuesday Time/P	Wednesday Time/P	Thursday Time/P	Friday Time/P	Saturday Time/P
Out of bed								
First contact with another person								
Start work/school/ volunteer/family care								
Dinner								
To bed								
Rate mood daily from −5 (very depressed) to +5 (very elated)								

*P = Number of people present

Note: Adapted from Frank, E. (2005). *Treating bipolar disorder: A clinician's guide to interpersonal and social rhythm therapy.* New York: Guilford.

of a student pulling an all-nighter, for example, and provoking a manic episode (Frank, Swartz, & Kupfer, 2000). IPSRT does not attempt to treat mania once it has arisen—when patients are unlikely to listen to or collaborate with therapists—but rather to prevent its recurrence.

The depressive phase of bipolar illness is treated much as it is for unipolar depression. The usual concomitants of depression arise with complicated bereavement, role disputes, and role transitions associated with depressive episodes. An added interpersonal focus is "grief for the lost healthy self." This concept encompasses the reality that patients may remit from a severe manic or depressive episode to find their lives in shambles. They need to grieve and come to terms with the effect their illness has wrought on their lives. This would seem to be a special case of a role transition.

A new facet of the ISPRT approach is the development of a smartphone app to help patients chart the connections between their mood, sleep, and interpersonal activity (Matthews et al., 2016).

CASE EXAMPLE: TAMING THE ROLLER COASTER

Rebecca, a 28-year-old woman, presented for treatment with bipolar II disorder. She felt depressed much of the time and became hypomanic under stress, resulting in impulsive behavior and mild overspending. On presentation, her Hamilton Rating Scale for Depression score was 23 (moderately severely depressed). Stressors in her life included job pressures and a conflicted sexual relationship of two years with Charles, an older, married celebrity. Her work in a publishing house prompted frequent all-nighters to meet copy deadlines, a pattern that disrupted her sleep schedule and mood. Rebecca reported that her mother had been diagnosed with manic depression and had responded well to lithium. She herself had seen psychiatrists in the past but had been put off by their emphasis on medication, which she feared taking.

Her therapist gave Rebecca the diagnosis of bipolar II disorder and explained its risks and potential treatments. The therapist pointed out that bipolar II was a lifelong but treatable illness; he suggested a twelve-week IPSRT treatment with likely maintenance treatment if acute treatment proved beneficial. He also emphasized that, while acute treatment was important, the goal of therapy was the general stabilization of mood and reduction of both depressive and hypomanic episodes over time, what the patient termed "taming the roller coaster."

Rebecca was reluctant to take lithium like her mother but did accept another medication, which seemed to provide partial relief of her symptoms; nonetheless, she remained depressed much of the time and still reported a tendency toward hypomania. Using the Social Rhythm Metric (see Table 18.1), she and her therapist reviewed her erratic sleep schedule and discussed good "sleep hygiene": slowing down in the evening, avoiding caffeine and alcohol, conducting only relaxing activities in the hours before bedtime, and going to bed and arising at the same regular hours. They discussed what work options Rebecca had to avoid all-nighters, which she decided she could minimize by spacing out her work assignments and not procrastinating.

In the meantime, the therapist noted that Rebecca's depression often seemed related not to her work, which she loved, but to her relationship with her "VIP lover," Charles. They defined this as a role dispute. Rebecca tended to take a subservient role in this relationship but felt neglected and misunderstood. Taking the standard role dispute approach, both patient and therapist explored Rebecca's positive and negative feelings about Charles and their relationship, what she wanted from it, and how she could achieve her wishes. Except during hypomanic moments, Rebecca was extremely passive in the relationship and had great difficulty either expressing her needs or setting limits with Charles.

Using the Social Rhythm Metric, Rebecca was able to organize and regularize her sleep and activity schedule. She had initially been skeptical of how helpful this would be, but she now conceded that it made a difference in her mood and energy level. With considerable role playing, she was able to express her wishes to Charles more fully; he was not entirely receptive but respected her opinions and met her halfway on some wishes, such as taking a vacation together, which the patient considered a huge achievement. Her Ham-D score had fallen to 9 by the end of twelve sessions. Rebecca then contracted for two years of monthly maintenance sessions (see Chapter 9), through which she remained minimally depressed and without hypomanic episodes. She then recontracted for another two years, during which she has generally remained well.

CONCLUSION

Supported by growing evidence, ISPRT appears to be an important development in the treatment of bipolar I disorder as an adjunct to mood-stabilizing medication, and possibly as a monotherapy for bipolar II disorder. Frank et al. (2005) treated patients for two years, but bipolar illness is lifelong, and continual treatment is indicated. IPSRT warrants further study.

Adaptations of IPT
for Non-Mood Disorders

19

Substance-Related and Addictive Disorders

OVERVIEW

Substance-related and addictive disorders comprise misuse of or dependence upon substances such as alcohol, opiates, cocaine, and nicotine. Substance use and dependence are prevalent, debilitating conditions. These DSM-5 disorders often leave a trail of broken relationships and eroded social skills. The state of sobriety is a role transition that might fit the IPT model, as it requires the rebuilding of social skills, relationships, and life roles that substance use has devastated (Cherry & Markowitz, 1996). The available data do not allow us to recommend IPT as a treatment for patients whose focus of the treatment is a substance use disorder. There have been promising pilot studies, mainly for alcohol dependence comorbid with depression (Gamble et al., 2013; Johnson & Zlotnick, 2012; Johnson et al., 2015; Markowitz et al., 2008), as well as several negative trials for other substance use. Despite the small database, one group has argued the rationale for pursuing trials in the area (Brache, 2012), and the government of Scotland is supporting IPT as a treatment for incarcerated women with depression and substance abuse.

There have been several negative IPT trials with patients with substance use disorders. The first study added IPT to a standard drug program psychosocial intervention to reduce psychopathology among seventy-two methadone-maintained, opiate-dependent patients (Rounsaville, Glazer, Wilber, Weissman, & Kleber, 1983). Both treatment groups improved, but there was no advantage found for adding IPT. Because all of the patients were already receiving good substance abuse treatment and psychotherapy, this raises the issue of a ceiling effect; it is hard to show differences between effective treatments.

IPT was also ineffective in helping intravenous cocaine–dependent patients in achieving cocaine abstinence (Carroll, Rounsaville, & Gawin, 1991). In that twelve-week study, IPT was compared to a behavioral therapy. Both were characterized by a high dropout rate and poor response; there was no suggestion of an advantage for IPT.

A small randomized pilot study comparing sixteen weeks of IPT to brief supportive therapy for patients with DSM-IV dysthymic disorder suffering from secondary alcohol abuse or dependence found that both treatments showed improved depressive symptoms and alcohol abstinence (Markowitz et al., 2008). IPT had a large and brief supportive therapy a moderate effect size in depression, whereas the opposite was true for days abstinent from alcohol. The sample was too small to draw conclusions but suggested that IPT may have greater efficacy in treating depression but no advantage in treating the comorbid alcohol abuse/dependence. Both treatments recommended attendance at Alcoholics Anonymous, but few patients actually attended.

An open pilot study adding eight sessions of IPT to thrice-weekly addiction treatment assessed fourteen alcohol-dependent women with co-occurring depression up to thirty-two weeks. The outcomes showed feasibility, high treatment satisfaction, and decreased drinking behavior, depressive symptoms, and impaired functioning sustained over the follow-up (Gamble et al., 2013). A controlled trial of group IPT compared to an attention-matched control for thirty-eight incarcerated women with major depression who were also attending separate substance use treatment found significantly lower depressive symptoms at the end of eight weeks in the group IPT (Johnson & Zlotnick, 2012) than the control group after release from prison. The results suggest that the rapid effects of IPT on depression may reduce some of the serious interpersonal consequences of prison.

The third study by Johnson, Williams, and Zlotnick (2015) included twenty-two female prisoners experiencing depression and substance misuse disorder and tested the feasibility of a Sober Network (http://www.sobernetwork.com) IPT intervention that supported women through the transition from prison to community re-entry. All participants received twenty-four seventy-five-minute group sessions of Sober Network IPT over eight weeks plus one pre-group, one mid-group, and one post-group individual sessions. Six of the twenty-four sessions were explicitly focused on establishing and building a sober network (a network of positive social supports that did not misuse substances). In addition to group sessions, each woman was given a "sober phone" prior to her release from prison. Upon release, women received thirty-two telephone appointments over a three-month period. The use of cell phones was a novel feature of the study. The study reported that participants' depressive symptoms and substance use had significantly decreased by the end of the intervention, but results did not demonstrate a significant increase in social and sober supports.

The Scottish government is investing in testing IPT as an early intervention for women in the criminal justice system with depression. The large majority have substance use disorders. Twelve weekly sessions for seventeen women yielded remission in 76.5 percent of women and increases in perceived social supports, and only one of the seventeen had a further offense on follow-up. Information on substance use was not reported. IPT is now part of routine service delivered in the prison system for women in Scotland (Black, 2016).

The level of evidence for IPT is (no stars; negative findings). IPT has been found to be no better than a control condition. However, some small studies in process are more optimistic for its use in narrowly defined samples.

ADAPTATION

The rationale for using IPT with patients who have substance-related disorders was the assumption that such disorders represent an attempt to compensate for inadequate interpersonal relationships or have negative consequences on existing relationships. The goal was to help patients resolve interpersonal problems and to develop new skills to alleviate stress and obviate the need for substance use. It was also hoped that patients for whom methadone reduced opiate craving would be more likely to engage in psychotherapy.

IPT was used as an adjunctive treatment with methadone-maintained patients and as a sole intervention or combined treatment to achieve abstinence in the treatment of cocaine abusers. Adaptations to IPT were minor. The content of the sessions was geared to the particular problems of patients with substance abuse, and the focus was switched from treating depression to the reduction or elimination of substance abuse and the development of better social and interpersonal coping strategies.

Patients were encouraged to accept the need to stop drugs, manage impulsivity, and recognize the context of drug use and supply. The interpersonal inventory explored the history of drug use, the family's reaction to it, and the influence of drugs on both the patient's interpersonal behavior and the behaviors necessary to obtain and finance drug use, as well as the illegal behaviors and risks accompanying it. The usual IPT problem areas were employed. As these applications of IPT have not worked, we cannot recommend their use for the treatment of patients with substance-related disorders.

Many reasons have been suggested for the failure of IPT to show benefit in this treatment population. Substance use disorders are notoriously difficult to treat. There were problems in recruiting and retaining patients for the studies, and the patients did not seem to find the interpersonal focus relevant to their problems. It was important to stabilize the patients on methadone in the first study to relieve their cravings and dysphoria before trying to interest them in psychotherapy. It is possible that the serious consequences of drug abuse responded to the use of sustained methadone maintenance and the accompanying comprehensive drug treatment program, which already included group psychotherapy. The effect of IPT by itself, without a pharmacotherapy program, has not been tested. Regarding the Carroll et al. study, Najavits and Weiss (1994) argued that IPT was helpful for patients who met criteria for depression and low-severity cocaine addiction.

In the dysthymic disorder and alcohol abuse study, IPT therapists focused on achieving sobriety as a role transition. Therapists presented alcohol abuse, like depression, as a medical illness, a treatable condition that was not the patient's fault. Therapists tried to link drinking episodes to interpersonal stresses, both of which patients recorded in a diary. It was usually possible to link both mood shifts and drinking behavior to life circumstances. Patients were encouraged to attend Alcoholics Anonymous meetings, although they rarely did. Participants showed some gains, and there was a suggestion of greater antidepressant effect in the IPT condition than in supportive therapy. Statistical power was limited, and IPT did not show a significant advantage on the Hamilton Rating Scale for Depression, the primary outcome measure, but did result in significantly greater improvement than brief supportive psychotherapy on the Beck Depression self-report inventory (Markowitz et al., 2008).

CONCLUSION

It has long been clinically acknowledged that substance abuse interferes with many psychotherapeutic approaches. Based on the published literature, approaches other than IPT that focus on sobriety or relapse prevention may be preferable for patients with substance use disorders (e.g., CBT, motivational interviewing, Alcoholics Anonymous or other twelve-step support groups, detoxification, and rehabilitation when appropriate). However, it is possible to prematurely abandon a treatment approach based on limited negative data. One should not overlook the findings in incarcerated women with depression and substance use problems, or the suggestion by Brache (2012) for more specific adaptation of IPT to substance-related disorders. If developing meaningful roles in society, encouraging social bonding with non-substance users, and using the therapeutic relationship for self-soothing are built in, then shouldn't IPT have some benefit?

Once sober, such patients might benefit from IPT techniques to rebuild their lives and relationships (Miller & Carroll, 2006), but the benefits of IPT for such patients at this point are speculative. IPT has never been intended as a treatment for all patients with all conditions, and substance abuse may be an area where its application has limited utility.

20

Eating Disorders

The most common eating disorders are anorexia nervosa (AN), bulimia nervosa (BN), and binge eating disorder (BED). The DSM-5 recommends assigning only one of these diagnoses during a single episode. Obesity is not a DSM-5 mental disorder, although it is robustly associated with several mental health disorders, including other eating disorders. IPT has been tested in studies of BED for prevention of obesity. The assumption for testing IPT with eating disorders is that they occur in response to distress at poor social and interpersonal functioning and consequent negative mood, to which the patient responds with maladaptive eating behaviors (Rieger et al., 2010).

DIAGNOSIS

Anorexia Nervosa

For AN, a condition for which no outpatient treatments have shown great benefit, few data provide evidence for the benefit of IPT. One study from New Zealand compared twenty weeks of CBT, IPT, or supportive psychotherapy used in clinical practice to fifty-six women with anorexia nervosa followed up over six years (Carter et al., 2010). About half the patients had a good outcome defined on a four-point global assessment rating scale. No significant differences were found between treatments at follow-up on any of the outcomes. Among patients who remained in the study both at end of twenty-week treatment and at follow-up, the percentage of patients with good outcome for the different treatments was 75 percent for supportive psychotherapy, 33 percent for CBT, and 15 percent for IPT (McIntosh et al., 2005) based on a small number of patients. At the six-year follow-up, the results remained stable for CBT (41 percent), improved for IPT (64 percent), and decreased for supportive psychotherapy (42 percent). The authors interpreted these findings to suggest that a stepped-care approach focusing on targeting eating disorders and restoring weight, followed by IPT focusing on a broader context, may be useful (Kass et al., 2013). The small sample size was underpowered to detect small to moderate effects.

Bulimia Nervosa

The first trial using IPT for BN compared it with CBT, which was the standard treatment for BN, and behavior therapy (BT), a dismantled version of CBT that excluded reference to the patient's concern about her shape or weight and focused on normalization of eating habits. All IPT trials for BN have used individual treatment. IPT was adapted for BN by formulating the patient's eating disorder in interpersonal terms; however, to avoid overlap with CBT, IPT therapists had to avoid discussing the patient's eating habits or attitudes about shape and weight as well as role playing, which are important techniques in both IPT and CBT (Fairburn et al., 1991).

Seventy-five patients with BN entered the study, receiving sessions twice weekly for the first month, weekly for the next two months, and every other week until termination at eighteen weeks. CBT was more effective than IPT or BT in modifying disturbed attitudes toward shape, weight, and extensive attempts to diet. An eight-month follow-up, however, found no difference between CBT on the behavioral features because the IPT patients continued to improve. There was considerable post-treatment relapse in the BT group over the eight months (Fairburn et al., 1993).

A larger, two-center study (N = 220) using the same CBT and IPT protocol replicated these findings. CBT was superior to IPT at the end of treatment but at the eight- and twelve-month follow-ups, the two were equivalent (Agras et al., 2000; see Murphy et al., 2012, for clinical description).

Fairburn et al. (2015) again compared CBT to IPT using a transdiagnostic individual therapy approach that included patients with various eating disorders (not anorexia) and a body mass index (BMI) over 17.5 and under 40; the treatment lasted twenty weeks, with a one-year follow-up. Unlike previous studies, the IPT protocol included role playing and discussion of the eating disorder. Results resembled those in previous studies, with significantly faster improvement by twenty weeks in CBT relative to IPT and equivalent improvement in the IPT remission rate over the one year of follow-up.

Efforts to find predictors or moderators of response to CBT or IPT in the Fairburn et al. (2015) study were disappointing (Cooper et al., 2016). Patients who had a longer duration of bulimia or who overvalued body shape were less likely to benefit from either treatment. It was not possible to identify subgroups of patients who differentially responded to treatment.

Mitchell et al. (2000) entered 62 out of 194 patients with BN who had not responded to CBT into either IPT or medication management. The dropout and withdrawal rates (about 40 percent) were high, and the response rate was low. The authors concluded that offering sequential treatments had little value. The IPT used was the modification originally designed by Fairburn et al. (1993), eliminating discussion of eating problems and role play in order to avoid overlap with CBT.

Eating disorders are common among women college students. Wilfley and Eichen (in press) are testing a briefer form of individual IPT (ten sessions) for bulimia nervosa in counseling centers on several college campuses. They are also testing high- versus low-intensity training strategies for implementing IPT for eating and mood disorders at twenty-six college counseling centers and appointing 230 therapists (Wilfley, personal communication, 2016). A guided online training program with telephone-based simulation assessment of clinician fidelity is being tested (Wilfley & Van Buren, personal communication, 2016).

Binge Eating Disorder

Wilson et al. (2010) compared IPT to behavioral weight loss (BWL) and to a guided self-help treatment based on CBT (CBTgsh) in the treatment of 205 overweight men and women with binge eating. Patients received twenty sessions of IPT or BWL or ten sessions of CBTgsh over six months. At the six-month and one-year follow-ups there were no differences in treatment outcome. At the two-year follow-up, both IPT and CBTgsh were associated with greater remission from binge eating than BWL, but CBTgsh had a higher attrition rate (30 percent) than IPT (7 percent). Wilson (2011) noted that IPT showed the best results in patients who reported the most binge eating, shape and weight concerns, compensatory behaviors, and negative affect. In a separate study, Cooper et al. (2016) did not find subgroups of patients with eating disorders who differentially responded to CBT or IPT.

Rapid responders (defined as a 70 percent reduction in binge eating in four weeks) in the Wilson study in the CBT group, but not in the IPT or BWL group, showed significantly greater remission for BED compared to non-rapid responders. IPT had comparable efficacy for both rapid and non-rapid responders, whereas non-rapid response in CBT and both rapid and non-rapid response in BWL were associated with the lowest rates of remission. These findings suggested the value of IPT as a second-level treatment for binge eaters who did not respond to CBTgsh.

Cooper et al. (2016) did not find subgroups of patients with BED who differentially responded to CBT or IPT.

Note that all these studies used the Fairburn et al. (1993) IPT adaptation that avoided discussion of eating disorders so as not to overlap with CBT. This exclusion may have hindered IPT because symptom discussion is part of IPT for other disorders.

Wilfley et al. (2002) treated 162 overweight subjects with BED, randomizing them to twenty weeks of group IPT or CBT and assessing them up to one year following treatment. Two independent clinics were involved. Recovery rates were equivalent for group CBT (64 [79 percent] of 81) and group IPT (59 [73 percent] of 81) at posttreatment and at the one-year follow-up (48 [59 percent] of 81 vs. 50 [62 percent] of 81). Binge eating increased slightly during follow-up but remained significantly below pretreatment levels. Across treatments, patients had similarly significant reductions in associated eating disorders and psychiatric symptoms and maintenance of gains through follow-up. Dietary restraint decreased more quickly in the CBT group, but the IPT subjects had equivalent levels by later follow-ups. Patients' relative weight decreased with statistical significance, but in absolute terms only slightly, with the greatest reduction among patients sustaining recovery from binge eating from posttreatment to the one-year follow-up.

The authors concluded that group IPT is a viable alternative to group CBT for the treatment of overweight patients with BED. Although lack of a nonspecific control condition limits the conclusions that can be made about treatment specificity, both treatments showed initial and long-term efficacy for the core and related symptoms of BED. Predictors of differential treatment response at one year found that greater interpersonal problems prior to and at mid-treatment or greater concern about shape predicted a poor response at the end of treatment and at follow-up for both group therapies (Hilbert et al., 2007).

A four-year follow-up of 90 of the original 162 patients found substantial long-term recovery and partial remission and significant improvement (58 percent of patients in both treatments; Hilbert et al., 2012). BMI remained stable and did not increase. The IPT group demonstrated greater improvement (abstinence from binge eating) in eating disorder symptoms and the CBT group displayed a worsening, but these results did not reach statistical significance at any time point during follow-up. The fact that less than 60 percent of the sample participated weakens the generalizability of findings.

Binge Eating and Excessive Weight Gain in Adolescents

Binge eating is a common abnormal behavior among obese adults, and adolescent obesity is a strong predictor of adult obesity (Tanofsky-Kraff et al., 2007). To prevent obesity, Tanofsky-Kraff et al. initiated an IPT pilot study as part of standard health education for teens at high risk for adult obesity (BMI in the 75th to 97th percentile; see Tanofsky-Kraff et al., 2016). Thirty-eight girls ages 12 to 17 were randomized to group IPT versus standard health education for twelve weeks, with eight- and twelve-month follow-ups. Girls in the IPT group reported fewer loss-of-control episodes at posttreatment, and at one year they were less likely to increase their BMI as might have been expected by age (Tanofsky-Kraff et al., 2010).

The same group repeated this study in a larger trial (Tanofsky-Kraff et al., 2014) with 113 adolescents using the same entrance criteria and design but more precise outcome measures of BMI. No treatment differences were found after twelve weeks in terms of BMI, episodes of loss-of-control eating, or depressive or anxiety symptoms. However, as in the pilot study, teens with loss-of-control binge eating had lower BMI, adiposity, and mood symptoms over one year (Tanofsky-Kraff et al., 2014).

The level of evidence of IPT for AN is no stars (IPT has been found to be no better than a control condition). The level of evidence for individual and group IPT for BN and BED is **** (four stars; treatment has been validated by at least two randomized, controlled trials demonstrating the efficacy of IPT compared to a control condition). IPT is included as a recommended, evidence-based treatment for BN and BED in treatment guidelines in Australia, Canada, the United Kingdom, Scotland, Japan, Spain, and the United States (Clinical Practices Guideline, 2016). The level of evidence of IPT for prevention of obesity in adolescents with high BMI is * (one star; the evidence is suggestive but weak).

ADAPTATIONS

Partly because the researchers conducting the early trials wanted to contrast elements of IPT with CBT, they made several changes in IPT for bulimia for research purposes. First, whereas IPT therapists frequently emphasize that depression is an illness—because depressed patients tend to forget this and blame themselves, confusing themselves with their illness—bulimic patients have no such difficulty. They need no reminders to know they have bulimia and eating difficulties. Therefore, rather than focusing on bulimia as an illness, IPT therapists in Fairburn's studies mentioned the diagnosis at the start of treatment but thereafter avoided discussing food, eating, body image, and so forth—the usual topics of their patients' conversation (Fairburn et al., 1991). Whereas CBT therapists focused on such matters, IPT therapists interrupted their patients when they raised eating topics and steered them back to examining their discomfort with feelings and relationships that might trigger binge episodes. Thus, IPT focused not directly on the eating symptoms, but on their affective and interpersonal context.

Second, because role playing is also a CBT technique, IPT therapists were asked not to use it in Fairburn's studies. This represents the loss of a potentially powerful aspect of IPT. In clinical practice, we do not recommend that IPT therapists avoid role play in treating bulimia. The subsequent Fairburn et al. (2015) study, however, did not exclude role playing and yielded similar results.

The Wilfley studies linked interpersonal problems to eating disorder symptoms and changes in body weight. The trajectory of therapy depended on the specific type of eating disorder being treated. To treat these patients, Wilfley et al. redefined the confusing term "interpersonal deficits." Depressed individuals with the IPT focal problem area of interpersonal deficits have traditionally been conceptualized as having few to no social ties and no current life events; the category is generally only used in the absence of other life event foci. In eating disorders, however, "interpersonal deficits" became a focal problem area for patients who experience poor-quality social ties or chronically unfulfilling relationships (Tanofsky-Kraff & Wilfley, 2012; Wilfley et al., 2002). Thus, a clinician working with a patient with eating disorders on "interpersonal deficits" focuses on helping the patient develop more satisfying relationships rather than (or more than) initiating new ones. The liberal use of interpersonal deficits in an eating disorders group provides a common theme for patients in the group, avoiding the potential confusion in group process of having some patients address grief and others role disputes. Thus, IPT for eating disorders gives the term "interpersonal deficits" a different function than it has in individual IPT for depression.

IPT for eating disorders (IPT-ED) conceptualizes symptoms as recurring and chronic, and connected to interpersonal factors that maintain as well as trigger eating disorder symptoms. IPT-ED uses a timeline to chart interpersonal events, eating disorder symptoms, and weight change over time to enhance the interpersonal inventory. This provides the clinician with the opportunity to concretely depict the connections between the patient's interpersonal ups and downs and the waxing and waning of eating disorder symptoms (see Markowitz & Weissman [2012] for clinical descriptions).

Wilfley et al. (1993) combined two initial individual sessions with subsequent group IPT sessions. The individual visits allowed the therapist to develop a therapeutic alliance with each patient and prepare the patient for the group while determining the patient's history, symptoms, and IPT formulation. That constituted the first phase. Once the group began, therapists sent patients home with feedback specific to their own cases. The other adaptations followed those used in individual IPT-ED.

With these changes, group IPT functions much like individual IPT. The overall structure of initial, middle, and termination sessions persists. The focus remains on the connection between feelings and life situations, and patients identify common themes and work together to help one another solve their interpersonal problems (Tanofsky-Kraff & Wilfley, 2012).

Arcelus et al. (2009, 2012) have explored a form of IPT modified with some cognitive elements for treating BN and found some initial promise in a case series. Fairburn has described a hybrid treatment beginning and ending with CBT but including an interval of IPT for bulimic patients. The latter approach is intriguing but complex, requiring patients and therapists to shift focus in midstream, then switch back. Data on these adaptations are limited (Fairburn, personal communication, 2015).

CASE EXAMPLE: OBESITY IN HER THOUGHTS

Gail, a 27-year-old single assistant editor at a publishing firm, presented with bulimia nervosa. Her chief complaint was "I'm embarrassed to say I can't control my eating."

Gail reported a history of bingeing and vomiting since age 14. She tended to eat little, and then periodically binged on huge quantities of pound cake or sweets. She was muscular and thin, worked out frequently at the gym, but felt "grossly obese" in ways that "other people can't see" and obsessively checked herself in the mirror for flaws in her figure. Similarly, she weighed herself several times a day and forced herself to vomit if her weight was unacceptable. She threw up at least once a day, a pattern she saw as a necessary ritual. She had social contacts but confided in no one because she was sure that they would be "grossed out" by her eating behavior or turned off by her mood. She kept a similar distance from her family and her roommate. She had had numerous sexual liaisons but declared with negative bravado that she had never had more than three dates with a man. She felt men were "for some reason" attracted to her but that they quickly figured out her ugly side.

Gail had gotten little benefit from two adequate trials of serotonin reuptake inhibitors, which she felt caused weight gain. She had undergone two courses of psychodynamic psychotherapy, each lasting about two years, with little benefit. She presented with worsening bulimia in the wake of "being dumped" by an Internet date and increased pressure at work. Symptoms included worsening binges, a three-pound weight gain, and subsequently increased purging and exercise. She also reported moderate depressive symptoms (Hamilton Rating Scale for Depression score = 18).

The therapist gave her the diagnosis of bulimia nervosa. He noted that her eating behavior might be related to her life situation and wondered whether she might be curious about this connection. Picking up on her concern about relationships, he suggested that they spend the next sixteen weeks working on understanding the connection between her interpersonal functioning and her symptoms and on building new interpersonal skills. He described this as a role transition in the wake of her latest breakup of a relationship. She agreed.

Although Gail often drifted into the topic of food, the therapist would seek the context of her concern: If she had binged, how had she been feeling at that time? Had something happened, or was she anxious about something that was about to occur? What were her feelings? The therapist worked hard to normalize those feelings, which the patient tended to regard as "weird" or abnormal. Once she had begun to acknowledge disappointment and anger and to recognize patterns of these feelings arising in interpersonal contexts, they began to explore options for putting them into words and expressing them to other people:

> What might you say? . . . How did that sound? Is that saying what you want to say? How comfortable are you in saying "no"?

Gail had difficulties in asserting herself at work and on dates and in setting limits with other people. In her effort to please, she frequently ignored her own wishes, with predictably unhappy results. After a date in which she had felt pawed or a work assignment had been dumped upon her, she frequently felt helpless, a feeling that almost inevitably led to a briefly soothing but soon distressing binge and then to vomiting, which made her feel like a "disgusting freak." She began tentatively to express her feelings, first by defining her hours and job responsibilities with her work colleagues, which relieved some deadline pressures, and then by taking the seemingly riskier step of telling dates what she wanted and did not like on their dates. Initially skeptical that expressing her feelings would do any good, she was surprised by successes in both settings and noted that her eating and mood symptoms had both decreased.

By the end of the sixteen-week treatment, Gail was infrequently bingeing and had not vomited in four weeks. Her Ham-D score had returned to the normal range. Moreover, she recognized for the first time the important connection between her interpersonal life and her bulimic symptoms. The therapist congratulated her on her gains, and they agreed to a once-a-month maintenance treatment, during which she has remained almost asymptomatic for two and a half years. She is now in a sustained relationship for the first time and engaged to be married.

THERAPIST NOTE

Whether or not associated it is with comorbid depression, bulimia is treatable with IPT. Gail not only mastered her eating symptoms but also did so through grappling with the perhaps still more important arena of her interpersonal life. Like many bulimic patients, Gail's obsession with her eating had obscured for her its connection with her feelings and relationships.

CONCLUSION

Little evidence supports the treatment of AN with IPT (or with any psychotherapy). There is strong evidence that CBT is the most effective psychotherapy for BN; individual IPT might be as effective but is slower to achieve improvements. Including the handling of eating disorder symptoms in the initial phase of IPT might add to or accelerate the improvement achieved in IPT by focusing purely on interpersonal issues. Group IPT for BED is an efficacious treatment in both the short and the long term, but may be slower in the short term than CBT for dietary restraints. IPT is considered a viable option for treatment of BN and BED and is recommended in numerous guidelines.

21

Anxiety Disorders

Social Anxiety Disorder and Panic Disorder

BACKGROUND

The psychotherapeutic treatment of anxiety disorders has been best established for cognitive and behavioral therapies, and indeed for some time appeared to be predominantly the domain of CBT (Markowitz et al., 2014). Some of the DSM-5 diagnostic criteria resonate with cognitive thinking, and research has shown that forms of CBT frequently benefit patients with a spectrum of anxiety disorders. Yet not all patients respond to any treatment modality, and while some patients work comfortably within the CBT framework, others have trouble accepting it. In recent years, IPT researchers have begun to approach anxiety disorders, including social anxiety disorder (also known as social phobia) and panic disorder. As many anxiety disorders are comorbid with major depression and tend to complicate its treatment (Frank et al., 2011; Milrod et al., 2014), it would reassure IPT therapists focusing on the latter to know whether IPT effectively treats anxiety disorders. Indeed, the meta-analysis by Cuijpers et al. (2016), based on eight randomized trials, suggests efficacy for anxiety disorders: "In anxiety disorders, IPT had large effects compared with control groups, and there is no evidence that IPT was less effective than CBT."

The level of evidence for IPT varies by disorder; in general, research is in an early stage. But we can still assign it a rating of *** (three stars; encouraging findings in one or more open trials or in pilot studies with small samples).

THERAPIST NOTE

Posttraumatic stress disorder (PTSD), a DSM-IV anxiety disorder that was moved to a trauma disorder section in DSM-5, is discussed in Chapter 22.

ADAPTATIONS

Anxiety and depression frequently overlap, and the focal IPT problem areas fit both categories of syndromes. Like depressed patients, anxious individuals are often risk-averse: inhibited in expressing anger, confronting people, and asserting themselves. At least several of the DSM anxiety disorders have important interpersonal aspects. Thus, the general IPT approach has seemed to need little overhaul for anxiety disorders: the usual focal problem areas and approaches still apply, simply linking life events and interpersonal circumstances to anxiety states rather than to mood states.

SOCIAL ANXIETY DISORDER (SOCIAL PHOBIA)

Like persistent depressive disorder/dysthymia (Chapter 17), social anxiety disorder is a chronic syndrome. Individuals with social anxiety disorder fear humiliation in social situations from saying or doing the wrong thing, blushing, or otherwise looking foolish or incompetent in the eyes of others. They feel judged by others. As a result, they avoid social interactions and close relationships and tend to have few social supports. Research has documented these relationship difficulties, impaired intimacy, fewer friendships, and lower likelihood of marriage (Markowitz et al., 2014). Thus, the central pathology of social phobia seems an appropriate interpersonal target for IPT.

Because social phobia is a chronic syndrome, Lipsitz, Fyer, Markowitz, and Cherry (1999) applied the idea of an *iatrogenic role transition* to social phobia in the same way that it has been used with dysthymic patients. By exploring new interpersonal options, patients alter maladaptive social interactions, function more effectively, and feel better. As they do, they begin to recognize that the long-standing pattern they had considered a part of who they were was a treatable illness rather than an integral aspect of themselves. Treatment itself thus becomes a therapist- and patient-initiated role transition to health. Lipsitz and Markowitz (2006) substituted the more benign term "role insecurity" as an alternative to the awkward formulation of "interpersonal deficits" for highly isolated socially anxious patients. The intervention emphasizes that the patient has an illness, not a personality disorder; that is, a chronic, treatable symptom, not a (more pejorative and hopeless-sounding) deficit.

Like persistently depressed patients, those with social phobia have been chronically demoralized about their social functioning and need considerable encouragement, support, and role playing to enter new social situations. In general, however, the usual IPT approach for depression seems helpful for these patients as well.

There have now been pilot open trials of social phobia and four randomized clinical trials. Lipsitz et al., having found encouraging results in an open fourteen-week IPT trial of nine patients with social phobia (Lipsitz et al., 1999), conducted a small randomized trial comparing IPT to brief supportive psychotherapy for seventy additional patients (Lipsitz et al., 2008). As in some other trials (e.g., Markowitz et al., 2005, 2008), brief supportive psychotherapy proved an active control condition, and methodological difficulties complicated the interpretation of the results. In any event, both treatments showed clinically meaningful, statistically significant, but similar pretreatment-to-posttreatment improvement (Lipsitz et al., 2008). A secondary analysis suggested that higher therapist adherence to IPT yielded better outcomes (Sinai et al., 2012).

A Norwegian research group completed a randomized trial comparing residential group IPT and CBT as a ten-week treatment for eighty unmedicated patients with treatment-resistant social anxiety disorder. They found both treatments equally efficacious (Borge et al., 2008; Hoffart et al., 2007). The entire sample showed continuing improvement at the one-year follow-up. The findings that chronically socially avoidant, highly comorbid, treatment-resistant patients responded to a relatively brief residential treatment without concomitant medication are very encouraging and deserve replication. The question is how much improvement was specific to either group psychotherapy, and how much to the overall milieu effect of the treatment (Hoffart et al., 2009).

Stangier et al. (2011) in Germany conducted a randomized controlled trial comparing CBT, IPT, and a waiting list condition for 106 patients with social anxiety disorder. Patients in CBT or IPT received sixteen weekly sessions plus a booster session. Although IPT showed superiority to the waiting list condition ($d = 0.79$–0.95) and had lower attrition (11 percent) than CBT (18 percent), it also had a lower response rate: 42 percent versus 66 percent for CBT. We have argued that aspects of this study may have been affected by researcher allegiance favoring CBT (Markowitz et al., 2014).

Dagöö et al. (2014) in Sweden compared a previously tested mobile-phone version of CBT to "a guided self-help treatment based on" IPT delivered by computer and smartphone for nine weeks to fifty-two patients with social anxiety disorder. They found the CBT approach far more efficacious than the IPT approach. The authors warn that the mobile-IPT results deserve cautious interpretation (Dagöö et al., 2014, p. 415). (See Chapter 25 for discussion of IPT in telephone format.)

Thus, IPT, at least as a face-to-face, in-person treatment, has emerged as a potentially efficacious if underbruited treatment for social anxiety disorder. IPT had large treatment effects, ranging from $d = 0.60$ to 1.73, across these studies, and potentially could have greater impact with some tinkering to more specifically adapt it to patients with this disorder (Markowitz et al., 2014).

CASE EXAMPLE: SCARED TO TALK

Henry, a 35-year-old single businessman, presented for treatment with a lifelong history of social anxiety that emerged most dramatically in public speaking situations. Henry had grown up with a stutter that he conquered with speech "lessons and great effort. Schoolmates had made fun of his speech, and a teacher had once humiliated him in junior high school during a class presentation. To his credit, he had joined his college debate team and felt he had mastered this important area of his life.

Having joined a business firm that required presentations in front of large groups of colleagues and customers, Henry was then appalled when, in the setting of his father's illness and a romantic disappointment, he blanked, froze, and then completely fell apart with panic symptoms during an important pitch. He subsequently felt intimidated at meetings; worried about blushing, sweating, or having his voice break when talking; and generally retreated from what had been an active and successfully developing career. He felt particularly intimidated by his superior, whom he felt had always been critical of him before, and more so since this incident. This had been a problem for months.

Henry had always been "shy," always tentative about relationships outside his family of origin. He was close to his parents and his older sister but had few close friends. Dating was torture: he became so anxious in the presence of women that he could barely speak. He stammered, sweated, blushed, and retreated. He had finally begun a tentative relationship with a coworker some months before the big presentation but felt frightened by her interest and responsiveness and pulled back, then felt humiliated when she subsequently snubbed him.

Henry's IPT therapist diagnosed him as having social anxiety disorder with both generalized and specific (public speaking) features. He defined this as a chronic illness that was treatable, not Henry's fault, and related to his interpersonal discomfort in social situations. Treatment was formulated as a role dispute with his boss, although they acknowledged that his dating breakup was also a treatment issue. They agreed to a sixteen-week treatment.

Therapy focused on Henry's feelings at work and how his interpersonal behavior might communicate or miscommunicate his wishes and needs. He initially discussed talking with coworkers and having lunch with Mike, a colleague whom he liked but whom he feared disliked him. Henry was uncertain about approaching Mike but agreed with his therapist that it was okay in principle to ask him to have lunch. The therapist validated his wish to have friends, discussed the importance of having social supports, and role played his saying, "Hey, wanna grab something to eat?" They fine-tuned his words and tone of voice until he was able to do this.

Lunch was planned and went well, as Henry admitted even while relating his indigestion afterward. Further social successes with coworkers made him increasingly comfortable and less worried about blushes and stammers. With this gain in confidence, he was willing to address the still uncomfortable dispute with his boss, Rod. On careful analysis, it appeared that Henry was reacting more strongly than might have been warranted to the behavior of his superior, a domineering type who gave little quarter to anyone.

The therapist and Henry talked about whether he should take Rod's criticism personally. They again discussed what he wanted from the situation and what options he had to achieve this. Henry decided to arrange a meeting to talk over how he was doing and even—with some trepidation—the debacle of his presentation. He approached this meeting sweating, tremulous, and anxious but was able to tell Rod how important his job was to him and that he hoped he had not damaged his chances with the presentation flub. As Henry and his therapist had discussed, Rod actually saw the event as far less serious than Henry had. What felt like an eternity of silence to Henry had only seemed a long pause to him. Rod gruffly told him his future chances were "as good as anyone's."

This greatly relieved Henry. His symptoms continued to recede, but he remained nervous about making public presentations. When, near the end of treatment, the opportunity arose to give another pitch, he was quite nervous. He and his therapist discussed and role played contingencies, including what he would say if (when) he felt uneasy giving his talk. Was it okay to acknowledge some nervousness about speaking, if this arose, rather than fighting to appear perfectly calm? The therapist described anxiety symptoms as symptoms, rather than some personal defect. The talk went fairly well: Henry was nervous but got through it successfully.

After sixteen weeks his social anxiety disorder was under good control. Henry and his therapist then contracted for a year of monthly maintenance therapy, during which Henry continued to do well at work, made several successful big presentations, and began to work on dating, too.

THERAPIST NOTE

For many patients, the structure of a work role, with its built-in job description, makes it easier to address than the uncharted dangers of social life. Once patients have gained confidence in the work arena, they may feel willing to risk the social scene. Henry's case illustrates this.

PANIC DISORDER

Patients with panic disorder experience their paralyzing episodic physical attacks as coming "out of the blue," yet research suggests that panic attacks reflect a response to interpersonal events: one study found that three-quarters of panic patients had had an interpersonal loss within six weeks of panic onset (Klass et al., 2009). Individuals with panic disorder are highly sensitive to interpersonal separation (Milrod et al., 2014). Other affect-focused therapies also benefit panic patients (Milrod et al., 2016). Thus, IPT seems an intuitively reasonable intervention that takes a very different approach from somatically focused forms of CBT for these patients.

Lipsitz, Gur, Miller, Vermes, and Fyer (2006) conducted a small pilot open trial of fourteen weeks of IPT for twelve patients with panic disorder, finding marked improvement in most of the patients. This trial applied the standard IPT approach for depression to panic disorder. They focused on pervasive, more prolonged interpersonal problems associated with onset and maintenance of panic disorder. Most of the patients fit formulations for either role transition or role dispute. Vos et al. (2012) in the Netherlands compared twelve weekly sessions of IPT versus CBT in a randomized trial for ninety-one patients with panic disorder. From a protracted (nine-year) trial with possible allegiance problems (Falkenström et al., 2013) and idiosyncratic outcome measures (Markowitz et al., 2014), the authors report overall improvements, but better outcome in CBT than IPT; however, IPT had a lower attrition rate (21 percent) than CBT (31 percent) (Vos et al., 2012).

The level of evidence varies by disorder; in general, research is in an early stage. But we can still assign it a rating of *** (three stars; encouraging findings in one or more open trials or in pilot studies with small samples).

OTHER APPLICATIONS

Chung (2015) has reported a case of postnatal anxiety disorder successfully treated with IPT. This seems a natural extension of IPT as a perinatal treatment for depression (Chapter 13). Other anxiety disorders may also merit testing with adaptations of IPT. There has to date been no research on IPT as a treatment for generalized anxiety disorder.

CONCLUSION

The findings for IPT in anxiety disorders are encouraging but preliminary and need confirmation in controlled trials. The general IPT approach for mood disorders seems grossly translatable to these anxiety disorders with little adaptation of the IPT approach, yet further adaptation might add to its potency (Markowitz et al., 2014). It is noteworthy that social phobia and panic disorder contain strong interpersonal elements. IPT might be expected to be harder to apply to, and less effective for, a more internalized disorder such as obsessive-compulsive disorder. No trials have tested IPT for other anxiety disorders.

22

Trauma- and Stress-Related Disorders

Posttraumatic stress disorder (PTSD) has become a high-profile disorder since its formal definition in the DSM-III in 1980, a recognition of its widespread prevalence in U.S. Vietnam veterans. The explosion of traumas around the world in recent years has only increased its prominence and the need for effective treatments. PTSD is the only major psychiatric disorder defined by a life event. As IPT has always used a stress-diathesis model (Klerman et al., 1984), it seemed an appropriate target among the DSM-IV anxiety disorders for IPT treatment. One of the changes in the DSM-5 was to remove PTSD from the anxiety disorders section and place it in a new category entitled "trauma- and stressor-related disorders," which also includes adjustment disorders. We follow that classification here.

POSTTRAUMATIC STRESS DISORDER

Psychotherapies for PTSD have almost invariably focused on exposing patients to memories (imaginal) or concrete reminders (in vivo) of past traumas—the things they most fear. Some patients refuse or cannot tolerate this approach. As is the case for major depression, it may be helpful to have several effective psychotherapeutic approaches to PTSD. Accordingly, Bleiberg and Markowitz (2005) tested IPT as a treatment for patients with chronic PTSD that is not based on their exposure. Treatment focused not on the traumatic event but on its devastating interpersonal consequences. IPT focused not on patients' confronting and reconstructing trauma but on how they handled their daily social interactions—recognizing their feelings about, expressing their feelings to, and setting limits with other people. Therapists helped numbed patients to recognize that their feelings were not "bad" or dangerous but rather crucial interpersonal indicators of their day-to-day situations, noting that trauma had led the patients to mistrust and retreat from their social environment (Markowitz, 2016; Markowitz et al., 2009). Although therapists did not ask patients to expose themselves to traumatic reminders, as the patients improved, they frequently did so spontaneously. IPT is also appropriate for treating the comorbid depression many patients with PTSD describe.

Following this pilot study, Markowitz et al. (2015b) conducted a randomized controlled trial comparing a fourteen-week trial of IPT (as a non-exposure therapy) to Prolonged Exposure and Relaxation Therapy. All three treatments lowered PTSD symptoms, and IPT was non-inferior to Prolonged Exposure, the best-tested exposure therapy, on the Clinician-Administered PTSD Scale (CAPS). Moreover, patients preferred IPT (Markowitz et al., 2015b, 2016). Patients who had comorbid major depression were less likely to drop out of IPT than exposure therapy (Markowitz et al., 2015b), and patients with sexual trauma had a better outcome in IPT than the other two treatments (Markowitz et al., 2017). Personality disorder diagnoses resolved in many patients, across treatments, after fourteen weeks of PTSD-targeted therapy (Markowitz et al., 2015a). Moreover, patients who responded to IPT after fourteen weeks (>30 percent improvement in baseline CAPS score) remained improved at the three-month no-treatment follow-up. This study treated civilians, not military personnel, with PTSD and needs replication, but the findings suggest that a therapy focused on feelings and relationships rather than on exposure and fear avoidance may also benefit patients with PTSD.

Krupnick et al. (2016) have begun to test individual IPT for PTSD as a treatment for a veteran population. Ten of fifteen women veterans completed a twelve-week course of individual IPT, showing significant symptomatic improvement at posttreatment and at the three-month follow-up.

The level of evidence for IPT for PTSD is *** (three stars; treatment has been validated by at least one randomized, controlled trial demonstrating the efficacy of IPT compared to a control condition).

Adaptations

Individuals with PTSD withdraw socially because trauma has made their world feel dangerous and people untrustworthy. They become hypervigilant not only for trauma reminders in their environment, but of people generally. Internally, their emotions feel out of control, so they numb themselves. Yet feeling numb—ignoring one's own feelings—makes it hard to judge who is friend and who is foe.

The focus of IPT for PTSD is on helping patients to tolerate the strong affects, particularly the negative emotions that they desperately avoid, to relieve the numbness. The approach emphasizes what has always been central to IPT: interpersonal situations evoke emotions, and those emotions provide useful information about the encounters. IPT therapists work hard to normalize such emotions and help patients to verbalize them. The therapist says:

Feelings are powerful, but not dangerous—and in fact, you need them to decide whom you can trust. Expressing your feelings to another person may seem risky, but it provides a test of whether the other person is trustworthy or not. If

you feel angry and voice it to another person, the other person has the chance
either to apologize and change behavior, or to confirm that he or she is uncar-
ing or untrustworthy.

Thus, as much as the first half of the fourteen-session treatment focuses on affective attunement in daily life circumstances: for example, asking patients, "*How did*
you feel when [you were talking to your mother]?" Having regained better touch
with their emotions, patients can proceed to more usual IPT maneuvers, such as
solving a role transition. As patients gain comfort with their feelings, they handle interpersonal situations better, life feels safer, and they begin spontaneously—
without IPT therapist encouragement—to face the situations and traumatic
reminders they have been avoiding.

Individuals with PTSD do not want to think about their traumas, and in IPT
they need not do so. After establishing that the patient has endured a trauma and
meets criteria for PTSD, the therapist clarifies that the treatment will focus not
on that trauma but on its interpersonal sequelae. The trauma explains why the
patient is struggling interpersonally, but receives no further direct discussion.

An advantage of treating PTSD using IPT is that every patient has suffered a life
event: by definition, PTSD encompasses a role transition. Hence there is no need
to invoke the interpersonal deficits category. A more detailed description of this
approach is available in an IPT PTSD manual (Markowitz, 2016).

CASE EXAMPLE: MUGGED IN THE SUBWAY

Andrew, a 37-year-old industrial worker, had been robbed at knifepoint by a teen-
ager in his neighborhood subway station two years before. He was horrified that he
had nearly died for a few dollars and had repeated flashbacks and nightmares about
the event. He began to avoid subways and buses and instead walked a long distance
to and from work. He retreated from friends, coworkers, and his wife of twelve years,
feeling he could not trust anything and that his world was shattered. He also felt
ashamed of having been robbed by a "kid" and hid this humiliating story from oth-
ers. His symptoms included insomnia, anxious and depressed mood, a pronounced
startle reaction, and a sense that his life was over. On presentation to treatment, he
met DSM-5 criteria for both PTSD and major depressive disorder (MDD).

The IPT therapist sympathized with what Andrew had been through, gave him
the diagnoses of PTSD and MDD, as well as the sick role, and defined the event
as a role transition. In recounting what had been lost, Andrew focused on his for-
merly close relationship with his wife. He now hid out from her in the bedroom.
He also restricted her activities outside the house as he feared that she, too, would
be attacked. Their sexual relationship had ended with the mugging, and he no
longer felt he could be close to or confide in her. Similarly, he had retreated from
his coworkers.

Therapist and patient agreed that the aftershock of the mugging on Andrew's
social functioning was "adding insult to injury." The therapist noted Andrew's former

interpersonal strengths and the loss of social supports following his attack. They discussed how he could "reclaim his life" and particularly his marriage. After discussion and role playing, he went home and had the most open discussion with his wife Cathy in years. He apologized to her for ruining their marriage and their lives. To his surprise, she was sympathetic, did not regard him as a weakling, and asked how they could make things better. He returned the next week to treatment feeling considerably better.

The couple's relationship continued to improve, and their sex life resumed. Emboldened, he began to risk fraternizing more with his coworkers. By the ninth of fourteen sessions, both his PTSD and MDD had remitted. In the termination phase, Andrew confided that he had resumed taking public transportation, including the subway, although this was not an issue on which therapy had focused. He remained asymptomatic at a six-month follow-up.

THERAPIST NOTE

Note that treatment did not focus on exposure or on symptoms such as flashbacks, but rather on interpersonal interactions and the rebuilding of social supports. By focusing on this one area, IPT seems to produce benefits that generalize to yield overall improvement and are not limited to the interpersonal area.

CASE EXAMPLE: DEFEATED SOLDIER

Captain Jana, a married 38-year-old military veteran, presented with PTSD related to military sexual trauma: she had been raped by her superior officer three years before. Symptoms included flashbacks of the event, nightmares, and insomnia; emotional numbness; and depressed and anxious mood; her CAPS score was 70, indicating severe PTSD. She reported a history of previous sexual trauma, including molestation by her father in childhood. Although she had entered the military to make herself stronger, she found herself beaten down both by the services hierarchy and in her social relationships, where she invariably deferred to the wishes of others. Captain Jana was married to a hard-drinking military officer who ordered her around and at times physically abused her. She acknowledged difficulty saying "no" to others, which meant that she generally went along with things she did not like. A previous course of exposure therapy and a serotonin reuptake medication trial had each been unavailing.

Her IPT therapist diagnosed PTSD, sympathizing that betrayal by one's colleagues is a horrible act and that it could only have confirmed her mistrust of others. He noted her history of such betrayals. Although the military rape constituted a role transition, the therapist suggested that they focus on the role dispute in her marriage. Jana agreed. They spent the first five or six of the fourteen treatment sessions focusing on her feelings. When asked how she felt during communication analysis about an interaction with her husband, or a friend or family member, Jana would answer: "I don't know. I didn't feel anything." The therapist let her sit with the benumbed feel-ings, from which would emerge: "I guess I felt a little upset when he said that."

> Therapist: What kind of upset?
> J: I don't know. . . . A little bothered. . . . Annoyed.
> Therapist: So that made you angry when he insulted you?
> J: I don't know. Anger is a strong word. I don't like to get angry.

Over time, Jana came to acknowledge a range of feelings, including negative emo-tions like anger, hurt, and sadness. The therapist normalized these emotions as useful signposts of what was happening in her relationships. They role played her expression of anger and how to fight—getting angry didn't have to mean drunken rages like her father's and husband's. By mid-treatment her CAPS score had fallen to 40, considerably improved although still symptomatic. After role play, she confronted her husband about his drinking and was increasingly successful in setting limits with him. She was initially very anxious about such encounters, but increasingly confi-dent as she discovered she had at least some control over her environment. She also spontaneously decided to file charges against the officer who had attacked her. By the end of treatment her CAPS score was 22, essentially remitted.

Group Format

Krupnick et al. (2008) at Georgetown conducted a randomized controlled trial comparing group IPT to a waiting list for forty-eight low-income women with chronic PTSD recruited from public primary care and gynecology clinics. Group IPT involved sixteen two-hour sessions with two therapists and three to five patients per group. Results were quite positive, despite limited IPT training among the IPT therapists, little specific adjustment of the IPT approach, and the fact that the study patients had not been seeking psychiatric treatment. Campanini et al. (2010) added this group approach to pharmacotherapy for forty patients (six to eight per group) who had not responded to a twelve-week adequate trial of phar-macotherapy for chronic PTSD. Patients' CAPS scores fell from 72.3 (SE = 4.4) to 36.5 (5.4) (Campanini et al., 2010).

The level of evidence for group IPT is *** (three stars; treatment has been vali-dated by at least one randomized, controlled trial demonstrating the efficacy of IPT compared to a control condition).

ADJUSTMENT DISORDERS

Adjustment disorders are symptomatic responses to recent stressors that do not meet threshold criteria for a disorder such as major depression. In general, milder symptomatology responds to IPT at least as well as more severe presentations (Elkin et al., 1995). Thus, the same IPT model that works for major depression is very likely to benefit an adjustment disorder with depressed mood. Both IPT and interpersonal counseling (IPC), a trimmed, more scripted version of IPT intended for use by non-mental health professionals (Chapter 16), can benefit patients with adjustment disorders. In the same way that the demonstration that IPT treats major depression suggests its applicability to milder, subthreshold adjustment disorders with depressed mood, the emerging benefits of IPT for PTSD suggest its utility for adjustment disorders with anxious mood.

CONCLUSION

The limited research on IPT for PTSD has had exciting outcomes: it's good to have alternatives to exposure therapy, which is effective but unwelcomed by many patients and some therapists. Use of IPT in this area is still new, however, and more research is needed to understand its efficacy in veterans and other traumatized populations.

Borderline Personality Disorder

DIAGNOSIS

IPT has generally targeted what DSM-IV called Axis I and explicitly *not* Axis II disorders: that is, psychiatric illnesses, like major depression, rather than personality disorders. Its brief time frame and its attention to relatively acute symptoms lend itself to this Axis I focus.[1] Yet extension of the acute IPT model to chronic Axis I syndromes such as persistent depressive disorder/dysthymia (Chapter 17), bipolar disorder (Chapter 18), and social anxiety disorder (Chapter 21) suggests that IPT might benefit more chronically ill psychiatric patients. Indeed, social anxiety disorder overlaps significantly with avoidant personality disorder. Can IPT treat personality disorders?

Borderline personality disorder (BPD) is a prevalent, debilitating syndrome. Patients with BPD are heavy users of mental health services and have historically had a poor prognosis. This disorder is closely associated with mood disorders; indeed, mood instability is a key dimension of the BPD syndrome. Other features of BPD are identity diffusion, cognitive distortions, and, of interest to IPT therapists, interpersonal impairment. BPD is associated with high rates of suicidal ideation, parasuicidal gestures, and completed suicide.

In recent years, research has determined that treatments as diverse as dialectical behavioral therapy (DBT; Linehan, Armstrong, Suárez, Allmon, & Heard, 1991) and psychodynamic approaches (Bateman & Fonagy, 2001, 2009; McMain et al., 2012) are effective in patients with BPD (Cristea et al., 2017). Further, careful longitudinal studies have demonstrated that this diagnosis, which was once considered nearly hopeless, may remit over time with, or perhaps even without, treatment (Gunderson et al., 2011; Shea et al., 2002; Zanarini et al., 2014). What may be crucial is to avoid causing iatrogenic damage with unhelpful treatment (Fonagy & Bateman, 2006).

---

1. DSM-5 (2013) dispensed with the previous multiaxial system that separated disorders like major depression from personality disorders. Nonetheless, the distinction of Axis I ("state") disorders from Axis II ("trait") disorders has some conceptual utility.

Although IPT has not been nearly as well studied as a treatment for personality disorders as some of the approaches mentioned above, some research on its application to BPD has appeared. In a small, unpublished trial partly confounded by medication use, Angus and Gillies (1994) felt that twelve weekly sessions of IPT held promise as a treatment for patients with BPD. Markowitz, Skodol, and Bleiberg (2006) at Columbia University conducted a small open trial of an eight-month adaptation of IPT for patients with BPD who were in interpersonal crisis. Their impression was that BPD overlaps meaningfully with mood disorder and produces a host of interpersonal difficulties, and that IPT benefitted most of the patients in their small (N = 11) sample (Markowitz et al., 2007).

Ten women and one man with DSM-IV BPD who reported an interpersonal crisis entered the trial. (Thus the trial did not recruit patients who met the borderline diagnosis but presented with "interpersonal deficits," no current life events.) Schizotypal and schizoid personality disorders were also exclusion criteria. One patient was married, two were divorced, and eight had never married. Three worked full-time, two worked part-time, and six were unemployed. Six were white, three Hispanic, and two African American. All had active comorbid Structured Clinical Interview for DSM-IV (SCID) diagnoses: 100 percent current or lifetime mood disorders, 82 percent histories of substance abuse/dependence, and 64 percent histories of eating disorders. Overlapping personality disorders were avoidant (n = 4), paranoid (n = 4), obsessive-compulsive (n = 2), passive-aggressive, and narcissistic (Markowitz, 2012).

Three patients dropped out during the eighteen-session, four-month acute phase; a fourth, with comorbid anorexia nervosa, chronic depression, and substance abuse in reported remission, was removed for worsening symptoms and substance use. The remaining seven subjects entered the second sixteen-week phase, which all but one completed. Six of the seven no longer met DSM-IV criteria for BPD. The patients' scores dropped from 18.3 to 8.8 on the Hamilton Rating Scale for Depression and from 17.8 to 12.8 on the Beck Depression Inventory. Symptom Checklist (SCL-90) scores fell from 219 to 188. These encouraging findings hint at the feasibility of this shortest of psychotherapies for BPD, but they clearly need replication and further development (Markowitz, 2012).

Bellino et al. (2006) in Turin, Italy, randomly assigned thirty-nine patients with DSM-IV BPD and comorbid major depressive disorder (MDD) to twenty-four weeks of either fluoxetine 20 to 40 mg daily alone, or fluoxetine 20 to 40 mg daily plus weekly IPT. Although the two groups did not differ on all measures, the combined IPT/fluoxetine group had better depression outcomes on the Ham-D, higher patient satisfaction, and improvement on some Inventory of Interpersonal Problems scales. This study again provides encouragement but does not demonstrate the specific benefit of IPT relative to another psychotherapy in patients with BPD, and the researchers did not re-evaluate the BPD diagnosis at the end of the trial.

Taking the next step, Bellino et al. (2007) compared IPT to CBT, each combined with fluoxetine, in a twenty-four-week randomized trial of thirty-five patients with comorbid MDD and BPD. Both groups had high rates of depressive remission among treatment completers. Unsurprisingly given the small sample size, no between-group differences appeared on the major measures. The authors again did not re-evaluate BPD status after twenty-four weeks.

In a subsequent study, this same group returned to testing fluoxetine alone versus fluoxetine combined with IPT in a trial of fifty-five patients with MDD and BPD, this time using the thirty-two-week Columbia adaptation of IPT for BPD (Bellino et al., 2010). Eleven patients (20%) dropped out due to noncompliance. Among treatment completers, depressive symptoms again improved in both groups, without significant between-group difference in remission rates. The combined treatment showed advantages on some secondary measures, such as the Hamilton Anxiety Rating Scale. Gains were generally maintained at the two-year follow-up (Bozzatello & Bellino, 2016). Unfortunately, this comparison still lacked the power to show treatment differences and could not determine the specificity of IPT relative to other psychotherapies.

This is the state of research on IPT as a treatment for BPD: tantalizing but fragmentary, in need of a larger and more definitive trial. Bateman (2012), a clinical researcher who is an expert in IPT but more associated with mentalization (Bateman & Fonagy, 2006) as a treatment, has been encouraging about the prospects of IPT for BPD.

The level of evidence for IPT for BPD is ** (two stars; there are encouraging findings in one or more open trials or in pilot studies with small samples [less than 12 subjects]).

ADAPTATION

The Columbia adaptation involves changes in standard IPT relating to (1) the conceptualization and (2) chronicity of the disorder, (3) difficulties in forming and maintaining the treatment alliance, (4) length of treatment, (5) suicide risk, (6) termination, and (7) choice of subjects within the BPD spectrum of diagnosis (Markowitz, 2005; Markowitz, Skodol, & Bleiberg, 2006). The value of these adaptations and of IPT as a treatment for BPD will depend on the outcome of such studies.

The therapist presents BPD to the patient as a poorly named syndrome that has a significant depressive component. A major difference between MDD and BPD is that while depressed patients often have difficulty expressing any anger, patients with BPD often do the same much of the time but then periodically explode with excessive anger, which reinforces their tendency to avoid expressing anger whenever possible. The goals of treatment are, as is usually the case in IPT, to link mood (including anger) to interpersonal situations, to find better ways of handling such situations, and to build better social supports and skills. Psychoeducation about BPD includes clarification of the current versus the historical meanings of the diagnosis.

The chronicity of the BPD diagnosis links it to IPT approaches for both dysthymic disorder and social phobia, in which longstanding behavioral patterns become associated with one's sense of self. By defining such patterns as part of the illness rather than part of the person, the therapist can help to make them ego alien and help the patient to change.

The treatment alliance is more fragile and complex in working with patients with BPD than in those with MDD. Whereas IPT typically avoids a direct focus on therapist–patient interactions, this becomes unavoidable when problems arise in the alliance. When such problems crop up, the therapist addresses them in a here-and-now, interpersonal fashion rather than making psychodynamic interpretations (see the case example below).

Treatment has been conceptualized as having two phases: first, eighteen sessions in sixteen weeks, with a focus on building a strong treatment alliance, providing a formulation, and introducing IPT concepts. Assuming this initial phase goes well, the second phase comprises sixteen additional sessions in as many weeks, or a total of eight months of more or less weekly psychotherapy. In addition, therapists may check in with patients for once-a-week, ten-minute telephone checks.

Self-destructive behavior and suicide risk are concerns for BPD as for MDD. Close monitoring of suicidality is warranted with such patients. Suicidal behavior has not been a frequent problem in the trial thus far.

Because patients with BPD are extremely sensitive to abandonment, termination is discussed early and often in the treatment. Using this approach, termination has been sad but successful for these patients, who have generally found treatment helpful.

CASE EXAMPLE: BEYOND THE RAGE

Bob, a 38-year-old unemployed man, presented with BPD and paranoid personality disorder. He described a long history of alcohol dependence but was now sober. His principal affect was rage, and he had run through seven sponsors in Alcoholics Anonymous. Despite the therapist's attempts to focus on his daily life outside the therapy office, Bob's hypersensitivity to his interaction with the therapist led to frequent disruptions. He noticed and objected if the tape recorder had been moved a few inches from one session to the next. He objected to the therapist's jewelry and stylish clothing. Once angered, he would storm out of the office, slamming the door and announcing he would not return. Yet return he did—to repeat the scenario.

The therapist, despite doubts about whether treatment could proceed, persevered. She noted that anger was the problem that had brought Bob to treatment and that it was a key symptom of BPD. It was just what they needed to work on. She apologized for upsetting Bob and explored his options for expressing his feelings about relationships. Note that the therapeutic alliance was addressed in interpersonal terms in the here and now, not with psychodynamic interpretations. As soon as things were mended in the office, the therapist tried to focus on anger difficulties in outside relationships: at AA, in his neighborhood, and in potential job leads.

Although the angry pattern continued, it changed over time. With the therapist's tolerance and support, Bob began to stay longer in sessions where he felt enraged, at first fuming silently. Later in treatment, he was able not only to remain in the room but also to voice his feelings. The treatment focus then shifted back to outside relationships. He began to discuss his related fears of abandonment and of dropping his guard lest others reject him.

Once the therapeutic alliance had been stabilized, the focus on outside relationships began in earnest. Bob continued to have difficulties with his AA sponsor. He was devoted to him but also felt as though his sponsor had frequently betrayed him. The therapist was able to validate some of his anger and help Bob choose more muted expressions of it in role playing. Encounters with the sponsor were successful, and that relationship was maintained whereas previous sponsorships had failed.

By the end of the eight-month therapy, Bob was more active in AA, was friendlier with people there and in his neighborhood, and seemed on the verge of getting a job after two years of unemployment. He no longer met criteria for BPD and was far less depressed. He was even able to haltingly tell his therapist he had learned a lot in treatment and would miss her. [This case example has been adapted, with the publisher's permission, from Markowitz, Skodol, & Bleiberg, 2006.]

CONCLUSION

There has been no IPT research on the treatment of personality disorders other than BPD, although some research suggests that apparent personality disorders associated with MDD (Cyranowski et al., 2004) and posttraumatic stress disorder (Markowitz et al., 2015a) may regress with IPT treatment of the "Axis I" disorder.

Special Topics, Training, and Resources

24

IPT Across Cultures and in Resource-Poor Countries

OVERVIEW

Although psychiatric disorders exist worldwide, the cultures within which they arise differ considerably. IPT has been successfully disseminated to a variety of cultures within and outside the United States. IPT has been used in Australia, Austria, Brazil, Canada, China, Congo, the Czech Republic, Denmark, Ethiopia, Finland, France, Germany, Greece, Haiti, Hungary, Iceland, India, Ireland, Israel, Italy, Japan, Jordan, Lebanon, the Netherlands, New Zealand, Norway, Portugal, Romania, Spain, Sweden, Switzerland, Thailand, Turkey, Uganda, and the United Kingdom, and the number of cultures continues to grow. Versions of the IPT manual have been translated into numerous languages (see Chapter 26).

In the United States, IPT has been used successfully in clinical trials with cultural adjustments in patients with African American and Hispanic backgrounds (e.g., Frank et al., 2014; Markowitz et al., 2009). In developing countries, the largest clinical trials have been carried out in Uganda (Bass et al., 2006; Bolton et al., 2003, 2007; Verdeli et al., 2003). Much of the use of IPT in developing countries has been its adaptation, implementation, and small clinical trials for humanitarian crises following civil war, refugee crisis, or natural disaster. Little systematic work has examined differences in how IPT is practiced in treating patients from these varied cultural environments. Adaptations have focused on treating major depressive disorder (MDD) or subsyndromal depression, and more recently on posttraumatic stress disorder (PTSD).

This chapter begins by describing the International Society of Interpersonal Psychotherapy and the activities of the World Health Organization (WHO) in disseminating IPT around the world. The chapter focuses on experiences in low- and middle-income countries. The outcomes of clinical trials in high-income countries do not vary by ethnic and racial makeup and are included in the reviews of specific diagnostic adaptations.

INTERNATIONAL SOCIETY OF INTERPERSONAL PSYCHOTHERAPY (ISIPT)

The ISIPT, a multidisciplinary, nonprofit, noncommercial international organization, is committed to the advancement of IPT through research, training, and dissemination. The ISIPT is an important factor in the growth and dissemination of IPT worldwide. The ISIPT includes members from over thirty countries; holds a biennial international meeting; and has a multinational board, a very active listserv (isipt-list@googlegroups.com), a website (https://www.interpersonalpsychotherapy.org/), and Facebook page (https://www.facebook.com/InterpersonalPsychotherapy) that distribute information about IPT training, education, and research. The ISIPT distributes information and maintains connections among IPT clinicians, researchers, and local IPT organizations around the world. The organization holds a biennial international research and clinical meeting.

WORLD HEALTH ORGANIZATION (WHO)

The WHO has helped to increase interest in IPT. In response to requests for guidance on psychological interventions, the WHO developed its mental health Gap Action Programme Intervention Guide (mhGAP-IG; WHO, 2016). The mhGAP seeks to spread care for various mental, neurological, and substance use conditions more widely. An mhGAP priority condition was moderate to severe depressive disorder. The mhGAP-IG recommended psychological interventions for this disorder but did not describe in sufficient detail what these are or how to implement them. However, in 2015 an independent WHO Guidelines Development Committee agreed on the following recommendations for the management of moderate to severe depressive disorder:

1. As first-line therapy, health-care providers may select psychological treatments such as behavioral activation, CBT, and IPT, or antidepressant medication such as selective serotonin reuptake inhibitors and tricyclic antidepressants.
2. The possible adverse effects associated with antidepressant medication, the ability to deliver interventions (clinician expertise and/or treatment availability), and individual preferences need consideration in treatment selection.
3. Different psychotherapy formats considered include individual and group face-to-face psychological treatments, delivered by professionals or supervised lay therapists (WHO, 2015).
4. WHO (2015) recommends evidence-based psychological interventions such as IPT and CBT as the first-line treatment for pregnant and breastfeeding women with moderate to severe depressive disorder, and for adults with mild depressive disorder. The guidelines noted that

antidepressant medication should be avoided where possible for these two groups. This makes the accessibility of IPT or CBT essential around the world.

As part of this effort, following the outcome of the Ugandan IPT clinical trials (e.g., Bolton et al., 2003, 2007), WHO sponsored the development and dissemination of a group IPT manual for depression. WHO launched this work in Geneva in October 2016. The manual is available online at no cost (http://www.who.int/mental_health/mhgap/interpersonal_therapy/en/).

WHO further sponsored the development of an individual IPT manual for refugees in Lebanon. A simplified interpersonal counseling (IPC) manual for primary care patients in Muslim countries is under development by Weissman and Verdeli in consultation with Khalid Saeed from Egypt.

PRINCIPLES OF CULTURAL ADAPTATION

The principles of adapting IPT to cultural issues are straightforward, although their implementation may pose challenges for both the clinician and patient (Lewis-Fernandez, 2015). In the spirit of IPT's focus on the effects of environment, IPT clinicians must proceed carefully in approaching cultures to which they do not belong. We outline some essential elements here:

1. Include at least one person familiar with the culture as a member of the team assisting in any adaptation.
2. Understand how the symptoms of the targeted disorder present clinically and are interpreted in the culture.
3. Determine what interventions will be acceptable in the patient's culture. Those deemed appropriate in mainstream American culture may seem insensitive or disrespectful in other cultures.
4. Differentiate between the problem areas (grief, disputes, etc.) of IPT, which may be universal triggers for depression, and the specific techniques used to achieve change or resolution, which may be culturally bound.

    The cultural context of the problem areas also requires understanding. For example, marital disputes may arise in the context of marital infidelity, which has a different meaning in a culture where marriage is uncommon or where having more than one wife is the norm. The range of acceptable responses to this situation may similarly differ across cultures. Yet the emotional issues in a marital dispute of betrayal, fear of abandonment, and concern about economic security for oneself and one's children may be the same across these cultural contexts. Developing a depressive episode in the context of role disputes, as well as the nature of the disputes, whether at an impasse, in negotiation, or in dissolution, also may not differ by culture. The therapist must recognize and respect culturally appropriate options for resolving disputes (i.e., strategies used for achieving resolution): directly verbally expressing opinions in parts of the United States; cooking a bad meal to signal displeasure in Uganda; or gaining the support of relatives in some Latino cultures.

5. When dealing with issues of family engagement and privacy, recognize that the desire for and expectations of privacy may vary considerably by culture. In some countries, family members essentially always accompany the patient to the treatment; hence you must make accommodation to include the family. Although as the therapist you should consult the patient about having family members present, in some cases it is a given; consider the patient's family member as part of a system in which each influences the other member's behavior. These concepts are familiar to any IPT therapist but will be shaded by cultural context and may have greater importance in cultures where family treatments are the norm.

Beyond custom or curiosity, family members who have legitimate reasons for attending the treatment deserve understanding and respect. Reasons might include concern about patient safety, protection of patient and family, concern that the therapist is competent and treatment is helpful from their perspective, interest in clarification about the situation and advice about how to help, to provide information, and concern about blame. Therapists can identify these reasons during the assessment phase or treatment with simple questions such as "*What help would you like for ___?*" and "*What are your concerns about the treatment? The patient? The family?*"

The relative ease in using IPT in diverse cultures probably reflects that the focal IPT problem areas—death of a loved one, disagreements with important persons in one's life, life changes that disrupt close attachments, loneliness and isolation—are intrinsic, universal elements of the human condition, transcending culture. The experience of using IPT in diverse cultures suggests the conservation of these triggers of depression and disruptions of human attachment across cultures (Miller, 2006).

THE UGANDAN EXPERIENCE

We present our experience in modifying and testing IPT in Uganda as this experience may be relevant to much cross-cultural treatment.

Epidemiological studies conducted in the past quarter-century have found that the prevalence of depression in Uganda is about 21 percent (Bolton et al., 2003). Local people considered depression a consequence of the HIV epidemic in Uganda, which has one of the highest rates of HIV infection in the world. Interviewed in a 2000 survey, many traditional healers in these communities felt unable to treat depression using traditional methods. The dearth and cost of physicians and medication preempted the use of antidepressant medications, especially in rural areas. Psychotherapy was deemed a viable treatment option so long as there was evidence of its effectiveness. However, psychotherapy could not require highly trained mental health providers, due to their scarcity, and required a group format to conform to the cultural norm, increase access, and reduce cost.

The project team selected IPT because of its evidence base; because it could be administered in a group format; and because Bolton, the clinician directing the work, was familiar with Uganda and felt IPT was compatible with a culture in which people consider themselves part of a family and a community before they see themselves as individuals, and where interpersonal relations are extremely important.

The Ugandan adaptation of IPT retained its basic structure but simplified the language and included detailed scripts for use by non-clinicians (Clougherty, Verdeli, & Weissman, 2003; Verdeli et al., 2002, 2003). The simplification resembles IPC (Chapter 16), but in group, not individual, format. Grief was called the "death of a loved one." Role disputes were termed "disagreements," and transitions became "life changes." The interpersonal deficits category was dropped during the training, as the local workers felt it culturally irrelevant. Because all Ugandan life takes place in groups, people are never alone. This situation might not apply in other communities. Modifications to improve cultural relevance were made on site, based on information from the trainee group leaders, college-educated non-mental health workers who had grown up and lived in the participating districts. Two IPT experts from the United States conducted training in English, assisted by two mental health professionals who had lived and worked in the area and spoke the language.

Efficacy of the Ugandan Trials

There have been two large clinical trials of group IPT in Uganda. The first randomized thirty villages in rural Uganda and randomly assigned 248 depressed adults, males and females in separate groups, to sixteen weeks of either group IPT or treatment as usual. Results showed a highly significant reduction of depressive symptoms and improvement in functioning in IPT versus controls. After sixteen weeks. 6.5 percent of the IPT group and 54.7 percent of the controls met criteria for MDD (Bolton et al., 2003). The differences were maintained six months later (Bass et al., 2006).

A second controlled clinical trial for depression treated 314 depressed adolescent survivors of war and displacement in northern Uganda (Bolton et al., 2007). This time the interventions were group IPT, creative play treatment, or waitlist control. Groups were again divided by sex. In the girls receiving IPT treatment, depressive symptoms improved significantly more than in the waitlist arm, and IPT treatment was significantly better than creative play. Improvement among boys was not significant. Depression was not significantly improved in the creative play and waitlist groups. No treatment improved conduct problems or anxiety for boys.

Implementation of IPT in Uganda

In 2013, Strong Minds, led by Sean Mayberry, undertook a mission to improve the mental health of African women, focusing on depression. Strong Minds is the only organization focused on depression in the developing world. The stated goal is to treat two million depressed African women by 2025, restoring these mentally ill individuals and their families to healthy, productive, and satisfying lives. They planned to expand services and treat additional mental illnesses throughout Africa. By 2014 they had treated 514 women in forty-six groups for twelve weeks in a pilot study, working with trainers from the original Ugandan clinical trials and externally auditing participant depression scores over time. They are now testing a model of peer support groups based on IPT principles and using graduates of the IPT groups. By June 2016, 4,100 women had completed IPT and a program had been started for 2,000 depressed adolescents. They report that 82 percent of the first cohort of women remains free from depression (https://strongminds.org/). They are developing partnerships with relief agencies, presented results at the WHO World Bank meeting in April 2016, and are undertaking a study to measure the social and economic impact of the treatment. Strong Minds plans to eventually include men in the project.

Basic Group Structure

Each group comprised eight to ten participants with MDD. Men and women attended separate groups as it was felt that patients would not talk freely in coed groups. A trained group leader conducted two individual and sixteen weekly group sessions of ninety minutes each. There were four treatment phases:

1. Two pre-group individual sessions, in which the leader learned the participant's symptoms, made diagnoses, explained depression as a medical illness, and began to formulate the individual's interpersonal problem focus associated with symptom onset. Using the standard first phase of IPT (Chapter 4), leaders elicited information about triggers of the depressive episode and determined one or two problem areas to work on. The leader individually explained how the group would work:

   Everyone in the group will be asked to talk about the problems that brought out their depression, listen to the problems of others, and find new ways of understanding and handling these problems in order to feel less depressed.

   The leader then detailed the frequency and length of meetings and confirmed that the person wanted to join the group.

2. Beginning group (four sessions): The group members learned each other's symptoms and problems. The leader explained how the group would work: that the group was a place to learn and practice skills that would help participants manage interpersonal problems that had led to their depression. During the sessions, group members were encouraged to talk about their depressive symptoms and the social situations that worsened the depression or brought it about; to listen to and help each other; to suggest ways of handling problems; and to practice new ways of coping.

3. Working (ten sessions): In the middle phase, members discussed their problems and feelings and tried to make changes in their lives.

4. Ending (two sessions): These group sessions summarized changes in symptoms and problems, and discussed why participants had improved and possible new problems that might bring about depression. Time was allotted to express feelings about ending the group and to explore how the participants could continue to help one another.

The process did not differ from group IPT conducted in the United States (see Chapter 25). We considered the treatment IPC rather than IPT, as group therapists were not mental health workers and had written scripts for guidance. The leader was nonjudgmental and discussed confidentiality with group members. Because of the country's prior experience with nongovernmental organizations (NGOs), it was important in the initial phase to clarify that the group leader did not provide participants with material goods.

The Ugandan trainees were familiar with the state of depression but used different words to describe it (Verdeli et al., 2003). These terms were compatible with common depressive signs and symptoms such as sadness, poor sleep and appetite, self-neglect, suicidality, jitteriness, low energy, and feelings of worthlessness. Regarding confidentiality, group members were asked not to disclose the content of the group meetings outside the group. However, such secrecy risked being misconstrued as conspiracy, perhaps suggesting that the village was starting a new political movement or encouraging women to use birth control. The leader therefore encouraged group members to generally describe the group's purpose to the community and to relatives but to avoid discussing specific content. Meetings were held in community centers, churches, and open spaces as available. Scheduling was flexible, to accommodate community events such as funerals or weddings in which the whole village participated. Interruptions (e.g., relatives of group members wanting to talk to someone, breastfeeding children crying for their mothers) were expected.

The IPT problem areas fit well the reality of problems the Ugandan community experienced. The death of a family member or close friend that produced grief was often due to AIDS. Because of cultural intolerance of any negative mention of the dead, evinced in the popular saying, "The dead are living among us," the closest formulation of a question aimed at capturing negative experiences with the deceased was "*Were there times in your life together when you felt disappointed?*"

Disagreements (role disputes) included arguments with neighbors about property boundaries or stolen animals, political fights, family members claiming privileges that traditionally belonged to other members, wives protesting the husband's bringing in a second wife, or acceding—out of fear—to an HIV-infected husband's refusal to use condoms. The issue here was how to communicate one's feelings indirectly. Whereas Westerners might state their expectation of another person directly, in Uganda such directness would be deemed inappropriate and disrespectful.

A woman who was angry at her husband could not confront him directly but could start cooking bad meals, which would signal to him that something was wrong. An indirect way of addressing disagreements was to engage relatives in helping to resolve disputes, or to encourage a woman to discuss the prospect of her children becoming orphans rather than invoking her own health when pleading with an HIV-infected man to use protection. If that failed, she could enlist the help of a medical person or a traditional healer whom the husband could trust without suspicion that another man was seducing his wife.

Another challenge involved finding culturally appropriate options for resolving a dispute. For example, when exploring options available to an infertile wife, trainees responded that she could ask her sister or another woman to marry her husband, so that the new wife would be an ally and they could raise the children together.

Life changes (role transitions) included becoming sick with AIDS and other illnesses, unemployment, marriage and moving to the husband's house, and dealing with the husband's decision to marry a new wife, which inevitably altered the first wife's position in the household and reduced the resources available to her children. In working on a role transition in standard IPT, the therapist helps the patient to recognize positive and negative aspects of the old and the new roles. For many experiences in Uganda—the devastation of war, tyrannical regimes, torture, AIDS, and hunger—finding positive aspects of the life change was difficult. Instead, the trainees identified and focused on elements that were under the individuals' control, and worked on building skills and identifying options such as persuading potential advocates for assistance.

Acceptance of the approach was high. Attendance was excellent, and the dropout rate from the groups was low (7.8 percent). Evidence of efficacy was impressive (Bolton et al., 2003). The groups actually continued to meet on their own after the official termination.

Themes reflecting the culture included the centrality of the extended family (including polygamy) and the extended community (the village), and the avoidance of direct confrontation, which could lead to unforgivable statements and the loss of the relationship. Variations on these themes arise in many cultures. Even with considerable cultural differences between Uganda and the United States, the researchers found that the adaptations required to translate IPT from one place to the other were surprisingly minor, and the predicaments of depressed individuals continents apart were quite similar.

HUMANITARIAN AND TRAINING EFFORTS

Varied humanitarian efforts sponsored by multiple relief agencies are using IPT to train health workers. These are mainly implementation activities, although some have a research component and small clinical trials. Verdeli, Clougherty, and Weissman are adapting IPT for Syrian refugees living in Lebanon. After the 2010 earthquake in Haiti, Verdeli worked with a local health-care organization to train psychologists, social workers, and community health workers in IPT offered as part of a collaborative care model (see Verdeli et al., 2016). Grand Challenge of Canada in 2015 awarded $1 million to scale up this program nationally. Weissman and Verdeli, assisted by Saeed in Egypt, are adapting a WHO-sponsored IPC manual for use in primary care in Muslim countries, as noted above.

Verdeli led training in Bogotà to implement IPC for internally displaced women exposed to life threats, kidnapping, sexual assaults, and torture, treating depression, anxiety, and PTSD (Ceballos et al., 2016). Gomes et al. (2016) illustrated the cultural adaptation of IPT to treat common mental disorders in primary care in Goa, India. The case study was part of a controlled clinical trial testing a stepped-care intervention. Six to twelve sessions of IPT were only added if the patient had not responded to earlier steps or if symptomatology was severe (Gomes et al., 2016). Health outcomes from the study in a public facility improved and were significantly cost-effective; health outcomes in a private facility did not differ but were less costly with IPT.

Meffert trained workers to use IPT to treat Darfur refugees in Cairo, Egypt, and earthquake survivors in Sichuan, China. In Cairo, a small randomized clinical trial of the refugees with PTSD compared IPT to waitlist control for six sessions using community workers with no mental health background (Meffert et al., 2014). IPT predicted a significant decrease in PTSD, anger, and depression and is ongoing. In China, a small, twelve-week clinical trial compared IPT and treatment as usual to usual treatment alone for forty-nine adults with PTSD and MDD. Investigators found significant reductions in both PTSD and MDD for IPT (51.9 percent and 30 percent, respectively) versus usual treatment (3.4 percent and 3.4 percent), with treatment gains maintained at the six-month follow-up (Jiang et al., 2014). Meffert is leading an ongoing study addressing depression in the context of HIV and domestic violence in Kenya. Three hundred women with HIV and MDD or PTSD will receive either IPT and usual treatment versus usual treatment alone, provided by non-specialists (Onu et al., 2016; Zunner et al., 2015).

A four-session course of group IPT was compared to narrative exposure therapy in a small trial with twenty-six Rwandan genocide orphans with PTSD. There were no differences at the end of treatment, but at six months only 25 percent of the narrative exposure therapy participants and 71 percent of the IPT participants still had PTSD, suggesting lesser effectiveness for IPT (Schaal et al., 2009). In contrast, in a program for victims of violence in Sao Paulo, Brazil, thirty-three patients who were not responsive to medication participated in group IPT for twelve weeks in an open trial; they showed significantly improved depressive and anxiety symptoms and quality of life (Campanini et al., 2010; Chapter 22).

Ravitz, a Canadian psychiatrist, led an educational collaboration between Addis Ababa University and the University of Toronto Department of Psychiatry to develop psychiatric residency training in Ethiopia, including IPT training. Ravitz conducted a month-long, intensive, interactive, didactic, and clinically contextualized IPT course for psychiatry residents. A key task was to culturally and structurally adapt IPT to the Ethiopian context. The curriculum reviewed the clinical presentation and epidemiology of depression in Ethiopia (Kedebe & Alem, 1999), the nature of associated local life stressors (Alem, Destal, & Araya, 1995), and cultural perspectives and case formulation in psychotherapy (Lo & Fung, 2003). To facilitate the transfer of knowledge to practice and to reinforce learning, laminated pocket cards summarizing IPT practice principles provided trainees quick reminders. IPT was found to provide helpful clinical guidelines to assist in assessment and case formulation of psychiatric patients in acute treatment; to resolve interpersonal crises in inpatient and outpatient treatment settings; and to facilitate more effective discharge planning, including contingency and aftercare considerations. IPT was deemed more feasible using less frequent (less than weekly) or shorter sessions. Therapists commonly faced somatic presentations of psychiatric illness and needed sensitive awareness of at times politicized ethnic diversity. Ethnic groups differ in language and in cultural, religious, and social practices, so it was essential not to assume what constituted culturally accepted social practices. As in Uganda, indirect communication was common and potentially effective; therapists needed to explore all options when conducting communication and decisional analyses with patients.

Ravitz concluded that the program established the clinical relevance and feasibility of IPT in Ethiopia for diverse psychiatric patients (Ravitz et al., 2014). Whether such projects produce sustained changes in practice and improved patient outcomes deserves study.

The level of evidence for IPT for MDD in Uganda is **** (four stars). The evidence is excellent that group IPT for MDD is efficacious in Uganda based on two large clinical trials (Bolton et al., 2003, 2007). The evidence for the efficacy of IPT in low- or middle-income countries for depression or PTSD is based on a few small clinical trials. Implementation of IPT for humanitarian reasons is growing at an impressive pace.

CONCLUSION

The spread of IPT from its American origin is exciting. As IPT proved easily transplantable to Uganda, it is likely to fit into many cultures with relatively minor adjustment. Dutch clinicians who initially saw IPT as an overly optimistic, American "can-do" therapy that would not work under the cloudy skies in the Netherlands were impressed by its efficacy in their own hands (Blom et al., 2007; Peeters et al., 2013). IPT apparently required little adaptation in Holland, Scandinavia (Ekeblad et al., 2016; Karlsson et al., 2011; Saloheimo et al., 2016), Puerto Rico (Rossello & Bernal, 1999), and Brazil (de Mello et al., 2001). Again, in order to produce positive experiences, therapists must be familiar with the culture.

25

Group, Conjoint, Telephone, and Internet Formats

IPT was developed as an individual, face-to-face psychotherapy, but its principles work flexibly in other formats. This chapter briefly describes adaptations of IPT to other formats. Throughout the book, we have presented examples of these adaptations for different disorders.

GROUP IPT

Group therapy has flourished in the last decade and has several evident advantages for IPT. It reduces interpersonal isolation by providing an environment in which to discuss and resolve interpersonal problems. It allows patients to see that others share their illness, validating the IPT sick role. Patients may also feel gratified to find that they can help other group members. Group psychotherapy allows a therapist to treat larger numbers of patients, making it a potentially cost-effective alternative or a more viable treatment when patient volume is high and resources are limited.

Group therapy has potential disadvantages as well. Patients receive less individual attention from the therapist. Difficulties in assembling adequate numbers of patients to form a group may delay treatment. More specific to IPT, group therapy raises the risk of confusion if patients present with different focal interpersonal problem areas. Inasmuch as a strength of IPT is the precision of its focus, group IPT risks diminishing that organizing clarity. Finally, in some cultures the potential breach of confidentiality and stigma preclude group treatment: Hankerson (personal communication, 2016), in his work in African American churches in New York City, learned this through church focus groups.

Wilfley et al. (1993) were the pioneers in group IPT. They developed the first group IPT adaptation in a study of nonpurging bulimic patients (Chapter 20; see Welch et al., 2012, for detailed discussions of this model). The approach combined two initial individual sessions with subsequent group sessions. The individual visits allowed the therapist to develop a therapeutic alliance with each patient and prepare the patient for the group while determining the patient's history, symptoms, and IPT formulation. That constituted the first phase. Once the group began, therapists sent patients home with feedback specific to their own cases.

Wilfley et al. (1993) addressed the issue of contrary IPT foci by giving all of the group patients in treatment for eating disorders the formulation of interpersonal deficits. This is interesting: in depression, the term "interpersonal deficits" implies an absence of precipitating life events and the presence of social isolation, with likely difficulties in group interactions. The term clearly meant something different for bulimic patients, who could interact at a superficial level in group but had difficulty in revealing intimate feelings. The shared interpersonal formulation provided a helpful homogeneity to the group, just as the shared diagnosis of bulimia did.

With these changes, group IPT functions much like individual IPT. The overall structure of initial, middle, and termination sessions persists. The focus remains on the connection between feelings and life situations, and patients identify common themes and work together to help one another solve their interpersonal problems.

The first adaptation of group IPT for depression in adults was the Ugandan study (Chapter 24). In October 2016, the World Health Organization, as part of its mental health Gap Action Program (mhGAP) to scale up services for mental health disorders in low- and middle-income countries, distributed an eight-session group IPT (Chapter 24). It is sufficiently detailed to allow training of non-specialized health-care providers. It derives from the Ugandan study group IPT manual, which in turn derives from the interpersonal counseling (IPC) manual and contains even more detailed scripts. Verdeli, Clougherty, and Weissman have added monitoring forms and directions. Although this may be considered a form of IPC, it is called "group interpersonal *therapy*," not "psychotherapy," to avoid credentialing issues in some countries. The manual is available in hard copy though the WHO and online for free (http://apps.who.int/iris/bitstream/10665/250219/1/WHO-MSD-MER-16.4-eng.pdf?ua=1).

In various adaptations, several studies have compared group IPT to treatment as usual to treat or prevent recurrence of postpartum depression, with positive results out to the two-year follow-up in one study (Klier et al., 2001; Mulcahy et al., 2010; Reay et al., 2012; see Chapter 13). Group IPT has also been adapted and tested with depressed adolescents (Mufson et al., 2004; Rosselló & Bernal, 1999; Rosselló et al., 2008; Young et al., 2006; Chapter 14). One study compared group IPT to group CBT for treatment-resistant social anxiety disorder in a Norwegian residential setting (Chapter 21).

Considerable effort has been made to test and implement group IPT for bipolar disorder (Bouwkamp et al., 2013; Hoberg et al., 2013; Chapter 18) across different levels of care in routine practice by Pittsburgh investigators. For bipolar patients, some groups required an adaptation to group Interpersonal and Social Rhythm Therapy, meeting weekly for twelve to sixteen ninety-minute sessions. Implementation on an inpatient unit proved difficult because of the heterogeneity of the patient population, length of stay, and lack of experienced therapists. The researchers adapted the group for inpatients by including a broad range of bipolar spectrum diagnoses, limiting the social rhythm focus, and simplifying the intervention in order to train less experienced clinicians (Swartz et al., 2011). They excluded patients with highly acute illness and included performance measures. While staff and patients expressed high levels of satisfaction and the feasibility of the adaptation was demonstrated, efficacy data are not yet available (Swartz et al., 2011).

Group IPT has been implemented for posttraumatic stress disorder (PTSD; Campanini et al., 2010; Krupnick et al., 2008; Chapter 22) and for substance abuse in female prisoners (Johnson & Zlotnick, 2008; Chapter 19) and is being implemented for PTSD in low-income countries (Chapters 22, 24). Sample sizes in these studies are relatively small.

Therapists undertaking group IPT should have experience with the group format, the target diagnosis, and the culture. Efforts should be made to maximize homogeneity: while we have recommended in the past that patients share a diagnosis, the experience with group IPT in inpatient units suggests that this may not be necessary or always feasible (Swartz et al., 2011). It may be useful to organize groups around an interpersonal problem area, such as complicated bereavement. No research has yet compared group with individual IPT; thus, although group IPT has efficacy, we do not know how it compares with individual IPT.

The level of evidence for the efficacy of group IPT in patients with bulimia is **** (four stars; validated by at least two randomized controlled trials demonstrating the superiority of group IPT to a control condition for bulimia). The level of evidence for depression is **** (four stars; validated by two randomized trials for depression in Uganda in adults and adolescents, three randomized controlled studies of adolescents in the United States, and two postpartum depression studies).

CONJOINT (COUPLES) IPT

IPT and couples therapy share an interest in interpersonal interactions. Indeed, individual IPT treatment focusing on role disputes often has the feel of a unilateral "couples" therapy, helping the patient to resolve a marital impasse. Only one small pilot study has researched conjoint IPT, comparing it to individual IPT in treating depressed married women, half of whose husbands were assigned to participate with them in conjoint IPT (Foley et al., 1989). Conjoint and individual IPT improved depressive symptoms equally, but patients in conjoint IPT reported greater marital satisfaction.

Carter et al. (2010) have suggested applying conjoint IPT to postpartum depression. An important aspect of conjoint IPT for depression is the need to diagnose both parties. People are generally attracted to individuals like themselves. In couples therapy, both spouses may be depressed. (Indeed, treating depressed husbands may have contributed to the greater marital satisfaction found in conjoint

IPT.) The therapist should interview each partner separately before beginning conjoint treatment.

Conjoint IPT starts as an individual treatment of the identified patient, with the spouse brought in to assist. Role transitions and especially role disputes are prominent.

The level of evidence for the efficacy of couples IPT is * (one star; only one pilot study with a small treatment sample [fewer than 12 subjects]).

THERAPIST NOTE

This approach is intuitively appealing, and the one small study that was conducted had encouraging findings. Nonetheless, this continues to be a relatively neglected area of IPT research. Therapists using this approach should be familiar with both couples therapy and the target diagnosis.

TELEPHONE IPT

The telephone is a powerful mode of communication that has been increasingly used as a vector for psychotherapy. It may provide convenient access for patients who are homebound, are unable to arrange childcare, or live in remote locales far from therapists. Some patients may prefer the relative anonymity and distance of a telephone contact. Tradeoffs for the therapist are the inability to see the patient's demeanor and facial reactions and the difficulty in intervening if the patient reports an acute suicidal risk. There is also the potential for loss of confidentiality on an open telephone line. (The same issues apply to psychotherapy conducted over the Internet.) The increasing use of Skype and Facetime, although yet not reported in any studies, may overcome some of these problems once the confidentiality of the medium is ensured.

A few small studies have used telephone IPT (IPT-T) as a treatment. In these projects, patients generally reported that they liked the approach, some even stating that they preferred it to face-to-face contact. The telephone approach uses standard IPT. Most treatments begin with an in-person interview to determine the patient's diagnosis and degree of suicidality, after which treatment takes place by telephone.

Donnelly et al. (2000) piloted this approach in treating patients receiving high doses of chemotherapy for cancer who were homebound or were too ill to come to in-person sessions. Their level of depression was unclear. Miller and Weissman (2002) treated by telephone for twelve weeks thirty depressed patients in partial remission who had difficulty attending clinics due to family obligations or finances. Compared to a waitlist, the IPT patients reported improved functioning and fewer symptoms. Eighty-three percent expressed a wish to continue with telephone treatment if they needed it. Note that these telephone trials limited the patients' severity of depressive symptomatology and suicide risk.

Neugebauer et al. (2006) at Columbia University randomized twenty-six women with recent miscarriage and minor depression to interpersonal counseling by telephone or usual care and found reduction in symptoms in the patients who received treatment by telephone. In a subsequent trial, certified nurse-midwives in obstetrical clinics treated forty-one women with postpartum depression with eight telephone IPT sessions and compared these patients to twenty women referred for usual medical care (Posmontier et al., 2016). Patients receiving telephone IPT had lower depression scores at week 8 ($p = .047$) and at week 12 follow-up ($p = .029$).

Gao (2010) in China examined the effects of an IPT childbirth psychoeducation intervention on postnatal depression, psychological well-being, and satisfaction with interpersonal relationships in first-time mothers. The intervention consisted of two ninety-minute antenatal classes and a telephone follow-up within two weeks after delivery. One hundred ninety-four first-time pregnant women were randomly assigned to the intervention group (N = 96) or usual care consisting of routine childbirth education (N = 98). Women receiving the IPT-based intervention had significantly better psychological well-being, fewer depressive symptoms, and better interpersonal relationships six weeks postpartum than those in the usual care group.

A pilot study examined whether brief IPT-T reduced psychiatric distress among persons living with HIV-AIDS in rural areas of the United States (Ransom et al., 2008). Seventy-nine participants were assigned randomly to usual care or to six sessions of IPT-T. Patients in the IPT-T group continued to receive standard services available to them in the community. Patients receiving IPT-T evidenced greater reductions in depressive symptoms and in overall levels of psychiatric distress compared with those in the control group. Nearly one-third of patients receiving IPT-T reported clinically meaningful reductions in psychiatric distress from pre- to post-intervention. The same group replicated these findings in a randomized trial of 162 rural depressed HIV patients spread across twenty-eight states. Patients were assigned to either nine sessions of IPT-T or standard care. Patients in the IPT-T group (N = 70) ended with lower depression and interpersonal problem scores, with 22 percent of IPT-T and only 4 percent of standard care patients achieving a priori response criterion of at least 50 percent depressive symptom reduction (Heckman et al., 2016).

Therapists using telephone IPT should be experienced in IPT and in treating the target diagnosis. Patients should ideally be seen in person before beginning therapy to determine their suitability for this "long-distance" treatment. This decision will depend upon clinical judgment; patients at high risk of impulsivity, violence, or suicide are probably not optimal candidates for this approach. If the therapist cannot actually see the patient, a proxy visit with a nearby clinician (e.g., a family doctor) might be indicated. Telephone IPT sessions may also be conducted as part of standard IPT if a patient or the therapist leaves town but wishes to maintain momentum in the treatment.

The level of evidence for IPT-T is *** (three stars; validation by at least one randomized controlled trial or equivalent to a reference treatment of established efficacy). The data are limited but certainly encouraging.

INTERNET IPT—SELF-GUIDED IPT

While electronic IPT training programs for therapists exist (Chapter 26), electronic versions of IPT that allow direct self-guided use by patients have been slower to develop. Some are underway. Donker et al. (2013) conducted an automated, three-arm, fully self-guided, online noninferiority trial comparing IPT (n = 620) and CBT (n = 610) to an active control treatment (MoodGYM: n = 613) over a four-week period in the general population. Depressive symptoms on the CES-D and the Client Satisfaction form were completed immediately following treatment and at a six-month follow-up. Completer analyses showed a significant reduction in depressive symptoms at posttest and follow-up for both CBT and IPT, and the results were noninferior to MoodGYM. Within-group effect sizes were medium to large for all groups. There were no differences in clinically significant change between the programs. Reliable change was shown at posttest and follow-up for all programs, with consistently higher rates for CBT. Participants allocated to IPT showed significantly lower treatment satisfaction compared to CBT and MoodGYM. There was a 70 percent dropout rate at posttest, highest for MoodGYM. Intention-to-treat analyses confirmed these findings.

Despite the high dropout rate and lower satisfaction scores, this study suggests that Internet-delivered self-guided IPT may have promise in reducing depressive symptoms, and may be noninferior to MoodGYM. Completion rates for IPT and CBT were higher than for MoodGYM, indicating some progress in refining Internet-based self-help. Internet-delivered treatment options available for people suffering from depression now include IPT. Weissman and Donker are developing an electronic version of brief IPT.

An online version of IPSRT called RAY (Rhythms And You) is under development and beginning testing (Swartz et al., 2016). This online version of Interpersonal and Social Rhythm Therapy, a psychotherapy treatment specific to bipolar disorder, uses a problem-solving approach to help individuals regularize their social rhythms in order to entrain underlying disturbances in circadian and sleep/wake regulation. RAY comprises twelve weekly modules covering such topics as mood and daily rhythms, bipolar disorder and physical health, sleep, and relationships and rhythms. It uses animations and other tools. A twelve-week, primary care feasibility trial is underway comparing supported and unsupported administrations of RAY (administered with and without coaching from a clinical helper) compared with a control condition (online, written psychoeducation about bipolar disorder).

26

Training and Resources

TRAINING

Evidence-based psychotherapies like IPT are increasingly being offered to patients, and patients are requesting them as information filters into the popular press and social media. In the United States, psychiatric residency training programs require "competence" in certain psychotherapeutic approaches. Based on its evidential support and inclusion in treatment guidelines, IPT should be listed among the required psychotherapies, but it is not yet. Nor do most American psychologists, social workers, or nurses in training get much exposure to IPT. While some training programs are incorporating IPT, progress is slow (Lichtmacher, Eisendrath, & Haller, 2006; Weissman, Verdeli, et al., 2006). In the meantime, whether you are in or out of training, how do you become a skillful IPT practitioner?

CERTIFICATION

Many practicing clinicians interested in further training would like to receive formal certification. Such certification has become an increasing point of controversy. IPT began as a research psychotherapy (Markowitz & Weissman, 2012), with researchers training clinicians to levels of competence and adherence in order to treat patients in their studies (Rounsaville et al., 1986). When, based on the research success of IPT, clinicians began learning it in various sorts of postgraduate training courses, many asked about diplomas and certification. The answer was that none existed. The status of certification now varies by country. The United Kingdom has constructed detailed accreditation requirements for different levels of training (http://www.iptuk.net/). In the United States, by contrast, some trainers offer workshop attendees diplomas, but their value is unclear: there is really no such thing as being an "accredited" IPT therapist in the United States. The International Society of Interpersonal Psychotherapy (ISIPT; https://www.interpersonalpsychotherapy.org/; https://www.facebook.com/InterpersonalPsychotherapy/) is wrestling with this issue, but at present there is no global consensus. If you work in a region with a local IPT organization, check its standards.

From our perspective, so long as you have clinical credentials, certification is less important than that you develop clinical expertise in IPT as a treatment modality. The course is relatively easy if you already have basic training in psychotherapy, including how to listen and talk to patients; express empathy and warmth, holding back your own reactions and opinions; formulate a problem; maintain a therapeutic alliance; understand the limits of confidentiality; and maintain professional boundaries and ethical practice. A basic familiarity with clinical psychiatric diagnosis is essential. Learning IPT involves discovering how to take your basic psychotherapy training and modify it for use with a specific set of strategies. Most training consists of three elements, as has been true since Klerman and Weissman trained the first IPT therapists for the first studies in the 1970s:

- Read the IPT manual.
- Attend an IPT training workshop.
- Obtain clinical supervision on training cases.

Read the IPT Manual

We have designed the manual you are reading to highlight the basic elements of IPT and take you through the strategies. The manual should provide you with both an overview of how to approach treating a patient and specific tactics to encourage a good outcome. Any good manual also should have prohibitions: in order to ensure you are doing pure IPT, the version on which the evidence of its efficacy is based, you should avoid using other therapeutic modalities that might muddy the water and confuse a patient. IPT avoids cognitive behavioral and psychodynamic techniques, among others. This does not mean we would not refer patients to such treatment, when appropriate; however, when you treat a patient, you should treat purely and avoid eclecticism (see Chapter 1).

Attend an IPT Training Workshop

Continuing medical education (CME) courses are given at many of the annual meetings of professional organizations. The American Psychiatric Association, for example, has at least two workshops on IPT at its annual meeting. These are usually half- or full-day courses and are primarily didactic. Such courses may reinforce your IPT reading and allow clarifications of questions you may have about IPT.

Some academic centers offer two- to four-day workshops that are much more intensive and provide some practical (hands-on) training. These have been held throughout the world, particularly in England, Canada, New Zealand, and recently France. Since the sites change, the best way to learn about workshops and supervision is through the International Society of Interpersonal Psychotherapy https://www.interpersonalpsychotherapy.org/).

Obtain Clinical Supervision on Training Cases

We learn psychotherapy by practicing it; simply taking a workshop does not suffice (Davis et al., 1999). To guide you through initial cases, you can use this manual. We recommend that you conduct *a minimum of two time-limited, diagnosis-focused IPT cases* to gain comfort with the structure and techniques of the treatment.

Get the patient's written permission to audio- or videotape these sessions, explaining that the focus of such taping is your technique, and that this is in essence a quality control for the therapy. Tell the patient that you are concerned about maintaining confidentiality, so the tape will be locked up and only be used for supervision, and then erased after an interval. (All of this should be described in the written release.) Having a record of the actual session is a huge educational benefit, alerting you to what you do and don't do during the treatment. It also frees you from taking process notes during the session, which are a distraction from engaging the patient. If you wish, you may use a rating scale such as the CSPRS-6 (Hollon, 1984; Markowitz et al., 2000) to check your IPT adherence.

Use a rating scale such as the Hamilton Rating Scale for Depression at the start of treatment and repeat it at regular intervals during treatment. This allows you and the patient to gauge the patient's progress in the treatment.

The best assurance that you are learning IPT is to get supervision from an experienced IPT clinician who already knows it. Supervision can take place in individual or group format, in person or over the phone. (Phone supervision requires sending the supervisor an encrypted copy of the treatment session ahead of time.) Group supervision has the advantage of allowing you to follow the progress of other therapists' cases. In cases where no experienced IPT therapist was available, several groups have conducted peer supervision, successfully training themselves using the IPT manual and taped sessions as guides.

RESOURCES

Associated Manuals

Clougherty, K. F., Verdeli, H., & Weissman, M. M. (2003). *Interpersonal psychotherapy adapted for a group in Uganda (IPT-G-U).* Unpublished manual available from M. M. Weissman, New York State Psychiatric Institute, 1051 Riverside Drive, Unit 24, New York, NY 10032 (mmw3@columbia.edu).

Frank, E. (2005). *Treating bipolar disorder: A clinician's guide to interpersonal and social rhythm therapy.* New York: Guilford.

Hinrichsen, G. A., & Clougherty, K. F. (2006). *Interpersonal psychotherapy for depressed older adults.* Washington, DC: American Psychological Association.

Hoffart, A., Abrahamsen, G., Bonsaksen, T., Borge, F. M., Ramstad, R., & Markowitz, J. C. (2007). *A residential interpersonal treatment for social phobia.* New York: Nova Science Publishers.

Klerman, G. L., Weissman, M. M., Rounsaville, B., & Chevron, E. (1984). *Interpersonal psychotherapy of depression.* New York: Basic Books.

Law, R. (2013). *Defeating depression—Using the people in your life to open the door to recovery.* London: Constable and Robinson.

Law, R. (2016). *Defeating teenage depression—Getting there together.* London: Little Brown Books.

Lipsitz, J. D., & Markowitz, J. C. (2006). *Manual for interpersonal psychotherapy for social phobia (IPT-SP).* Unpublished manual available from Joshua D. Lipsitz, Ph.D., Anxiety Disorders Clinic, New York State Psychiatric Association, 1051 Riverside Drive, Unit 69, New York, NY 10032.

Markowitz, J. C. (1998). *Interpersonal psychotherapy for dysthymic disorder.* Washington, DC: American Psychiatric Publishing.

Markowitz, J. C. (2016). *Interpersonal psychotherapy for posttraumatic stress disorder.* New York: Oxford University Press.

Markowitz, J. C., & Weismann, M. M. (Eds.). (2012). *Casebook of interpersonal psychotherapy.* New York: Oxford University Press.

Mufson, L., Pollack Dorta, K., Moreau, D., & Weissman, M. M. (2011). *Interpersonal psychotherapy for depressed adolescents* (2d ed.). New York: Guilford Press.

Pilowsky, D., & Weissman, M. M. (2005). *Interpersonal psychotherapy with school-aged depressed children.* Unpublished manual available from Dan Pilowsky, Ph.D., 1051 Riverside Drive, Unit 24, New York, NY 10032.

Spinelli, M. G. (1999). *Manual of interpersonal psychotherapy for antepartum depressed women (IPT-P).* Unpublished manual, College of Physicians and Surgeons of Columbia University, New York State Psychiatric Institute, 1051 Riverside Drive, Box 123, New York, NY 10032.

Weissman, M. M. (2005). *Mastering depression through interpersonal psychotherapy: Monitoring forms.* New York: Oxford University Press.

Weissman, M. M., & Klerman, G. L. (1986). *Interpersonal counseling (IPC) for stress and distress in primary care settings.* Unpublished manual available through M. M. Weissman, Ph.D., 1051 Riverside Drive, Unit 24, New York, NY 10032 (mmw3@columbia.edu).

Weissman, M. M., Markowitz, J. C., & Klerman, G. L. (2000). *Comprehensive guide to interpersonal psychotherapy.* New York: Basic Books.

Weissman, M. M., Markowitz, J. C., & Klerman, G. L. (2007). *Clinicians' quick guide to interpersonal psychotherapy.* New York: Oxford University Press.

Wilfley, D. E., Mackenzie, K. R., Welch, R., Ayres, V., & Weissman, M. M. (Eds.). (2000). *Interpersonal psychotherapy for group.* New York: Basic Books.

World Health Organization (2016). *Group interpersonal therapy (IPT) for depression.* http://www.who.int/mental_health/mhgap/interpersonal_therapy/en/

IPT Manual Translations

Translations of: Klerman, G. L., Weissman, M. M., Rounsaville, B., & Chevron, E. S. (1984). *Interpersonal psychotherapy of depression*. New York: Basic Books.

> Spanish: *Afronta tu depresion con psicoterapia interpersonal*, translated by Juan Garcia Sanchez and Pepa Palazon Rodriguez, published by Desclee De Brouwer, 2010.
> German: *Interpersonelle Psychotherapie bei Depressionen und anderen psychischen Storungen*, translated by Elisabeth Schramm, published by Schattauer GMbH (Stuttgart New York), 1996.
> German: *Interpersonelle Psychotherapie*, translated by Elisabeth Schramm, published by Schattauer GmbH, 2010,
> Italian: *Psicoterapia Interpersonale Della Depressione*, translated by Pina Galeazzi, published by Bollati Boringhieri, 1989,
> Japanese: *Interpersonal Psychotherapy of Depression*, translated by Yutaka Omo and Hiroko Mizoshima, Japanese translation rights arranged with Basic Books, Inc. through Tuttle-Mori Agency, Inc., Tokyo, 1997.

Translations of Weissman, M. M., Markowitz, J. C., & Klerman, G. L. (2000). *Comprehensive guide to interpersonal psychotherapy*. New York: Basic Books.

> French: *Guide to psychotherapie interpersonnelle*, translated by Simon Patry, M.D., FRPC, DFAPA, published by Basic Books, 2006.
> Japanese: *Comprehensive Guide to Interpersonal Psychotherapy*, Japanese translation rights arranged with Basic Books, Inc. through Tuttle-Mori Agency, Inc., Tokyo.
> Spanish: *Manual de Psicoterapia interpersonal*, translated and edited by Josep Solé Puig, published by Editorial Grupo 5, Madrid, 2013.

Translations of Weissman, M. M., Markowitz, J. C., & Klerman, G. L. (2007). *A clinician's quick guide to interpersonal psychotherapy*. New York: Oxford University Press.

> Danish: *Interpersonal Psykoterapi Praksisvejledning*, translated by Dorte Herdolt Silver, published by Dansk Psykologisk Forlag, 2009.
> German: *Interpersonelle Psychotherapie*, translated by Barbara Preschl, published by Hogrefe Verlag GmbH & Co. KG, 2009.
> Portuguese: *Psicoterapie Interpesoal guia practico do terapeuta*, translated by Sandra Maria Mallmann da Rosa, published by Artmed, 2009.
> Japanese: translated by Hiroko Mizushima, published by arrangement with Oxford University Press.
> Korean: *Clinician's quick guide to interpersonal psychotherapy*

Other Non-English Manuals

French
Rahioui, H. (2016). *La Thérapie Interpersonnelle*. Presses Universitaires de France.
Hovaguimian, T., & Markowitz, J. C. (2002). *La Psychothérapie Interpersonnelle de la Dépression*. Genève: Editions Médecine & Hygiène Société (2nd ed., 2014).

German
Weissman, M. M., Markowitz, J. C., & Klerman, G. L. (2009). *Interpersonelle Psychotherapie: Ein Behandlungsleitfaden*. Göttingen: Hogrefe.

Italian
Pergami, A., Grassi, L., & Markowitz, J. C. (1999). *Il Trattamento Psicologico della Depressione nell'Infezione da HIV—La Psicoterapia Interpersonale*. Milan: Franco Angeli.

Japanese
Klerman, G. L., Weissman, M. M., Rounsaville, B. J., & Chevron, E. S. (1997). *Interpersonal psychotherapy of depression*, trans. H. Mizushima, M. Shimada, & Y. Ono. Tokyo: Iwasaki Gakujyutsa.

Hamilton Rating Scale for Depression

Department of health education and welfare Public Health Service Alcohol, Drug abuse and Mental Health Administration NIMH-PRE Collaborative Study of Maintenance Drug Therapy in Affective Illness **HAMILTON PSYCHIATRIC RATING SCALE FOR DEPRESSION**	RATER: _____ DATE: _____	PATIENT'S ID# WEEK	**PHASE** SCORE

For each item select the "cue" which best characterizes the patient's state in the past week

1. DEPRESSED MOOD (Sadness, hopeless, helpless, worthless)	0 Absent 1 These feeling states indicated only on questioning 2 These feeling states spontaneously reported verbally 3 Communicates feeling states non-verbally – i.e., through facial expression, voice, posture, tendency to weep 4 Patient reports VIRTUALLY ONLY these feeling states in his spontaneous verbal and non-verbal communication
2. FEELINGS OF GUILT	0 Absent 1 Self-reproach, feels he has let people down 2 Ideas of guilt or rumination over past errors or sinful deeds 3 Present illness is a punishment. Delusions of guilt 4 Hears accusatory or denunciatory voices and/or experiences threatening visual hallucinations
3. SUICIDE	0 Absent 1 Feels life is not worth living 2 Wishes he were dead or any thoughts of possible death to self 3 Suicide ideas or gesture 4 Attempts at suicide (any serious attempt rates 5)
4. INSOMNIA EARLY	0 No difficulty falling asleep 1 Complains of occasional difficulty falling asleep – i.e., more than ½ hour 2 Complains of nightly difficulty falling asleep

5. INSOMNIA MIDDLE	0 No difficulty 1 Patient complains of being restless and disturbed during the night 2 Waking during the night – any getting out of bed rates 3 *(except for purposes of voiding)*
6. INSOMNIA LATE	0 No difficulty 1 Waking in early hours of the morning but goes back to sleep 2 Unable to fall asleep again if gets out of bed
7. WORK AND ACTIVITIES	0 No difficulty 1 Thoughts and feeling of incapacity, fatigue or weakness related to activities, work or hobbies 2 Loss of interest in activity; hobbies or work – either directly reported by patient, or indirectly in listlessness, indecision and vacillation *(feels he has to push self to work or activities)* 3 Decrease in actual time spent in activities or decrease in productivity. In hospital, rate 4 if patient does not spend at least three hours a day in activities *(hospital job, or hobbies)* exclusive of ward chores 4 Stopped working because of present illness, rate 5 if patient engages in no activities except ward chores, or if patient fails to perform ward chores unassisted
8. RETARDATION	0 Normal speech and thought 1 Slight retardation at interview 2 Obvious retardation at interview 3 Interview difficult 4 Complete stupor
9. AGITATION	0 None 1 "Playing with" hands, hair, moving about, can't sit still, etc. 2 Hand-wringing, nail-biting, hair-pulling, biting of lips
10. ANXIETY PSYCHIC	0 No difficulty 1 Subjective tension and irritability 2 Worrying about minor matters 3 Apprehensive attitude apparent in face or speech 4 Fears expressed without questioning
11. ANXIETY SOMATIC	0 Absent Physiological concomitants of anxiety, such as: 1 Mild Gastro-intestinal: dry mouth, wind, indigestion, diarrhea, cramps, belching 2 Moderate Cardio-vascular: palpitation, headaches 3 Severe Respiratory: Hyperventilation, sighing 4 Incapacitating Urinary frequency Sweating

12. SOMATIC SYMPTOMS GASTROINTESTINAL	0 None 1 Loss of appetite but eating without staff encouragement. Heavy feeling in abdomen 2 Difficulty eating without staff urging. Requests or requires laxatives or medication for bowels or medication for GI symptoms
13. SOMATIC SYMPTOMS GENERAL	0 None 1 Heaviness in limbs, back or head. Backache, headache, muscle ache. Loss of energy and fatigability 2 Any clear-cut symptom rates 2
14. GENITAL SYMPTOMS	0 Absent Symptoms such as: 1 Mild Loss of libido 2 Severe Menstrual disturbances
15. HYPOCHONDRIASIS	0 Not present 1 Self-absorption (bodily) 2 Preoccupation with health 3 Frequent complaints, requests for help, etc. 4 Hypochondriacal delusions
16. LOSS OF WEIGHT	A. WHEN RATING BY HISTORY 0 No weight loss 1 Probable weight loss associated with present illness 2 Definite (according to patient) weight loss B. WHEN ACTUAL WEIGHT CHANGES ARE MEASURED 0 Less than 1 lb. weight loss in week 1 Greater than 1 lb. weight loss in week 2 Greater than 2 lb. weight loss in week
17. INSIGHT	0 Acknowledges being depressed and ill 1 Acknowledges illness but attributes cause to bad food, climate, overwork, virus, need for rest, etc. 2 Denies being ill at all
18. DIURNAL VARIATION	AM PM 0 0 Absent If symptoms are worse in the morning or evening note which it is and 1 1 Mild rate severity of variation 2 2 Severe

19. DEPERSONALIZATION AND DEREALIZATION	0 Absent 1 Mild 2 Moderate Such as feeling of unreality – Nihilistic ideas 3 Severe 4 Incapacitating
20. PARANOID SYMPTOMS	0 None 1 Suspicious 2 Ideas of reference 3 Delusions of reference and persecution 4 Hallucinations, persecutory
21. OBSESSIONAL AND COMPULSIVE SYMPTOMS	0 Absent 1 Mild 2 Severe
22. HELPLESSNESS	0 Not present 1 Subjective feelings which are elicited only by inquiry 2 Patient volunteers his helpless feelings 3 Requires urging, guidance and reassurance to accomplish ward chores or personal hygiene 4 Requires physical assistance for dress, grooming, eating, bedside tasks or personal hygiene
23. HOPELESSNESS	0 Not present 1 Intermittently doubts that "things will improve" but can be reassured 2 Consistently feels "hopeless" but accepts reassurance 3 Expresses feelings of discouragement, despair, pessimism about future, which cannot be dispelled 4 Spontaneously and inappropriately perseverates. "I'll never get well" or its equivalent
24. WORTHLESSNESS	Ranges from mild loss of self-esteem, feelings of inferiority, self-deprecation to delusional notions of worthlessness 0 Not present 1 Indicates feelings of worthlessness (loss of self-esteem) only on questioning 2 Spontaneously indicates feelings of worthlessness (loss of self-esteem) 3 Different from 3 by degree: Patient volunteers that he is "no good," "inferior," etc. 4 Delusional notions of worthlessness – i.e., "I am a heap of garbage" or its equivalent

Patient Health Questionnaire (PHQ-9)

NAME:_____ DATE:_____

Over the *last 2 weeks,* how often have you been bothered
by any of the following problems? *(use "√" to indicate your answer)*

	Not at all	Several days	More than half the days	Nearly every day
1. Little interest or pleasure in doing things	0	1	2	3
2. Feeling down, depressed, or hopeless	0	1	2	3
3. Trouble falling or staying asleep, or sleeping too much	0	1	2	3
4. Feeling tired or having little energy	0	1	2	3
5. Poor appetite or overeating	0	1	2	3
6. Feeling bad about yourself—or that you are a failure or have let yourself or your family down	0	1	2	3
7. Trouble concentrating on things, such as reading the newspaper or watching television	0	1	2	3
8. Moving or speaking so slowly that other people could have noticed. Or the opposite—being so fidgety or restless that you have been moving around a lot more than usual	0	1	2	3
9. Thoughts that you would be better off dead, or of hurting yourself in some way	0	1	2	3

add columns: +   +

(Healthcare professional: For interpretation of TOTAL,   **TOTAL:**
please refer to accompanying scoring card.)

10. If you checked off any problems, how *difficult* have these problems made it for you to do your work, take care of things at home, or get along with other people?	Not difficult at all _____ Somewhat difficult _____ Very difficult _____ Extremely difficult _____

Fold back this page before administering this questionnaire

INSTRUCTIONS FOR USE

for doctor or healthcare professional use only

PHQ-9 QUICK DEPRESSION ASSESSMENT

For initial diagnosis:

1. Patient completes PHQ-9 Quick Depression Assessment on accompanying tear-off pad.
2. If there are at least 4 ✓s in the shaded gray section (including Questions #1 and #2), consider a depressive disorder. Add score to determine severity.
3. *Consider Major Depressive Disorder*

   —if there are at least 5 ✓s in the shaded gray section (one of which corresponds to Question #1 or #2)

   Consider Other Depressive Disorder

   —if there are 2 to 4 ✓s in the shaded gray section (one of which corresponds to Question #1 or #2)

Note: Since the questionnaire relies on patient self-report, all responses should be verified by the clinician and a definitive diagnosis made on clinical grounds, taking into account how well the patient understood the questionnaire, as well as other relevant information from the patient. Diagnoses of Major Depressive Disorder or Other Depressive Disorder also require impairment of social, occupational, or other important areas of functioning (Question #10) and ruling out normal bereavement, a history of a Manic Episode (Bipolar Disorder), and a physical disorder, medication, or other drug as the biological cause of the depressive symptoms.

TO MONITOR SEVERITY OVER TIME FOR NEWLY DIAGNOSED PATIENTS

or patients in current treatment for depression:

1. Patients may complete questionnaires at baseline and at regular intervals (eg, every 2 weeks) at home and bring them in at their next appointment for scoring or they may complete the questionnaire during each scheduled appointment.
2. Add up ✓s by column. For every ✓: Several days = 1
   More than half the days = 2   Nearly every day = 3

3. Add together column scores to get a TOTAL score.

4. Refer to the accompanying PHQ-9 Scoring Card to interpret the TOTAL score.

5. Results may be included in patients' files to assist you in setting up a treatment goal, determining degree of response, as well as guiding treatment intervention.

PHQ-9 SCORING CARD FOR SEVERITY DETERMINATION
for healthcare professional use only

SCORING— ADD UP ALL CHECKED BOXES ON PHQ-9

For every ✓: Not at all = 0;
Several days = 1; More than

half the days = 2;
Nearly every day = 3

INTERPRETATION OF TOTAL SCORE

Total Score Depression Severity

1-4	Minimal depression
5-9	Mild depression
10-14	Moderate depression
15-19	Moderately severe depression
20-27	Severe depression

Source: *www.agencymeddirectors.wa.gov/files/AssessmentTools/14-PHQ-9%20overview.pdf*

Interpersonal Psychotherapy Outcome Scale, Therapist's Version

IPT Problem Area Rating Scale

Rater: _____ Date:_____ Tape #:_____

Mark whether each problem area is present or absent, and check ALL appropriate explanatory items. At the end you will be asked to choose a primary focus for IPT with this subject based on the information available from the tape.

A. Interpersonal Problem Areas

1. Grief   present _____   absent _____
           uncomplicated _____   complicated _____

If grief is present, identify:
           a. deceased _____
           b. relationship to subject_____
           c. date of death _____
           d. number of months between death and onset of depression _____

2. Interpersonal Dispute   present _____ absent _____

If present, identify:
           a. significant other_____
           b. does an impasse exist? Yes_____ No_____
           c. predominant theme of dispute:
                   i.   authority/dominance _____
                   ii. dependence _____
                   iii. sexual issue _____
                   iv. child-rearing _____
                   v.   getting married/separation _____
                   vi. transgression _____
           d. Which theme checked in c. is primary? _____

Approximate duration of dispute in months _____

3. Role Transition   present _____   absent _____

If present, identify: a. geographic move _____
                                          b. marriage/cohabitation _____
                                          c. separation/divorce _____
                                          d. graduation/new job _____
                                          e. loss of job/retirement _____
                                          f. health issue _____
                                          g. other (specify): _____

If more than one checked, which predominates? _____

Number of months between event and onset of depression_____

4. Interpersonal Deficit   present _____ absent _____

If present, specify characteristics:
                                          a. avoidant _____
                                          b. dependent _____
                                          c. masochistic _____
                                          d. borderline _____
                                          e. schizoid _____
                                          f. lacks social skills _____
                                          g. other (specify): _____

If more than one checked, which predominates? _____

B. Formulation of Therapeutic Task

1. Rank interpersonal problem areas marked as "present" in order of their apparent impact on the subject's mood (1= most important, 2= secondary importance, 3= less important):

            Grief _____ Dispute _____ Transition _____ Deficit _____

2. Which problem areas would you use to formulate a treatment contract with the subject? (List up to 2, ranking 1= most important)

            Grief _____ Dispute _____ Transition _____ Deficit _____

3. What is the rationale for your answer to question 2?

_____

_____

_____

_____

4. Did the interviewer on the videotape bias your response by indicating his/her opinion of problem areas? (circle) Yes No

5. Did the videotape provide information adequate to formulate a problem area diagnosis? Yes No

6. Other comments _____

For scoring only:

APA Working Group on the Older Adult. (1998). What practitioners should know about working with older adults. *Professional Psychology: Research and Practice*, *29*, 413–427.

Agras, W. S., Walsh, T., Fairburn, C. G., Wilson, G. T., & Kraemer, H. C. (2000). A multicenter comparison of cognitive-behavioral therapy and interpersonal psychotherapy for bulimia nervosa. *Archives of General Psychiatry*, *57*, 459–466.

Alem, A., Destal, M., & Araya, M. (1995). Mental health in Ethiopia: EPHA expert group report. *Ethiopian Journal of Health Development*, *9*(1).

Alexopoulos, G. S., Katz, I. R., Bruce, M. L., Heo, M., Have, T. T., Raue, P., et al. (2005). Remission in depressed geriatric primary care patients: A report from the PROSPECT Study. *American Journal of Psychiatry*, *162*, 718–724.

Alexopoulos, G. S., Schultz, S. K., & Lebowitz, B. D. (2005). Late-life depression: a model for medical classification. *Biological Psychiatry*, *58*(4), 283–289.

Allen, J. P., Insabella, G., Porter, M. R., Smith, F. D., Land, D., & Phillips, N. (2006). A social-interactional model of the development of depressive symptoms in adolescence. *Journal of Consulting and Clinical Psychology*, *74*(1), 55–65.

American Psychiatric Association. (1994). *Diagnostic and statistical manual for mental disorders*, 4th ed. Washington, DC: American Psychiatric Association.

American Psychiatric Association. (2013). *Diagnostic and statistical manual of mental disorders*, 5th ed. Arlington, VA: American Psychiatric Association.

American Psychiatric Association & Rush, A. J., Jr. (2000). *Handbook of psychiatric measures*. Washington, DC: American Psychiatric Association.

American Psychiatric Association Workgroup on Major Depressive Disorder (2010). Practice guideline for the treatment of patients with major depressive disorder, 3rd ed. *American Journal of Psychiatry*, *167* (October supplement), S1–S152.

Angus, L., & Gillies, L. A. (1994). Counseling the borderline client: An interpersonal approach. *Canadian Journal of Counseling*, *28*, 69–82.

Arbuckle, T. Y., Nohara-LeClair, M., & Pushkar, D. (2000). Effect of off-target verbosity on communication efficiency in a referential communication task. *Psychology and Aging*, *15*, 65–77.

Arcelus, J., Whight, D., Brewin, N., & McGrain, L. (2012). A brief form of interpersonal psychotherapy for adult patients with bulimic disorders: a pilot study. *European Eating Disorders Review*, *20*, 326–330.

Arcelus, J., Whight, D., Langham, C., Baggott, J., McGrain, L., Meadows, L., & Meyer, C. (2009). A case series evaluation of a modified version of interpersonal psychotherapy

(IPT) for the treatment of bulimic eating disorders: a pilot study. *European Eating Disorders Review, 17,* 260–268.

Armor, D. J., & Klerman, G. L. (1968). Psychiatric treatment orientations and professional ideology. *Journal of Health and Social Behavior,* 243–255.

Armor, D. J., Klerman, G. L., Markowitz, J. C., & Weissman, M. M. (2012). IPT: past, present, and future. *Clinical Psychology and Psychotherapy, 19,* 99–105.

Badger, T., Segrin, C., Dorros, S. M., Meek, P., & Lopez, A. M. (2007). Depression and anxiety in women with breast cancer and their partners. *Nursing Research, 56*(1), 44–53.

Badger, T. A., Segrin, C., Figueredo, A. J., Harrington, J., Sheppard, K., Passalacqua, S, et al. (2011). Psychosocial interventions to improve quality of life in prostate cancer survivors and their intimate or family partners. *Quality of Life Research, 20*(6), 833–844.

Badger, T. A., Segrin, C., Figueredo, A. J., Harrington, J., Sheppard, K., Passalacqua, S., et al. (2013a). Who benefits from a psychosocial counselling versus educational intervention to improve psychological quality of life in prostate cancer survivors? *Psychology and Health, 28*(3), 336–354.

Badger, T. A., Segrin, C., Hepworth, J. T., Pasvogel, A., Weihs, K., & Lopez, A. M. (2013b). Telephone-delivered health education and interpersonal counseling improve quality of life for Latinas with breast cancer and their supportive partners. *Psychooncology, 22*(5), 1035–1042.

Badger, T., Segrin, C., Meek, P., Lopez, A. M., & Bonham, E. (2004). A case study of telephone interpersonal counseling for women with breast cancer and their partners. *Oncology Nursing Forum, 31*(5), 997–1003.

Badger, T., Segrin, C., Meek, P., Lopez, A. M., & Bonham, E. (2005a). Profiles of women with breast cancer: who responds to a telephone interpersonal counseling intervention. *Journal of Psychosocial Oncology, 23*(2-3), 79–99.

Badger, T., Segrin, C., Meek, P., Lopez, A. M., Bonham, E., & Sieger, A. (2005b). Telephone interpersonal counseling with women with breast cancer: symptom management and quality of life. *Oncology Nursing Forum, 32*(2), 273–279.

Barber, J. P., & Muenz, L. R. (1996). The role of avoidance and obsessiveness in matching patients to cognitive and interpersonal psychotherapy: Empirical findings from the treatment for depression collaborative research program. *Journal of Consulting and Clinical Psychology, 64,* 951–958.

Barth, J., Munder, T., Gerger, H., Nüesch, E., Trelle, S., Znoj, H et al. (2013). Comparative efficacy of seven psychotherapeutic interventions for patients with depression: a network meta-analysis. *PLoS Medicine, 10,* e1001454.

Bass, J., Neugebauer, R., Clougherty, K. F., Verdeli, H., Wickramaratne, P., Ndogoni, L., et al. (2006). Group interpersonal psychotherapy for depression in rural Uganda: 6-month outcomes: randomised controlled trial. *British Journal of Psychiatry, 188,* 567–573.

Bateman, A. W. (2012). Interpersonal psychotherapy for borderline personality disorder. *Clinical Psychology and Psychotherapy, 19,* 124–133.

Bateman, A., & Fonagy, P. (2001). Treatment of borderline personality disorder with psychoanalytically oriented partial hospitalization: An 18-month follow-up. *American Journal of Psychiatry, 158,* 36–42.

Bateman, A., & Fonagy, P. (2006). *Mentalization-based treatment for borderline personality disorder: a practical guide.* Oxford: Oxford University Press.

Bateman, A., & Fonagy, P. (2009). Randomized controlled trial of outpatient mentalization-based treatment versus structured clinical management for borderline personality disorder. *American Journal of Psychiatry, 166,* 1355–1364.

Beck, A. T. (1978). *Depression Inventory.* Philadelphia: Center for Cognitive Therapy.

Bellino, S., Rinaldi, C., & Bogetto, F. (2010). Adaptation of interpersonal psychotherapy to borderline personality disorder: a comparison of combined therapy and single pharmacotherapy. *Canadian Journal of Psychiatry, 55,* 74–81.

Bellino, S., Zizza, M., Rinaldi, C., & Bogetto, F. (2006). Combined treatment of major depression in patients with borderline personality disorder: a comparison with pharmacotherapy. *Canadian Journal of Psychiatry, 51,* 453–460.

Bellino, S., Zizza, M., Rinaldi, C., & Bogetto, F. (2007). Combined therapy of major depression with concomitant borderline personality disorder: comparison of interpersonal and cognitive therapy. *Canadian Journal of Psychiatry, 52,* 718–725.

Bhat, A., Grote, N. K., Russo, J., Lohr, M. J., Jung, H., Rouse, C. E., et al. [in press]. Collaborative care for perinatal depression among socioeconomically disadvantaged women: adverse neonatal birth events and treatment response. *Psychiatric Services.*

Black, S., Bowyer, D., Champion, L., Foreman, A., Graham, P., Irvine, L., et al. (2015). *Interpersonal psychotherapy as an early intervention strategy for female offenders.* Paper presented at the International Society for Interpersonal Psychotherapy Conference, London.

Bleiberg, K. L., & Markowitz, J. C. (2005). Interpersonal psychotherapy for posttraumatic stress disorder. *American Journal of Psychiatry, 162,* 181–183.

Blom, M. B., Spinhoven, P., Hoffman, T., Jonker, K., Hoencamp, E., Haffmans, P. M., & van Dyck, R. (2007). Severity and duration of depression, not personality factors, predict short term outcome in the treatment of major depression. *Journal of Affective Disorders, 104,* 119–126.

Bolton, P., Bass, J., Betancourt, T., Speelman, L., Onyango, G., Clougherty, K. F., et al. (2007). Interventions for depression symptoms among adolescent survivors of war and displacement in northern Uganda: a randomized controlled trial. *Journal of the American Medical Association, 298*(5), 519–527.

Bolton, P., Bass, J., Neugebauer, R., Verdeli, H., Clougherty, K. F., Wickramaratne, P., et al. (2003). Group interpersonal psychotherapy for depression in rural Uganda: a randomized controlled trial. *Journal of the American Medical Association, 289*(23), 3117–3124.

Borge, F.-M., Hoffart, A., Sexton, H., Clark, D. M., Markowitz, J. C., & McManus, F. (2008). Cognitive and interpersonal therapy for social phobia: a randomized clinical trial. *Journal of Anxiety Disorders, 22,* 991–1010.

Bouwkamp, C. G., de Kruiff, M. E., van Troost, T. M., Snippe, D., Blom, M. J., de Winter, R. F., et al. (2013). Interpersonal and social rhythm group therapy for patients with bipolar disorder. *International Journal of Group Psychotherapy, 63*(1), 97–115.

Bozzatello, P., & Bellino, S. (2016). Combined therapy with interpersonal psychotherapy adapted for borderline personality disorder: A two-years follow-up. *Psychiatric Research, 240,* 151–156.

Brache, K. (2012). Advancing interpersonal therapy for substance use disorders. *American Journal of Drug and Alcohol Abuse, 38*(4), 293–298.

Brandon, A. R., Ceccotti, N., Hynan, L. S., Shivakumar, G., Johnson, N., & Jarrett, R. B. (2012). Proof of concept: Partner-Assisted Interpersonal Psychotherapy for perinatal depression. *Archives of Women's Mental Health, 15*(6), 469–480.

Brendgen, M., Wanner, B., Morin, A. J., & Vitaro, F. (2005). Relations with parents and with peers, temperament, and trajectories of depressed mood during early adolescence. *Journal of Abnormal Child Psychology, 33*(5), 579–594.

British Columbia Ministry of Health. *Clinical Practice Guidelines for the BC Eating Disorders Continuum of Services*. British Columbia Ministry of Health.

Brody, A. L., Saxena, S., Stoessel, P., Gillies, L. A., Fairbanks, L. A., Alborzian, S., et al. (2001). Regional brain metabolic changes in patients with major depression treated with either paroxetine or interpersonal therapy: preliminary findings. *Archives of General Psychiatry, 58*, 631–640.

Brown, G. W., & Harris, T. (1978). *Social origins of depression*. New York: Free Press.

Browne, G., Steiner, M., Roberts, J., Gafni, A., Byrne, C., Dunn, E., et al. (2002). Sertraline and/or interpersonal psychotherapy for patients with dysthymic disorder in primary care: 6-month comparison with longitudinal 2-year follow-up of effectiveness and costs. *Affective Disorders, 68*, 317–330.

Bruce, M. L., Have, T. T., Reynolds, C. F., Katz, I. I., Schulberg, H. C., Mulsant, B. H., et al. (2004). Reducing suicidal ideation and depressive symptoms in depressed older primary care patients: A randomized controlled trial. *Journal of the American Medical Association, 291*, 1081–1091.

Campanini, R. F., Schoedl, A. F., Pupo, M. C., Costa, A. C., Krupnick, J. L., & Mello, M. F. (2010). Efficacy of interpersonal therapy-group format adapted to post-traumatic stress disorder: an open-label add-on trial. *Depression and Anxiety, 27*(1), 72–77.

Carreira, K., Miller, M. D., Frank, E., Houck, P. R., Morse, J. Q., Dew, M. A., et al. (2008). A controlled evaluation of monthly maintenance interpersonal psychotherapy in late-life depression with varying levels of cognitive function. *International Journal of Geriatric Psychiatry, 23*, 1110–1113.

Carroll, K. M., Rounsaville, B. J., & Gawin, F. H. (1991). A comparative trial of psychotherapies for ambulatory cocaine abusers: Relapse prevention and interpersonal psychotherapy. *American Journal of Drug and Alcohol Abuse, 17*, 229–247.

Carter, F. A., Jordan, J., McIntosh, V. V., Luty, S. E., McKenzie, J. M., Frampton, C. M., et al. (2010). The long-term efficacy of three psychotherapies for anorexia nervosa: a randomized, controlled trial. *International Journal of Eating Disorders, 44*(7), 647–654.

Carter, W., Grigoriadis, S., Ravitz, P., & Ross, L. E. (2010). Conjoint IPT for postpartum depression: literature review and overview of a treatment manual. *American Journal of Psychotherapy, 64*, 373–392.

Caspi, A., Sugden, K., Moffitt, T. E., Taylor, A., Craig, I. W., Harrington, H. L., et al. (2003). Influence of life stress on depression: moderation by a polymorphism in the 5-HTT gene. *Science, 301*, 386–389.

Ceballos, A. M. G., Andrade, A. C., Markowitz, T., & Verdeli, H. (2016). "You pulled me out of a dark well": a case study of a Colombian displaced woman empowered through interpersonal counseling (IPC). *Journal of Clinical Psychology, 72*, 839–846.

Cherry, S., & Markowitz, J. C. (1996). Interpersonal psychotherapy. In J. S. Kantor (Ed.), *Clinical depression during addiction recovery: Process, diagnosis, and treatment* (pp. 165–185). New York: Marcel Dekker.

Chung, J. P. (2015). Interpersonal psychotherapy for postnatal anxiety disorder. *East Asian Archives of Psychiatry, 25*, 88–94.

Clark, R., Tluczek, A., & Wenzel, A. (2003). Psychotherapy for postpartum depression: a preliminary report. *American Journal of Orthopsychiatry, 73*(4), 441–454.

Clougherty, K. F., Verdeli, H., & Weissman, M. M. (2003). *Interpersonal psychotherapy adapted for a group in Uganda (IPT-G-U)*. Unpublished manual available from M. M. Weissman, New York State Psychiatric Institute, 1051 Riverside Drive, Unit 24, New York, NY 10032.

Cohen, L. S., Altshuler, L. L., Harlow, B. L., Nonacs, R., Newport, D. J., Viguera, A. C., et al. (2006). Relapse of major depression during pregnancy in women who maintain or discontinue antidepressant treatment. *Journal of the American Medical Association*, *295*, 499–507.

Cooper, Z., Allen, E., Bailey-Straebler, S., Basden, S., Murphy, R., O'Connor, M. E., & Fairburn, C. G. (2016). Predictors and moderators of response to enhanced cognitive behaviour therapy and interpersonal psychotherapy for the treatment of eating disorders. *Behaviour Research and Therapy*, *84*, 9–13.

Cox, J. L., Holden, J. M., & Sagovsky, R. (1987). Detection of postnatal depression. Development of the 10-item Edinburgh Postnatal Depression Scale. *British Journal of Psychiatry*, *150*, 782–786.

Cristea, I. A., Gentili, C., Cotet, C. D., Palomba, D., Barbui, C., & Cuijpers, P. (2017). Efficacy of psychotherapies for borderline personality disorder: a systematic review and meta-analysis. *JAMA Psychiatry*, *74*, 319–328.

Cuijpers, P., Donker, T., Weissman, M. M., Ravitz, P., & Cristea, I. A. (2016). Interpersonal psychotherapy for mental health problems: a comprehensive meta-analysis. *American Journal of Psychiatry*, *173*, 680–687.

Cuijpers, P., Geraedts, A. S., van Oppen, P., Andersson, G., Markowitz, J. C., & van Straten, A. (2011). Interpersonal psychotherapy of depression: a meta-analysis. *American Journal of Psychiatry*, *168*, 581–592.

Cuijpers, P., Sijbrandij, M., Koole, S. L., Andersson, G., Beekman, A. T., & Reynolds, C. F. 3rd. (2013). The efficacy of psychotherapy and pharmacotherapy in treating depressive and anxiety disorders: a meta-analysis of direct comparisons. *World Psychiatry*, *12*, 137–148.

Cuijpers, P., van Straten, A., Andersson, G., & van Oppen, P. (2008). Psychotherapy for depression in adults: a meta-analysis of comparative outcome studies. *Journal of Consulting and Clinical Psychology*, *76*, 909–922.

Cyranowski, J. M., Frank, E., Winter, E., Rucci, P., Novick, D., Pilkonis, P., et al. (2004). Personality pathology and outcome in recurrently depressed women over 2 years of maintenance interpersonal psychotherapy. *Psychological Medicine*, *34*, 659–669.

Dagöö, J., Asplund, R. P., Bsenko, H. A., Hjerling, S., Holmberg, A., Westh, S., et al. (2014). Cognitive behavior therapy versus interpersonal psychotherapy for social anxiety disorder delivered via smartphone and computer: a randomized controlled trial. *Journal of Anxiety Disorders*, *28*, 410–417,

Davis, D., Thomson O'Brien, M. A., Freemantle, N., Wolf, F. M., Mazmanian, P., & Taylor-Vaisey, A. (1999). Impact of formal continuing medical education: Do conferences, workshops, rounds, and other formal traditional continuing education activities change physician behavior and health care outcomes? *Journal of the American Medical Association*, *282*, 867–874.

de Mello, M. F., Myczcowisk, L. M., & Menezes, P. R. (2001). A randomized controlled trial comparing moclobemide and moclobemide plus interpersonal psychotherapy in the treatment of dysthymic disorder. *Journal of Psychotherapy Practice and Research*, *10*(2), 117–123.

Dennis, C. L., & Hodnett, E. (2007). Psychosocial and psychological interventions for treating postpartum depression. *Cochrane Database of Systematic Reviews,* Oct 17;(4):CD006116.

Dietz, L. J., Mufson, L., Irvine, H., & Brent, D. A. (2008). Family-based interpersonal psychotherapy for depressed preadolescents: an open-treatment trial. *Early Intervention in Psychiatry. 2*(3). 154–161.

Dietz, L. J., Weinberg, R. J., Brent, D. A., & Mufson, L. (2015). Family-based interpersonal psychotherapy for depressed preadolescents: examining efficacy and potential treatment mechanisms. *Journal of the American Academy of Child and Adolescent Psychiatry, 54*(3), 191–199.

Donker, T., Bennett, K., Bennett, A., Mackinnon, A., van Straten, A., Cuijpers, P., et al. (2013). Internet-delivered interpersonal psychotherapy versus internet-delivered cognitive behavioral therapy for adults with depressive symptoms: randomized controlled noninferiority trial. *Journal of Medical Internet Research, 15*(5), e82.

Donnelly, J. M., Kornblith, A. B., Fleishman, S., Zuckerman, E., Raptis, G., Hudis, C. A., et al. (2000). A pilot study of interpersonal psychotherapy by telephone with cancer patients and their partners. *Psychooncology, 9*(1), 44–56.

Dugdale, D. C., Epstein, R., & Pantilat, S. Z. (1999). Time and the patient–physician relationship. *Journal of General Internal Medicine, 14*(Suppl 1), S34–S40.

Ekeblad, A., Falkenström, F., Andersson, G., Vestberg, R., & Holmqvist, R. (2016). Randomized trial of interpersonal psychotherapy and cognitive behavioral therapy for major depressive disorder in a community-based psychiatric outpatient clinic. *Depression & Anxiety, 33*, 1090–1098.

Elkin, I., Gibbons, R. D., Shea, M. T., Sotsky, S. M., Watkins, J. T., Pilkonis, P. A., & Hedeker, D. (1995). Initial severity and differential treatment outcome in the National Institute of Mental Health Treatment of Depression Collaborative Research Program. *Journal of Consulting and Clinical Psychology, 63*, 841–847.

Elkin, I., Shea, M. T., Watkins, J. T., Imber, S. D., Sotsky, S. M., Collins, J. F., et al. (1989). National Institute of Mental Health treatment of depression collaborative research program: General effectiveness of treatments. *Archives of General Psychiatry, 46*, 971–982.

Evans, D. L., Charney, D. S., Lewis, L., Golden, R. N., Gorman, J. M., Krishnan, K. R., et al. (2005). Mood disorders in the medically ill: scientific review and recommendations. *Biological Psychiatry, 58*(3), 175–189.

Fairburn, C. G., Bailey-Straebler, S., Basden, S., Doll, H. A., Jones, R., Murphy, R., et al. (2015). A transdiagnostic comparison of enhanced cognitive behaviour therapy (CBT-E) and interpersonal psychotherapy in the treatment of eating disorders. *Behavioural Research and Therapy, 70*, 64–71.

Fairburn, C. G., Jones, R., Peveler, R. C., Carr, S. J., Solomon, R. A., O'Connor, M. E., et al. (1991). Three psychological treatments for bulimia nervosa. A comparative trial. *Archives of General Psychiatry, 48*(5), 463–469.

Fairburn, C. G., Jones, R., Peveler, R. C., Hope, R. A., & O'Connor, M. (1993). Psychotherapy and bulimia nervosa: Longer-term effects of interpersonal psychotherapy, behavior therapy, and cognitive behavior therapy. *Archives of General Psychiatry, 50*, 419–428.

Falkenström, F., Markowitz, J. C., Jonker, H., Philips, B., & Holmqvist, R. (2013). Can psychotherapists function as their own controls? Meta-analysis of the "crossed therapist" design in comparative psychotherapy trials. *Journal of Clinical Psychiatry*, *74*, 482–491.

Fearon, R. M., Van Ijzendoorn, M. H., Fonagy, P., Bakermans-Kranenburg, M. J., Schuengel, C., & Bokhorst, C. L. (2006). In search of shared and nonshared environmental factors in security of attachment: a behavior-genetic study of the association between sensitivity and attachment security. *Developmental Psychology*, *42*, 1026–1040.

Feijò de Mello, M., Myczowisk, L. M., & Menezes, P. R. (2001). A randomized controlled trial comparing moclobemide and moclobemide plus interpersonal psychotherapy in the treatment of dysthymic disorder. *Journal of Psychotherapy Practice and Research*, *10*, 117–123.

Fisher, J., Cabral de Mello, M., Patel, V., Rahman, A., Tran, T., Holton, S., & Holmes, W. (2012). Prevalence and determinants of common perinatal mental disorders in women in low- and lower-middle-income countries: a systematic review. *Bulletin of the World Health Organization*, *90*(2), 139G–149G.

Foley, S. H., O'Malley, S., Rounsaville, B., Prusoff, B. A., & Weissman, M. M. (1987). The relationship of patient difficulty to therapist performance in interpersonal psychotherapy of depression. *Journal of Affective Disorders*, *12*, 207–217.

Foley, S. H., Rounsaville, B. J., Weissman, M. M., Sholomskas, D., & Chevron, E. (1989). Individual versus conjoint interpersonal psychotherapy for depressed patients with marital disputes. *International Journal of Family Psychiatry*, *10*, 29–42.

Fonagy, P., & Bateman, A. (2006). Progress in the treatment of borderline personality disorder. *British Journal of Psychiatry*, *188*, 1–3.

Frank, J. (1971). Therapeutic factors in psychotherapy. *American Journal of Psychotherapy*, *25*, 350–361.

Frank, E. (2005). *Treating bipolar disorder: A clinician's guide to interpersonal and social rhythm therapy*. New York: Guilford.

Frank, E., Cassano, G. B., Rucci, P., Thompson, W. K., Kraemer, H. C., Fagiolini, A., et al. (2011). Predictors and moderators of time to remission of major depression with interpersonal psychotherapy and SSRI pharmacotherapy. *Psychology in Medicine*, *41*, 151–162.

Frank, E., Kupfer, D. J., Buysse, D. J., Swartz, H. A., Pilkonis, P. A., Houck, P. R., et al. (2007). Randomized trial of weekly, twice-monthly, and monthly interpersonal psychotherapy as maintenance treatment for women with recurrent depression. *American Journal of Psychiatry*, *164*, 761–767.

Frank, E., Kupfer, D. J., Perel, J. M., Cornes, C. D., Jarrett, B., Mallinger, A. G., et al. (1990). Three-year outcomes for maintenance therapies in recurrent depression. *Archives of General Psychiatry*, *47*, 1093–1099.

Frank, E., Kupfer, D. J., Thase, M. E., Mallinger, A. G., Swartz, H., Fagiolini, A. M., et al. (2005). Two-year outcomes for interpersonal and social rhythm therapy in individuals with bipolar I disorder. *Archives of General Psychiatry*, *62*, 996–1004.

Frank, E., Kupfer, D. J., Wagner, E. F., McEachran, A. B., & Cornes, C. (1991). Efficacy of interpersonal psychotherapy as a maintenance treatment of recurrent depression: Contributing factors. *Archives of General Psychiatry*, *48*, 1053–1059.

Frank, E., Ritchey, F. C., & Levenson, J. C. (2014). Is interpersonal psychotherapy infinitely adaptable? A compendium of the multiple modifications of IPT. *American Journal of Psychotherapy*, *68*, 385–416.

Frank, E., Swartz, H. A., & Kupfer, D. J. (2000). Interpersonal and social rhythm therapy: Managing the chaos of bipolar disorder. *Biological Psychiatry*, *48*, 593–604.

Freud, S., & Strachey, J. E. (1964). *The standard edition of the complete psychological works of Sigmund Freud*. London: Hogarth Press.

Gallo, J. J., Bogner, H. R., Morales, K. H., Post, E. P., Have, T. T., & Bruce, M. L. (2005). Depression, cardiovascular disease, diabetes, and two-year mortality among older, primary-care patients. *American Journal of Geriatric Psychiatry*, *13*, 748–755.

Gamble, S. A., Talbot, N. L., Cashman-Brown, S. M., He, H., Poleshuck, E. L., Connors, G. J., & Conner, K. R. (2013). A pilot study of interpersonal psychotherapy for alcohol-dependent women with co-occurring major depression. *Substance Abuse*, *34*(3), 233–241.

Gao, L. L., Chan, S. W., Li, X., Chen, S., & Hao, Y. (2010). Evaluation of an interpersonal-psychotherapy-oriented childbirth education programme for Chinese first-time childbearing women: a randomised controlled trial. *International Journal of Nursing Studies*, *47*(10), 1208–1216.

Gao, L. L., Xie, W., Yang, X., & Chan, S. W. (2015). Effects of an interpersonal-psychotherapy-oriented postnatal programme for Chinese first-time mothers: a randomized controlled trial. *International Journal of Nursing Studies*, *52*(1), 22–29.

Garrity, M. Evolving models of behavioral health integration: evidence update 2010–2015. http://www.milbank.org/uploads/documents/evovling%20Models%20of%20BHF.pdf. Accessed August 2, 2016.

Gois, C., Dias, V. V., Carmo, I., Duarte, R., Ferro, A., Santos, A. L., et al. (2014). Treatment response in type 2 diabetes patients with major depression. *Clinical Psychology and Psychotherapy*, *21*(1), 39–48.

Goldstein, T. R., Fersch-Podrat, R., Axelson, D. A., Gilbert, A., Hlastala, S. A., Birmaher, B., & Frank, E. (2014). Early intervention for adolescents at high risk for the development of bipolar disorder: pilot study of interpersonal and social rhythm therapy (IPSRT). *Psychotherapy*, *51*, 180–189.

Gomes, M. F., Chowdhary, N., Vousoura, E., & Verdeli, H. (2016). "When grief breaks your heart": A case study of interpersonal psychotherapy delivered in a primary care setting. *Journal of Clinical Psychology*, *72*(8), 807–817.

González, H. M., Vega, W. A., Williams, D. R., Tarraf, W., West, B. T., & Neighbors, H. W. (2010). Depression care in the United States: too little for too few. *Archives of General Psychiatry*, *67*(1), 37–46.

Gonzalez, J. S., Safren, S. A., Cagliero, E., Wexler, D. J., Delahanty, L., Wittenberg, E., et al. (2007). Depression, self-care, and medication adherence in Type 2 diabetes: Relationships across the full range of symptom severity. *Diabetes Care*, *30*, 2222–2227.

Goodrich, D. E., Kilbourne, A. M., Nord, K. M., & Bauer, M. S. (2013). Mental health collaborative care and its role in primary care settings. *Current Psychiatry Reports*, *15*(8), 383.

Graham, P. (2006). *An adaptation of interpersonal psychotherapy for depression within primary care (IPT-Brief)*. Paper presented at the International Society for International Psychotherapy, Second International Conference, Toronto, Canada.

Grote, N. K., Bledsoe, S. E., Swartz, H. A., & Frank, E. (2004a). Culturally relevant psychotherapy for perinatal depression in low-income ob/gyn patients. *Clinical Social Work Journal*, *32*(3), 327–347.

Grote, N. K., Bledsoe, S. E., Swartz, H. A., & Frank, E. (2004b). Feasibility of providing culturally relevant, brief interpersonal psychotherapy for antenatal depression in an obstetrics clinic: A pilot study. *Research on Social Work Practice*, *14*, 397–407.

Grote, N. K., Katon, W. J., Russo, J. E., Lohr, M. J., Curran, M., Galvin, E., & Carson, K. (2015). Collaborative care for perinatal depression in socioeconomically disadvantaged women: a randomized trial. *Depression and Anxiety*, *32*, 821–834.

Grote, N. K., Katon, W. J., Russo, J. E., Lohr, M. J., Curran, M., Galvin, E., & Carson, K. (2016). A randomized trial of collaborative care for perinatal depression in socioeconomically disadvantaged women: the impace of comorbid posttraumatic stress disorder. *Journal of Clinical Psychiatry*, *77*(11), 1527–1537.

Grote, N. K., Swartz, H. A., Geibel, S. L., Zuckoff, A., Houck, P. R., & Frank, E. (2009). A randomized controlled trial of culturally relevant, brief interpersonal psychotherapy for perinatal depression. *Psychiatric Services*, *60*(3), 313–321.

Grote, N. K., Swartz, H. A., & Zuckoff, A. (2008). Enhancing interpersonal psychotherapy for mothers and expectant others on low incomes: adaptations and additions. *Contemporary Psychotherapy*, *38*, 23–33.

Grote, N. K., Zuckoff, A., Swartz, H., Bledsoe, S. E., & Geibel, S. (2007). Engaging women who are depressed and economically disadvantaged in mental health treatment. *Social Work*, *52*(4), 295–308.

Guffanti, G., Gameroff, M. J., Warner, V., Talati, A., Glatt, C. E., Wickramaratne, P., & Weissman, M. M. (2016). Heritability of major depressive and comorbid anxiety disorders in multi-generational families at high risk for depression. *American Journal of Medical Genetics B*, *171*, 1072–1079.

Gunderson, J. G., Stout, R. L., McGlashan, T. H., Shea, M. T., Morey, L. C., Grilo, C. M., et al. (2011). Ten-year course of borderline personality disorder: psychopathology and function from the Collaborative Longitudinal Personality Disorders Study. *Archives of General Psychiatry*, *68*, 827–837.

Hamilton, M. (1960). A rating scale for depression. *Journal of Neurology, Neurosurgery, and Psychiatry*, *25*, 56–62.

Heckman, T. G., Heckman, B. D., Anderson, T. I., Markowitz, J. C., Lovejoy, T., Shen, Y., & Sutton, M. (2016). Tele-interpersonal psychotherapy acutely reduces depressive symptoms in depressed HIV-infected rural persons: a randomized clinical trial. *Behavioral Medicine* April 26 [Epub ahead of print].

Hellerstein, D. J., Little, S. A. S., Samstag, L. W., Batchelder, S., Muran, J. C., Fedak, M., et al. (2001). Adding group psychotherapy to medication treatment in dysthymia. *Journal of Psychotherapy Practice and Research*, *10*, 93–103.

Hilbert, A., Bishop, M. E., Stein, R. I., Tanofsky-Kraff, M., Swenson, A. K., Welch, R. R., & Wilfley, D. E. (2012). Long-term efficacy of psychological treatments for binge eating disorder. *British Journal of Psychiatry*, *200*(3), 232–237.

Hilbert, A., Saelens, B. E., Stein, R. I., Mockus, D. S., Welch, R. R., Matt, G. E., & Wilfley, D. E. (2007). Pretreatment and process predictors of outcome in interpersonal and cognitive behavioral psychotherapy for binge eating disorder. *Journal of Consulting and Clinical Psychology*, *75*(4), 645–651.

Hinrichsen, G. A., & Clougherty, K. F. (2006). *Interpersonal psychotherapy for depressed older adults*. Washington, DC: American Psychological Association.

Hlastala, S. A., Kotler, J. S., McClellan, J. M., & McCauley, E. A. (2010). Interpersonal and social rhythm therapy for adolescents with bipolar disorder: treatment development and results from an open trial. *Depression and Anxiety*, *27*(5), 457–464.

Hoberg, A. A., Ponto, J., Nelson, P. J., & Frye, M. A. (2013). Group interpersonal and social rhythm therapy for bipolar depression. *Perspectives in Psychiatric Care, 49*(4), 226–234.

Hoffart, A., Abrahamsen, G., Bonsaksen, T., Borge, F. M., Ramstad, R., & Markowitz, J. C. (2007). *A residential interpersonal treatment for social phobia*. New York: Nova Science Publishers.

Hoffart, A., Borge, F. M., Sexton, H., & Clark, D. M. (2009). The role of common factors in residential cognitive and interpersonal therapy for social phobia: a process-outcome study. *Psychotherapy Research, 19*, 54–67.

Hoffer, M., Markowitz, J. C., & Blanco, C. (2012). Interpersonal psychotherapy for medically ill depressed patients. In J. C. Markowitz & M. M. Weissman (Eds.), *Casebook of interpersonal psychotherapy* (pp. 267–282). New York: Oxford University Press.

Hollon, S. D. (1984). *Final report: System for rating psychotherapy audiotapes*. Bethesda, MD: U.S. Department of Health and Human Services.

Holmes, A., Hodgins, G., Adey, S., Menzel, S., Danne, P., Kossmann, T., & Judd, F. (2007). Trial of interpersonal counselling after major physical trauma. *Australia and New Zealand Journal of Psychiatry, 41*(11), 926–933.

Holmes, T. H., & Rahe, R. H. (1967). The social readjustment rating scale. *Journal of Psychosomatic Research, 11*, 213–218.

Horowitz, J. L., Garber, J., Ciesla, J. A., Young, J. F., & Mufson, L. (2007). Prevention of depressive symptoms in adolescents: a randomized trial of cognitive-behavioral and interpersonal prevention programs. *Journal of Consulting and Clinical Psychology, 75*(5), 693–706.

IAPT; Institute of Medicine. (2015). *Psychosocial interventions for mental and substance use disorders: a framework for establishing evidence-based standards*. Washington, DC: National Academies Press.

Jacobson, C. M., & Mufson, L. (2012). Interpersonal psychotherapy for depressed adolescents adapted for self-injury (IPT-ASI): rationale, overview, and case summary. *American Journal of Psychotherapy, 66*(4), 349–374.

Jiang, R. F., Tong, H. Q., Delucchi, K. L., Neylan, T. C., Shi, Q., & Meffert, S. M. (2014). Interpersonal psychotherapy versus treatment as usual for PTSD and depression among Sichuan earthquake survivors: a randomized clinical trial. *Conflict and Health, 8*, 14.

Johnson, J. E., Williams, C., & Zlotnick, C. (2015). Development and feasibility of a cell phone-based transitional intervention for women prisoners with comorbid substance use and depression. *Prison Journal, 95*(3), 330–352.

Johnson, J. E., & Zlotnick, C. (2008). A pilot study of group interpersonal psychotherapy for depression in substance-abusing female prisoners. *Journal of Substance Abuse Treatment, 34*(4), 371–377.

Johnson, J. E., & Zlotnick, C. (2012). Pilot study of treatment for major depression among women prisoners with substance use disorder. *Journal of Psychiatric Research, 46*(9), 1174–1183.

Johnson, S. M., Hunsley, J., Greenberg, L., & Schindler, D. (1999). Emotionally focused couples therapy: status and challenges. *Clinical Psychology: Science and Practice, 6*, 67–79.

Judd, F. K., Piterman, L., Cockram, A. M., McCall, L., & Weissman, M. M. (2001). A comparative study of venlafaxine with a focused education and psychotherapy program versus venlafaxine alone in the treatment of depression in general practice. *Human Psychopharmacology*, 16(5), 423–428.

Judd, L. L., & Akiskal, H. S. (2000). Delineating the longitudinal structure of depressive illness: Beyond clinical subtypes and duration thresholds. *Pharmacopsychiatry*, 1, 3–7.

Judd, L. L., Akiskal, H. S., Maser, J. D., Zeller, P. J., Endicott, J., Coryell, W., et al. (1998). A prospective 12-year study of subsyndromal and syndromal depressive symptoms in unipolar major depressive disorders. *Archives of General Psychiatry*, 55, 694–700.

Judd, L. L., Rapaport, M. H., Yonkers, K. A., Rush, A. J., Frank, E., Thase, M. E., et al. (2004). Randomized, placebo-controlled trial of fluoxetine for acute treatment of minor depressive disorder. *American Journal of Psychiatry*, 161(10), 1864–1871.

Karlsson, H., Säteri, U., & Markowitz, J. C. (2011). Interpersonal psychotherapy for Finnish community patients with moderate to severe major depressive disorder and comorbidities: a pilot feasibility study. *Nordic Journal of Psychiatry*, 65, 427–432.

Karp, J. F., Scott, J., Houck, P., Reynolds, C. F., III, Kupfer, D. J., & Frank, E. (2005). Pain predicts longer time to remission during treatment of recurrent depression. *Journal of Clinical Psychiatry*, 66, 591–597.

Karyotaki, E., Smit, Y., Holdt Henningsen, K., Huibers, M. J., Robays, J., de Beurs, D., & Cuijpers, P. (2016). Combining pharmacotherapy and psychotherapy or monotherapy for major depression? A meta-analysis on the long-term effects. *Journal of Affective Disorders*, 194, 144–152.

Kass, A. E., Kolko, R. P., & Wilfley, D. E. (2013). Psychological treatments for eating disorders. *Current Opinion in Psychiatry*, 26(6), 549–555.

Katon, W. J. (2011). Epidemiology and treatment of depression in patients with chronic medical illness. *Dialogues in Clinical Neuroscience*, 13(1), 7–23.

Katon, W., Unützer, J., Wells, K., & Jones, L. (2010). Collaborative depression care: history, evolution and ways to enhance dissemination and sustainability. *General Hospital Psychiatry*, 32(5), 456–464.

Kebede, D., Alem, A., & Rashid, E. (1999). The prevalence and socio-demographic correlates of mental distress in Addis Ababa, Ethiopia. *Acta Psychiatrica Scandinavica Supplement*, 397, 5–10.

Kessler, R. G., Berglund, P., Demler, O., Jin, R., Merikangas, K. R., & Walters, E. E. (2005). Lifetime prevalence and age-of-onset distributions of DSM-IV disorders in the National Comorbidity Survey Replication. *Archives of General Psychiatry*, 62, 593–602.

Klass, E. T., Milrod, B. L., Leon, A. C., Kay, S., Schwalberg, M., & Markowitz, J. C. (2009). Does interpersonal loss preceding panic disorder onset moderate response to psychotherapy? *Journal of Clinical Psychiatry*, 70, 406–411.

Klerman, G. L. (1991). Ideological conflicts in integrating pharmacotherapy and psychotherapy. In B. D. Beitman & G. L. Klerman (Eds.), *Integrating Pharmacotherapy and Psychotherapy* (pp. 3–19). Washington, DC: American Psychiatric Press.

Klerman, G. L., Budman, S., Berwick, D., Weissman, M. M., Damico-White, J., Demby, A., & Feldstein, M. (1987). Efficacy of a brief psychosocial intervention for symptoms of stress and distress among patients in primary care. *Medical Care*, 25(11), 1078–1088.

Klerman, G. L., DiMascio, A., Weissman, M. M., Prusoff, B. A., & Paykel, E. S. (1974). Treatment of depression by drugs and psychotherapy. *American Journal of Psychiatry*, 131, 186–191.

Klerman, G. L., Weissman, M. M., Rounsaville, B., & Chevron, E. (1984). *Interpersonal psychotherapy of depression*. New York: Basic Books.

Klier, C. M., Muzik, M., Rosenblum, K. L., & Lenz, G. (2001). Interpersonal psychotherapy adapted for the group setting in the treatment of postpartum depression. *Journal of Psychotherapy Practice and Research, 10*(2), 124–131.

Kocsis, J. H., Gelenberg, A. J., Rothbaum, B. O., Klein, D. N., Trivedi, M. H., Manber, R., et al. (2009). Cognitive behavioral analysis system of psychotherapy (CBASP) and brief supportive psychotherapy for augmentation of antidepressant nonresponse in chronic depression: the REVAMP trial. *Archives of General Psychiatry, 66*, 1178–1188.

Kontunen, J., Timonen, M., Muotka, J., & Liukkonen, T. (2016). Is interpersonal counselling (IPC) sufficient treatment for depression in primary care patients? A pilot study comparing IPC and interpersonal psychotherapy (IPT). *Journal of Affective Disorders, 189*, 89–93.

Koszycki, D., Bisserbe, J. C., Blier, P., Bradwejn, J., & Markowitz, J. (2012). Interpersonal psychotherapy versus brief supportive therapy for depressed infertile women: first pilot randomized controlled trial. *Archive of Women's Mental Health, 15*(3), 193–201.

Kovacs, M., Obrosky, S., & George, C. (2016). The course of major depressive disorder from childhood to young adulthood: Recovery and recurrence in a longitudinal observational study. *Journal of Affective Disorders, 203*, 374–381.

Kroenke, K., Spitzer, R. L., & Williams, J. B. (2001). The PHQ-9: validity of a brief depression severity measure. *Journal of General Internal Medicine, 16*, 606–613.

Krupnick, J. L., Green, B. L., Stockton, P., Miranda, J., Krause, E., & Mete, M. (2008). Group interpersonal psychotherapy for low-income women with posttraumatic stress disorder. *Psychotherapy Research, 18*(5), 497–507.

Krupnick, J. L., Melnikoff, E., & Reinhard, M. (2016). A pilot study of interpersonal psychotherapy for PTSD in women veterans. *Psychiatry, 79*, 56–69.

Krupnick, J. L., Sotsky, S. M., Simmens, S., Moyer, J., Elkin, I., Watkins, J., & Pilkonis, P. A. (1996). The role of the therapeutic alliance in psychotherapy and pharmacotherapy outcome: findings in the National Institute of Mental Health Treatment of Depression Collaborative Research Program. *Journal of Consulting and Clinical Psychology, 64*, 532–539.

Lenze, S. N., & Potts, M. A. (2016). Brief interpersonal psychotherapy for depression during pregnancy in a low-income population: a randomized controlled trial. *Journal of Affective Disorders, 210*, 151–157.

Lespérance, F., Frasure-Smith, N., Koszycki, D., Laliberté, M. A., van Zyl, L. T., Baker, B., et al. (2007). Effects of citalopram and interpersonal psychotherapy on depression in patients with coronary artery disease: the Canadian Cardiac Randomized Evaluation of Antidepressant and Psychotherapy Efficacy (CREATE) trial. *Journal of the American Medical Association, 297*(4), 367–379. [Erratum in: *Journal of the American Medical Association*, 2007 Jul 4;298(1):40.]

Levenson, J. C., Frank, E., Cheng, Y., Rucci, P., Janney, C. A., Houck, P., et al. (2010). Comparative outcomes amont the problem areas of interpersonal psychotherapy for depression. *Depression and Anxiety, 27*, 434–440.

Lewis-Fernandez, R. (2015). *DSM-5(r) Handbook on the Cultural Formulation Interview*. Arlington, VA: American Psychiatric Publishing.

Lichtmacher, J. E., Eisendrath, S. J., & Haller, E. (2006). Implementing interpersonal psychotherapy into a psychiatry residency training program. *Academic Psychiatry, 30*, 385–391.

Linehan, M. M., Armstrong, H. E., Suárez, A., Allmon, D., & Heard, H. L. (1991). Cognitive-behavioral treatment of chronically parasuicidal borderline patients. *Archives of General Psychiatry, 48*, 1060–1064.

Lipsitz, J. D., Fyer, A. J., Markowitz, J. C., & Cherry, S. (1999). An open trial of interpersonal psychotherapy for social phobia. *American Journal of Psychiatry, 156*, 1814–1816.

Lipsitz, J. D., Gur, M., Miller, N., Vermes, D., & Fyer, A. J. (2006). An open trial of interpersonal psychotherapy for panic disorder (IPT-PD). *Journal of Nervous and Mental Disease, 194*(6), 440–445.

Lipsitz, J. D., Gur, M., Vermes, D., Petkova, E., Cheng, J., Miller, N., et al. (2008). A randomized trial of interpersonal therapy versus supportive therapy for social anxiety disorder. *Depression and Anxiety, 25*, 542–553.

Lipsitz, J. D., & Markowitz, J. C. (2006). *Manual for interpersonal psychotherapy for social phobia (IPT-SP)*. Available from Joshua D. Lipsitz, Ph.D., Anxiety Disorders Clinic, New York State Psychiatric Association, 1051 Riverside Drive, Unit 69, New York, NY 10032.

Lipsitz, J. D., & Markowitz, J. C. (2013). Mechanisms of change in interpersonal psychotherapy. *Clinical Psychology Review, 33*, 1134–1147.

Lo, H. T., & Fung, K. (2003). Culturally competent psychotherapy. *Canadian Journal of Psychiatry, 48*, 161–170.

London, P., & Klerman, G. L. (1982). Evaluating psychotherapy. *American Journal of Psychiatry, 139*, 709–717.

Maciejewski, P. K., Maercker, A., Boelen, P. A., & Prigerson, H. G. (2016). Prolonged grief disorder and persistent complex bereavement disorder but not complicated grief are one and the same diagnostic entity: an analysis of data from the Yale Bereavement Study. *World Psychiatry, 15*, 266–273.

Malm, H., Brown, A. S., Gissler, M., Gyllenberg, D., Hinkka-Yli-Salomäki, S., McKeague, I. W., et al. (2016). Gestational exposure to selective serotonin reuptake inhibitors and offspring psychiatric disorders: a national register-based study. *Journal of the American Academy of Child and Adolescent Psychiatry, 55*(5), 359–366.

Marcus, S. C., & Olfson, M. (2010). National trends in the treatment for depression from 1998 to 2007. *Archives of General Psychiatry, 67*, 1265–1273.

Markowitz, J. C. (1993). Psychotherapy of the postdysthymic patient. *Journal of Psychotherapy Practice and Research, 2*(2), 157.

Markowitz, J. C. (1998). *Interpersonal psychotherapy for dysthymic disorder*. Washington, DC: American Psychiatric Publishing.

Markowitz, J. C. (2005). Interpersonal therapy of personality disorders. In J. M. Oldham, A. E. Skodol, & D. E. Bender (Eds.), *Textbook of personality disorders* (pp. 321–338). Washington, DC: American Psychiatric Publishing.

Markowitz, J. C. (2012). Interpersonal psychotherapy for personality disorders. In T. Widiger (Ed.), *Oxford handbook of personality disorder* (pp. 751–766). New York: Oxford University Press.

Markowitz, J. C. (2016). *Interpersonal psychotherapy for posttraumatic stress disorder*. New York: Oxford University Press.

Markowitz, J. C., Bleiberg, K. L., Christos, P., & Levitan, E. (2006). Solving interpersonal problems correlates with symptom improvement in interpersonal psychotherapy: Preliminary findings. *Journal of Nervous and Mental Disease, 194,* 15–20.

Markowitz, J. C., Bleiberg, K. L., Pessin, H., & Skodol, A. E. (2007). Adapting interpersonal psychotherapy for borderline personality disorder. *Journal of Mental Health, 16,* 103–116.

Markowitz, J. C., Kocsis, J. H., Bleiberg, K. L., Christos, P. J., & Sacks, M. H. (2005). A comparative trial of psychotherapy and pharmacotherapy for "pure" dysthymic patients. *Journal of Affective Disorders, 89,* 167–175.

Markowitz, J. C., Kocsis, J. H., Christos, P., Bleiberg, K., & Carlin, A. (2008). Pilot study of interpersonal psychotherapy versus supportive psychotherapy for dysthymic patients with secondary alcohol abuse or dependence. *Journal of Nervous and Mental Disease, 196*(6), 468–474.

Markowitz, J. C., Kocsis, J. H., Fishman, B., Spielman, L. A., Jacobsberg, L. B., Frances, A. J., et al. (1998). Treatment of depressive symptoms in human immunodeficiency virus-positive patients. *Archives of General Psychiatry, 55,* 452–457.

Markowitz, J. C., Leon, A. C., Miller, N. L., Cherry, S., Clougherty, K. F., & Villalobos, L. (2000). Rater agreement on interpersonal psychotherapy problem areas. *Journal of Psychotherapy Practice and Research, 9,*131–135.

Markowitz, J. C., Lipsitz, J., & Milrod, B. L. (2014). A critical review of outcome research on interpersonal psychotherapy for anxiety disorders. *Depression and Anxiety, 31,* 316–325.

Markowitz, J. C., Meehan, K. B., Petkova, E., Zhao, Y., Van Meter, P. E., Neria, Y., et al. (2016). Treatment preferences of psychotherapy patients with chronic PTSD. *Journal of Clinical Psychiatry, 77,* 363–370.

Markowitz, J. C., & Milrod, B. (2011). The importance of responding to negative affect in psychotherapies. *American Journal of Psychiatry, 168,* 124–128.

Markowitz, J. C., & Milrod, B. L. (2015). What to do when a psychotherapy fails. *The Lancet Psychiatry, 2,* 186–190.

Markowitz, J. C., Milrod, B., Bleiberg, K. L., & Marshall, R. D. (2009). Interpersonal factors in understanding and treating posttraumatic stress disorder. *Journal of Psychiatric Practice, 15,* 133–140.

Markowitz, J. C., Neria, Y., Lovell, K., Van Meter, P. E., & Petkova, E. (2017). History of sexual trauma moderates psychotherapy outcome for posttraumatic stress disorder. *Depression and Anxiety.* Apr 4 [Epub ahead of print]

Markowitz, J. C., Patel, S. R., Balan, I., McNamara, M., Blanco, C., Brave Heart, M. Y. H., et al. (2009). Towards an adaptation of interpersonal psychotherapy for depressed Hispanic patients. *Journal of Clinical Psychiatry, 70,* 214–222.

Markowitz, J. C., Petkova, E., Biyanova, T., Ding, K., Suh, E. J., & Neria, Y. (2015a). Exploring personality diagnosis stability following acute psychotherapy for chronic posttraumatic stress disorder. *Depression and Anxiety, 32,* 919–926.

Markowitz, J. C., Petkova, E., Neria, Y., Van Meter, P., Zhao, Y., Hembree, E., et al. (2015b). Is exposure necessary? A randomized clinical trial of interpersonal psychotherapy for PTSD. *American Journal of Psychiatry, 172,* 430–440.

Markowitz, J. C., Skodol, A. E., & Bleiberg, K. (2006). Interpersonal psychotherapy for borderline personality disorder: Possible mechanisms of change. *Journal of Clinical Psychology, 62,* 431–444.

Markowitz, J. C., Svartberg, M., & Swartz, H. A. (1998). Is IPT time-limited psychodynamic psychotherapy? *Journal of Psychotherapy Practice and Research, 7*, 185–195.

Markowitz, J. C., & Swartz, H. A. (1998). Case formulation in interpersonal psychotherapy of depression. In T. D. Eells (Ed.), *Handbook of psychotherapy case formulation* (pp. 192–222). New York: Guilford.

Markowitz, J. C., & Swartz, H. A. (2007). Case formulation in interpersonal psychotherapy of depression. In T. D. Eells (Ed.), *Handbook of psychotherapy case formulation* (2nd ed., pp. 221–250). New York: Guilford Press.

Markowitz, J. C., & Weissman, M. M. (Eds.). (2012). *Casebook of interpersonal psychotherapy.* New York: Oxford University Press.

Markowitz, J. C., & Weissman, M. M. (2012). Interpersonal psychotherapy: past, present and future. *Clinical Psychology and Psychotherapy, 19*(2), 99–105.

Martin, S. D., Martin, E., Rai, S. S., Richardson, M. A., & Royall, R. (2001). Brain blood flow changes in depressed patients treated with interpersonal psychotherapy or venlafaxine hydrochloride: preliminary findings. *Archives of General Psychiatry, 58*, 641–648.

Matthews, M., Abdullah, S., Murnane, E., Voida, S., Choudhury, T., Gay, G., & Frank, E. (2016). Development and evaluation of a smartphone-based measure of social rhythms for bipolar disorder. *Assessment, 23*, 472–483.

McHugh, R. K., Whitton, S. W., Peckham, A. D., Welge, J. A., & Otto, M. W. (2013). Patient preference for psychological vs pharmacologic treatment of psychiatric disorders: a meta-analytic review. *Journal of Clinical Psychiatry, 74*(6), 595–602.

McIntosh, V. V., Jordan, J., Carter, F. A., Luty, S. E., McKenzie, J.M., Bulik, C. M., et al. (2005). Three psychotherapies for anorexia nervosa: A randomized, controlled trial. *American Journal of Psychiatry, 162*, 741–747.

McMain, S. F., Guimond, T., Streiner, D. L., Cardish, R. J., & Links, P. S. (2012). Dialectical behavior therapy compared with general psychiatric management for borderline personality disorder: clinical outcomes and functioning over a 2-year follow-up. *American Journal of Psychiatry, 169*, 650–661.

Meffert, S. M., Abdo, A. O., Alla, O. A. A., Elmakki, Y. O. M., Omer, A. A., Yousif, S., Metzler, T. J., & Marmar, C. R. (2014). A pilot randomized controlled trial of interpersonal psychotherapy for Sudanese refugees in Cairo, Egypt. *Psychological Trauma 6*(3), 240–249.

Menchetti, M., Bortolotti, B., Rucci, P., Scocco, P., Bombi, A., & Berardi, D.; DEPICS Study Group. (2010). Depression in primary care: interpersonal counseling vs selective serotonin reuptake inhibitors. The DEPICS Study. A multicenter randomized controlled trial. Rationale and design. *BMC Psychiatry, 10*, 97.

Menchetti, M., Rucci, P., Bortolotti, B., Bombi, A., Scocco, P., Kraemer, H. C., & Berardi, D.; DEPICS Group. (2014). Moderators of remission with interpersonal counselling or drug treatment in primary care patients with depression: randomised controlled trial. *British Journal of Psychiatry, 204*(2), 144–150.

Miklowitz, D. J., Otto, M. W., Frank, E., Reilly-Harrington, N. A., Kogan, J. N., Sachs, G. S., et al. (2007). Intensive psychosocial intervention enhances functioning in patients with bipolar depression: results from a 9-month randomized controlled trial. *American Journal of Psychiatry, 164*, 1340–1347.

Miller, L., & Weissman, M. M. (2002). Interpersonal psychotherapy delivered over the telephone to recurrent depressives: A pilot study. *Depression and Anxiety, 16*, 114–117.

Miller, M. D. (2009). *Clinician's guide to interpersonal psychotherapy in late life: Helping cognitively impaired or depressed elders and their caregivers.* New York: Oxford University Press.

Miller, M. D., & Reynolds, C. F. 3rd. (2007). Expanding the usefulness of interpersonal psychotherapy (IPT) for depressed elders with co-morbid cognitive impairment. *International Journal of Geriatric Psychiatry, 22*, 101–105.

Miller, W. R., & Carroll, K. M. (2006). *Rethinking substance abuse: What the science shows, and what we should do about it.* New York: Guilford Press.

Milrod, B. (2015). The IOM framework for developing evidence-based standards in the field of psychosocial interventions for mental illness and substance abuse: a dynamic researcher's perspective. Cause for concern. *Depression and Anxiety, 32*, 796–798.

Milrod, B., Chambless, D., Gallop, R., Busch, F. N., Schwalberg, M., McCarthy, K. S., et al. (2016). Psychotherapy for panic disorder: a tale of two sites. *Journal of Clinical Psychiatry, 77*, 927–935.

Milrod, B., Markowitz, J. C., Gerber, A. J., Cyranowski, J., Altemus, M., Shapiro, T., et al. (2014). Childhood separation anxiety and the pathogenesis and treatment of adult anxiety. *American Journal of Psychiatry, 171*, 34–43.

Miranda, J., & Cooper, L. A. (2004). Disparities in care for depression among primary care patients. *Journal of General Internal Medicine, 19*(2), 120–126.

Mitchell, J. E., Halmi, K., Wilson, G. T., Agras, W. S., Kraemer, H., & Crow, S. (2002). A randomized secondary treatment study of women with bulimia nervosa who fail to respond to CBT. *International Journal of Eating Disorders, 32*(3), 271–281.

Mossey, J. M., Knott, K. A., Higgins, M., & Talerico, K. (1996). Effectiveness of a psychosocial intervention, interpersonal counseling, for subdysthymic depression in medically ill elderly. *Journal of Gerontology Part A, 51*(4), M172–M178.

Mufson, L. (2010). Interpersonal psychotherapy for depressed adolescents (IPT-A): Extending the reach from academic to community settings. *Child and Adolescent Mental Health, 15*(2), 66–72.

Mufson, L., Dorta, K. P., Wickramaratne, P., Nomura, Y., Olfson, M., & Weissman, M. M. (2004). A randomized effectiveness trial of interpersonal psychotherapy for depressed adolescents. *Archives of General Psychiatry, 61*(6), 577–584.

Mufson, L., Gallagher, T., Dorta, K. P., & Young, J. F. (2004). A group adaptation of Interpersonal Psychotherapy for depressed adolescents. *American Journal of Psychotherapy, 58*(2), 220–237.

Mufson, L., Pollack Dorta, K., Moreau, D., & Weissman, M. M. (2004*). Interpersonal psychotherapy for depressed adolescents* (2d ed.). New York: Guilford.

Mufson, L. H., Pollack Dorta, K., Moreau, D., & Weissman, M. M. (2011). *Interpersonal psychotherapy for depressed adolescents* [paperback edition]. New York: Guilford.

Mufson, L., Weissman, M. M., Moreau, D., & Garfinkel, R. (1999). Efficacy of interpersonal psychotherapy for depressed adolescents. *Archives of General Psychiatry, 56*(6), 573–579.

Mufson, L., Yanes-Lukin, P., & Anderson, G. (2015). A pilot study of Brief IPT-A delivered in primary care. *General Hospital Psychiatry, 37*(5), 481–484.

Mulcahy, R., Reay, R. E., Wilkinson, R. B., & Owen, C. (2010). A randomised control trial for the effectiveness of group Interpersonal Psychotherapy for postnatal depression. *Archives of Women's Mental Health, 13*(2), 125–139.

Murphy, R., Straebler, S., Basden, S., Cooper, Z., & Fairburn, C. G. (2012). Interpersonal psychotherapy for eating disorders. *Clinical Psychology and Psychotherapy*, *19*(2), 150–158.

Najavits, L. M., & Weiss, R. D. (1994). The role of psychotherapy in the treatment of substance-use disorders. *Harvard Review of Psychiatry*, *2*(2), 84–96.

National Institute for Clinical Excellence. (2004). *Eating disorders: Core interventions in the treatment and management of anorexia nervosa, bulimia nervosa and related eating disorders* (clinical guideline 9). London, UK: National Institute for Clinical Excellence.

Neugebauer, R., Kline, J., Bleiberg, K., Baxi, L., Markowitz, J. C., Rosing, M., et al. (2007). Preliminary open trial of interpersonal counseling for subsyndromal depression following miscarriage. *Depression and Anxiety*, *24*(3), 219–222.

Neugebauer, R., Kline, J., Markowitz, J. C., Bleiberg, K., Baxi, L., Rosing, M., et al. (2006). Pilot randomized controlled trial of interpersonal counseling for subsyndromal depression following miscarriage. *Journal of Clinical Psychiatry*, *67*, 1299–1304.

Novalis, P. N., Rojcewicz, S. J., & Peele, R. (1993). *Clinical manual of supportive psychotherapy.* Washington, DC: American Psychiatric Press.

O'Connor, E., Rossom, R. C., Henninger, M., Groom, H. C., & Burda, B. U. (2016). Primary care screening for and treatment of depression in pregnant and postpartum women: Evidence report and systematic review for the US Preventive Services Task Force. *Journal of the American Medical Association*, *315*(4), 388–406.

O'Hara, M. W., Stuart, S., Gorman, L. L., & Wenzel, A. (2000). Efficacy of interpersonal psychotherapy for postpartum depression. *Archives of General Psychiatry*, *57*(11), 1039–1045.

Onu, C., Ongeri, L., Bukusi, E., Cohen, C. R., Neylan, T. C., Oyaro, P., et al. (2016). Interpersonal psychotherapy for depression and posttraumatic stress disorder among HIV-positive women in Kisumu, Kenya: study protocol for a randomized controlled trial. *Trials*, *17*, 64. Erratum in: *Trials*. 2016;17(1):151.

Oranta, O., Luutonen, S., Salokangas, R. K., Vahlberg, T., & Leino-Kilpi, H. (2010). The outcomes of interpersonal counselling on depressive symptoms and distress after myocardial infarction. *Nordic Journal of Psychiatry*, *64*(2), 78–86.

Oranta, O., Luutonen, S., Salokangas, R. K., Vahlberg, T., & Leino-Kilpi, H. (2011). The effects of interpersonal counselling on health-related quality of life after myocardial infarction. *Journal of Clinical Nursing*, *20*(23-24), 3373–3382.

Oranta, O., Luutonen, S., Salokangas, R. K., Vahlberg, T., & Leino-Kilpi, H. (2012). Depression-focused interpersonal counseling and the use of healthcare services after myocardial infarction. *Perspectives in Psychiatric Care*, *48*(1), 47–55.

Peeters, F., Huibers, M., Roelofs, J., Hollon, S., Markowitz, J. C., van Os, J., & Arntz, A. (2013). The effectiveness of treating depression with evidence-based interventions in routine daily practice: results from a pragmatic trial. *Journal of Affective Disorders*, *145*, 349–355.

Pilowsky, D., & Weissman, M. M. (2005*). Interpersonal psychotherapy with school-aged depressed children*. Unpublished manual available from Dan Pilowsky, MD, 1051 Riverside Drive, Unit 24, New York, NY 10032.

Pinsker, H. (1997). *A primer of supportive psychotherapy*. Hillsdale, NJ: Analytic Press.

Poleshuck, E. L., Gamble, S. A., Cort, N., Hoffman-King, D., Cerrito, B., Rosario-McCabe, L. A., & Giles, D. E. (2010a). Interpersonal psychotherapy for co-occurring depression and chronic pain. *Professional Psychology Research and Practice, 41*(4), 312–318.

Poleshuck, E. L., Talbot, N. E., Zlotnick, C., Gamble, S. A., Liu, X., Tu, X., & Giles, D. E. (2010b). Interpersonal psychotherapy for women with comorbid depression and chronic pain. *Journal of Nervous and Mental Disease, 198*(8), 597–600.

Posmontier, B., Neugebauer, R., Stuart, S., Chittams, J., & Shaughnessy, R. (2016). Telephone-administered interpersonal psychotherapy by nurse-midwives for post-partum depression. *Midwifery and Women's Health, 61,* 456–466.

Power, M. J., & Freeman, C. (2012). A randomized controlled trial of IPT versus CBT in primary care: with some cautionary notes about handling missing values in clinical trials. *Clinical Psychology and Psychotherapy, 19*(2), 159–169.

Ransom, D., Heckman, T. G., Anderson, T., Garske, J., Holroyd, K., & Basta, T. (2008). Telephone-delivered, interpersonal psychotherapy for HIV-infected rural persons with depression: a pilot trial. *Psychiatric Services, 59*(8), 871–877.

Ravitz, P., Wondimagegn, D., Pain, C., Araya, M., Alem, A., Baheretibeb, Y., et al. (2014). Psychotherapy knowledge translation and interpersonal psychotherapy: using best-education practices to transform mental health care in Canada and Ethiopia. *American Journal of Psychotherapy, 68,* 463–488.

Reay, R., Fisher, Y., Robertson, M., Adams, E., Owen, C., & Kumar, R. (2006). Group interpersonal psychotherapy for postnatal depression: a pilot study. *Archives of Women's Mental Health, 9*(1), 31–39. Erratum in: Arch Womens Ment Health. 2006 Mar;9(2):115.

Reay, R. E., Owen, C., Shadbolt, B., Raphael, B., Mulcahy, R., & Wilkinson, R. B. (2012). Trajectories of long-term outcomes for postnatally depressed mothers treated with group interpersonal psychotherapy. *Archives of Women's Mental Health, 15*(3), 217–228.

Reynolds, C. F. 3rd, Dew, M. A., Martire, L. M., Miller, M. D., Cyranowski, J. M., Lenze, E., et al. (2010). Treating depression to remission in older adults: a controlled evaluation of combined escitalopram with interpersonal psychotherapy versus escitalopram with depression care management. *International Journal of Geriatric Psychiatry, 25,* 1134–1141.

Reynolds, C. F., III, Dew, M. A., Pollock, B. G., Mulsant, B. H., Frank, E., Miller, M. D., et al. (2006). Maintenance treatment of major depression in old age. *New England Journal of Medicine, 354,* 1130–1138.

Reynolds, C. F., III, Frank, E., Dew, M. A., Houck, P. R., Miller, M., Mazumdar, S., et al. (1999). Treatment of 70(+)-year-olds with recurrent major depression: Excellent short-term but brittle long-term response. *American Journal of Geriatric Psychiatry, 7,* 64–69.

Reynolds, C. F., III, Frank, E., Perel, J. M., Imber, S. D., Cornes, C., Miller, M. D., et al. (1999). Nortriptyline and interpersonal psychotherapy as maintenance therapies for recurrent major depression: A randomized controlled trial in patients older than fifty-nine years. *Journal of the American Medical Association, 281,* 39–45.

Rieger, E., Van Buren, D. J., Bishop, M., Tanofsky-Kraff, M., Welch, R., & Wilfley, D. E. (2010). An eating disorder-specific model of interpersonal psychotherapy (IPT-ED): causal pathways and treatment implications. *Clinical Psychology Review, 30*(4), 400–410.

Rifkin-Graboi, A., Bai, J., Chen, H., Hameed, W. B., Sim, L. W., Tint, M. T., et al. (2013). Prenatal maternal depression associates with microstructure of right amygdala in neonates at birth. *Biological Psychiatry, 74*(11), 837–844.

Riso, L., du Toit, P. L., Blandino, J. A., Penna, S., Dacey, S., Duin, J. S., et al. (2003). Cognitive aspects of chronic depression. *Journal of Abnormal Psychology, 112,* 72–80.

Rosselló, J., & Bernal, G. (1999). The efficacy of cognitive-behavioral and interpersonal treatments for depression in Puerto Rican adolescents. *Journal of Consulting and Clinical Psychology, 67,* 734–745.

Rosselló, J., Bernal, G., & Rivera-Medina, C. (2008). Individual and group CBT and IPT for Puerto Rican adolescents with depressive symptoms. *Cultural Diversity and Ethnic Minority Psychology, 14*(3), 234–245.

Rounsaville, B. J., Chevron, E. S., Weissman, M. M., Prusoff, B. A., & Frank, E. (1986). Training therapists to perform interpersonal psychotherapy in clinical trials. *Comprehensive Psychiatry, 27,* 364–371.

Rounsaville, B. J., Glazer, W., Wilber, C. H., Weissman, M. M., & Kleber, H. D. (1983). Short-term interpersonal psychotherapy in methadone-maintained opiate addicts. *Archives of General Psychiatry, 40,* 629–636.

Rounsaville, B. J., Klerman, G. L., & Weissman, M. M. (1981). Do psychotherapy and pharmacotherapy for depression conflict? Empirical evidence from a clinical trial. *Archives of General Psychiatry, 38,* 24–29.

Rush, A. J., First, M. B., & Blacker, D. (Eds.). (2007). *Handbook of psychiatric measures* (2nd ed.). Arlington, VA: American Psychiatric Publishing.

Rush, A. J., Madhukar, H. T., Ibrahim, H. M., Carmody, T. J., Arnow, B., Klein, D. N., et al. (2003). The 16-item Quick Inventory of Depressive Symptomatology (QIDS) Clinician Rating (QIDS-C) and Self-Report (QIDS-SR): a psychometric evaluation in patients with chronic major depression. *Biological Psychiatry, 54,* 573–583.

Salisbury, A. L., O'Grady, K. E., Battle, C. L., Wisner, K. L., Anderson, G. M., Stroud, L. R., et al. (2016). The roles of maternal depression, serotonin reuptake inhibitor treatment, and concomitant benzodiazepine use on infant neurobehavioral functioning over the first postnatal month. *American Journal of Psychiatry, 173*(2), 147–157.

Saloheimo, H. P., Markowitz, J. C., Saloheimo, T. H., Laitinen, J. J., Sundell, J., Huttunen, M. O., et al. (2016). Psychotherapy effectiveness for major depression: a randomized trial in a Finnish community. *BMC Psychiatry, 16,* 131.

Schaal, S., Elbert, T., & Neuner, F. (2009). Narrative exposure therapy versus interpersonal psychotherapy. A pilot randomized controlled trial with Rwandan genocide orphans. *Psychotherapy and Psychosomatics, 78*(5), 298–306.

Schramm, E., Zobel, I., Dykierek, P., Kech, S., Brakemeier, E. L., Külz, A., & Berger, M. (2011). Cognitive behavioral analysis system of psychotherapy versus interpersonal psychotherapy for early-onset chronic depression: a randomized pilot study. *Journal of Affective Disorders, 129,* 109–116.

Schulberg, H. C., Block, M. R., Madonia, M. J., Scott, C. P., Rodriguez, E., Imber, S. D., et al. (1996). Treating major depression in primary care practice. Eight-month clinical outcomes. *Archives of General Psychiatry, 53*(10), 913–919.

Schulberg, H. C., Post, E. P., Raue, P. J., Have, T. T., Miller, M., & Bruce, M. L. (2007). Treating late-life depression with interpersonal psychotherapy in the primary care sector. *International Journal of Geriatric Psychiatry, 22,* 106–114.

Schulberg, H. C., Raue, P. J., & Rollman, B. L. (2002). The effectiveness of psychotherapy in treating depressive disorders in primary care practice: clinical and cost perspectives. *General Hospital Psychiatry, 24*, 203–212.

Schwenk, T. L. (2016). Integrated behavioral and primary care: What is the real cost? *Journal of the American Medical Association, 316*(8), 822–823.

Scocco, P., & Frank, E. (2002). Interpersonal psychotherapy as augmentation treatment in depressed elderly responding poorly to antidepressant drugs: A case series. *Psychotherapy and Psychosomatics, 71*, 357–361.

Scogin, F., & McElreath, I. (1994). Efficacy of psychosocial treatments for geriatric depression: A quantitative review. *Journal of Consulting and Clinical Psychology, 57*, 403–407.

Scotland: The Matrix. (2015). *A guide to delivering evidence-based psychological therapies in Scotland*. NHS Education for Scotland.

Shea, M. T., Sout, R., Gunderson, J., Morey, L. C., Grilo, C. M., McGlashan, T., et al. (2002). Short-term diagnostic stability of schizotypal, borderline, avoidant, and obsessive-compulsive personality disorders. *American Journal of Psychiatry, 159*, 2036–2040.

Shear, M. K., Reynolds, C. F. 3rd, Simon, N. M., Zisook, S., Wang, Y., Mauro, C., et al. (2016). Optimizing treatment of complicated grief: a randomized clinical trial. *JAMA Psychiatry, 73*, 685–694.

Sheeber, L. B., Davis, B., Leve, C., Hops, H., & Tildesley, E. (2007). Adolescents' relationships with their mothers and fathers: associations with depressive disorder and subdiagnostic symptomatology. *Journal of Abnormal Psychology, 116*(1), 144–154.

Sinai, D., Gur, M., & Lipsitz, J. D. (2012). Therapist adherence to interpersonal versus supportive therapy for social anxiety disorder. *Psychotherapy Research, 22*, 381–388.

Sinai, D., & Lipsitz, J. D. (2012). *Interpersonal counseling for frequent attenders of primary care: A telephone outreach study*. Paper presented at The 3rd Joint Meeting of the Society for Psychotherapy Research European and UK Chapters, Porto, Portugal.

Siu, A. L., Bibbins-Domingo, K., Grossman, D. C., Baumann, L. C., Davidson, K. W., Ebell, M., et al. (2016). Screening for depression in adults: US Preventive Services Task Force Recommendation Statement. *Journal of the American Medical Association, 315*(4), 380–387.

Sockol, L. E., Epperson, C. N., & Barber, J. P. (2011). A meta-analysis of treatments for perinatal depression. *Clinical Psychology Review, 31*(5), 839–849.

Spinelli, M. G. (1999). *Manual of interpersonal psychotherapy for antepartum depressed women (IPT-P)*. Unpublished manual, College of Physicians and Surgeons of Columbia University, New York State Psychiatric Institute, 1051 Riverside Drive, Box 123, New York, NY 10032.

Spinelli, M. G., & Endicott, J. (2003). Controlled clinical trial of interpersonal psychotherapy versus parenting education program for depressed pregnant women. *American Journal of Psychiatry, 160*, 555–562.

Spinelli, M. G., Endicott, J., Goetz, R. R., & Segre, L. S. (2016). Reanalysis of efficacy of interpersonal psychotherapy for antepartum depression versus parenting education program: initial severity of depression as a predictor of treatment outcome. *Journal of Clinical Psychiatry, 77*(4), 535–540.

Spinelli, M. G., Endicott, J., Leon, A. C., Goetz, R. R., Kalish, R. B., Brustman, L. E., et al. (2013). A controlled clinical treatment trial of interpersonal psychotherapy for depressed pregnant women at 3 New York City sites. *Journal of Clinical Psychiatry*, *74*(4), 393–399.

Stangier, U., Schramm, E., Heidenreich, T., Berger, M., & Clark, D. M. (2011). Cognitive therapy vs interpersonal psychotherapy in social anxiety disorder: a randomized controlled trial. *Archives of General Psychiatry*, *68*, 692–700.

Stewart, M. O., Raffa, S. D., Steele, J. L., Miller, S. A., Clougherty, K. F., Hinrichsen, G. A., & Karlin, B. E. (2014). National dissemination of interpersonal psychotherapy for depression in veterans: therapist and patient-level outcomes. *Journal of Consulting and Clinical Psychology*, *82*, 1201–1206.

Stice, E., Ragan, J., & Randall, P. (2004). Prospective relations between social support and depression: differential direction of effects for parent and peer support? *Journal of Abnormal Psychology*, *113*(1), 155–159.

Stuart, S., & Noyes, R., Jr. [in press]. Interpersonal psychotherapy for somatizing patients. *Psychotherapy and Psychosomatics*, *75*.

Stuart, S., & O'Hara, M. W. (1995). Interpersonal psychotherapy for postpartum depression: a treatment program. *Journal of Psychotherapy Practice and Research*, *4*(1), 18–29.

Swartz, H. A. (2015). IOM report on psychosocial interventions for mental and substance use disorders: the interpersonal psychotherapy perspective. *Depression and Anxiety*, *32*, 793–795.

Swartz, H. A., Cyranowski, J. M., Cheng, Y., Zuckoff, A., Brent, D., Markowitz, J. C., et al. (2016). Brief psychotherapy of maternal depression in very high risk families: impact on mothers and their psychiatrically ill children. *Journal of the American Academy of Child Psychiatry*, *55*, 495–503e2.

Swartz, H. A., Frank, E., O'Toole, K., Newman, N., Kiderman, H., Carlson, S., et al. (2011). Implementing interpersonal and social rhythm therapy for mood disorders across a continuum of care. *Psychiatric Services*, *62*(11), 1377–1380.

Swartz, H. A., Frank, E., Shear, M. K., Thase, M. E., Fleming, M. A., & Scott, J. (2004). A pilot study of brief interpersonal psychotherapy for depression among women. *Psychiatric Services*, *55*(4), 448–450.

Swartz, H. A., Frank, E., Zuckoff, A., Cyranowski, J. M., Houck, P. R., Cheng, Y., et al. (2008). Brief interpersonal psychotherapy for depressed mothers whose children are receiving psychiatric treatment. *American Journal of Psychiatry*, *165*(9), 1155–1162.

Swartz, H. A., Grote, N. K., & Graham, P. (2014). Brief interpersonal psychotherapy (IPT-B): overview and review of evidence. *American Journal of Psychotherapy*, *68*(4), 443–462.

Swartz, H. A., Levenson, J. C., & Frank, E. (2012). Psychotherapy for bipolar II disorder: the role of Interpersonal and Social Rhythm Therapy. *Professional Psychology, Research and Practice*, *43*, 145–153.

Swartz, H. A., Martin, S., & Silva, A. (2016). *Rhythms And You (RAY): Demonstrating a new online program for bipolar disorders*. 2nd Integrative Conference on Technology, Social Media, and Behavioral Health, Pittsburgh, PA.

Swartz, H. A., Rucci, P., Thase, M. E., Wallace, M., Carretta, E., et al. (2016). *Interpersonal and Social Rhythm Therapy as a treatment for bipolar II depression*. Presented as part of a panel Managing Bipolar II Disorder: Phenomenology, Treatments, and Future Directions (H. Swartz, chair) at the 2016 International Society for Bipolar Disorders/ International Society for Affective Disorders Annual Meeting, Amsterdam, Netherlands,

Swartz, H. A., Rucci, P., Thase, M. E., Wallace, M., Carretta, E., Celedonia, K. L., & Frank E [in press]. Psychotherapy alone and combined with medication as treatments for bipolar II depression: A randomized controlled trial. *Journal of Clinical Psychiatry.*

Swenson, S. L., Rose, M., Vittinghoff, E., Stewart, A., & Schillinger, D. (2008). The influence of depressive symptoms on clinician-patient communication among patients with type 2 diabetes. *Medical Care, 46*(3), 257–265.

Talati, A., Wickramaratne, P. J., Pilowsky, D. J., Alpert, J. E., Cerda, G., Garber, J., et al. (2007). Remission of maternal depression and child symptoms among single mothers. *Social Psychiatry and Psychiatric Epidemiology, 42*(12), 962–971.

Tang, T. C., Jou, S. H., Ko, C. H., Huang, S. Y., & Yen, C. F. (2009). Randomized study of school-based intensive interpersonal psychotherapy for depressed adolescents with suicidal risk and parasuicide behaviors. *Psychiatry Clinical Neuroscience, 63*(4), 463–470.

Tanofsky-Kraff, M., Shomaker, L. B., Wilfley, D. E., Young, J. F., Sbrocco, T., Stephens, M., et al. (2014). Targeted prevention of excess weight gain and eating disorders in high-risk adolescent girls: a randomized controlled trial. *American Journal of Clinical Nutrition, 100*(4), 1010–1018.

Tanofsky-Kraff, M., Shomaker, L. B., Young, J. F., & Wilfley, D. E. (2016). Interpersonal psychotherapy for the prevention of excess weight gain and eating disorders: A brief case study. *Psychotherapy, 53*(2), 188–194.

Tanofsky-Kraff, M., & Wilfley, D. E. *Interpersonal psychotherapy for the treatment of eating disorders.* Oxford Handbooks Online. 2012-09-18. Oxford University Press. Date of access October 19, 2016. http://www.oxfordhandbooks.com/view/10.1093/oxfordhb/9780195373622.001.0001/oxfordhb-9780195373622-e-020

Tanofsky-Kraff, M., Wilfley, D. E., Young, J. F., Mufson, L., Yanovski, S. Z., Glasofer, D. R., et al. (2010). A pilot study of interpersonal psychotherapy for preventing excess weight gain in adolescent girls at-risk for obesity. *International Journal of Eating Disorders, 43*(8), 701–706.

Tanofsky-Kraff, M., Wilfley, D. E., Young, J. F., Mufson, L., Yanovski, S. Z., Glasofer, D. R., & Salaita, C. G. (2007). Preventing excessive weight gain in adolescents: interpersonal psychotherapy for binge eating. *Obesity, 15*(6), 1345–1355. Erratum in: *Obesity.* 2007 Oct;15(10):2520.

Thase, M. E., Buysse, D. J., Frank, E., Cherry, C. R., Cornes, C. L., Mallinger, A. G., & Kupfer, D. J. (1997). Which depressed patients will respond to interpersonal psychotherapy? The role of abnormal EEG sleep profiles. *American Journal of Psychiatry, 154,* 502–509.

van Schaik, A., van Marwijk, H., Adèr, H., van Dyck, R., de Haan, M., Penninx, B., et al. (2006). Interpersonal psychotherapy for elderly patients in primary care. *American Journal of Geriatric Psychiatry, 14*(9), 777–786.

van Schaik, D. J., van Marwijk, H. W., Beekman, A. T., de Haan, M., & van Dyck, R. (2007). Interpersonal psychotherapy (IPT) for late-life depression in general practice: uptake and satisfaction by patients, therapists, and physicians. *BMC Family Practice, 8,* 52.

Verdeli, H., Clougherty, K. F., Bolton, P., Speelman, L., Ndogoni, L., Bass, J., et al. (2003). Adapting group interpersonal psychotherapy for a developing country: experience in rural Uganda. *World Psychiatry, 2,* 114–120.

Verdeli, H., Clougherty, K., Onyango, G., Lewandowski, E., Speelman, L., Betancourt, T. S., et al. (2008). Group interpersonal psychotherapy for depressed youth in IDP camps in Northern Uganda: adaptation and training. *Child and Adolescent Psychiatric Clinics of North America*, 17, 605–624.

Verdeli, H., Therosme, T., Eustache, E., Hilaire, O. S., Joseph, B., Sönmez, C. C., & Raviola, G. (2016). Community morms and human rights: supervising Haitian colleagues on interpersonal psychotherapy (IPT) with a depressed and abused pregnant woman. *Journal of Clinical Psychology*, 72(8), 847–855.

Vidair, H. B., Boccia, A. S., Johnson, J. G., Verdeli, H., Wickramaratne, P., Klink, K. A., et al. (2011). Depressed parents' treatment needs and children's problems in an urban family medicine practice. *Psychiatric Services*, 62(3), 317–321.

Vos, S. P., Huibers, M. J., Diels, L., & Arntz, A. (2012). A randomized clinical trial of cognitive behavioral therapy and interpersonal psychotherapy for panic disorder with agoraphobia. *Psychological Medicine*, 42, 2661–2672.

Wampold, B. E. (2001). *The great psychotherapy debate: models, methods, and findings.* Mahwah, NJ: Lawrence Erlbaum Associates.

Weikum, W. M., Oberlander, T. F., Hensch, T. K., & Werker, J. F. (2012). Prenatal exposure to antidepressants and depressed maternal mood alter trajectory of infant speech perception. *Proceedings of the National Academy of Sciences USA*, 109(Suppl 2), 17221–17227.

Weissman, M. M. (2005). *Mastering depression through interpersonal psychotherapy: Monitoring forms.* New York: Oxford University Press.

Weissman, M. M. (2006). A brief history of interpersonal psychotherapy. *Psychiatric Annals*, 36, 553–557.

Weissman, M. M. (2013) Psychotherapy: a paradox. *American Journal of Psychiatry*, 170(7), 712–715.

Weissman, M. M. (2016). What's a family? *Journal of the American Academy of Child and Adolescent Psychiatry*, 55, 927–928.

Weissman, M. M., Berry, O. O., Warner, V., Gameroff, M. J., Skipper, J., Talati, A., et al. (2016). A 30-year study of three generations at high risk and low risk for depression. *JAMA Psychiatry*, 73(9), 970–977.

Weissman, M. M., & Bothwell, S. (1976). Assessment of social adjustment by patient self-report. *Archives of General Psychiatry*, 33(9), 1111–1115.

Weissman, M. M., Hankerson, S. H., Scorza, P., Olfson, M., Verdeli, H., Shea, S., et al. (2014). Interpersonal counseling (IPC) for depression in primary care. *American Journal of Psychotherapy*, 68(4), 359–383.

Weissman, M. M., Klerman, G. L., Prusoff, B. A., Sholomskas, D., & Padian, N. (1981). Depressed outpatients: Results one year after treatment with drugs and/or interpersonal psychotherapy. *Archives of General Psychiatry*, 38, 52–55.

Weissman, M. M., Markowitz, J. C., & Klerman, G. L. (2000). *Comprehensive guide to interpersonal psychotherapy.* New York: Basic Books.

Weissman, M. M., Pilowsky, D. J., Wickramaratne, P., Talati, A., Wisniewski, S. R., Fava, M., et al. (2006). Remission of maternal depression is associated with reductions in psychopathology in their children: A Star*D-child report. *Journal of the American Medical Association*, 295, 1389–1398.

Weissman, M., & Verdeli, H. (2012). Interpersonal psychotherapy: evaluation, support, triage. *Clinical Psychology and Psychotherapy*, 19, 106–112.

Weissman, M. M., Verdeli, H., Gameroff, M. J., Bledsoe, S. E., Betts, K., Mufson, L., et al. (2006). A national survey of psychotherapy training in psychiatry, psychology, and social work. *Archives of General Psychiatry, 63*, 925–934.

Weissman, M. M., Wickramaratne, P., Gameroff, M. J., Warner, V., Pilowsky, D., Kohad, R. G., et al. (2016). Offspring of depressed parents: 30 years later. *American Journal of Psychiatry, 173*(10), 1024–1032.

Weissman, M. M., Wickramaratne, P., Pilowsky, D. J., Poh, E., Batten, L. A., Hernandez, M., et al. (2015). Treatment of maternal depression in a medication clinical trial and its effect on children. *American Journal of Psychiatry, 172*(5), 450–459.

Welch, R. R., Mills, M. S., & Wilfley, D. E. (2012). IPT for Group. In J. C. Markowitz & M. M. Weissman (Eds.), *Casebook of interpersonal psychotherapy.* New York: Oxford University Press.

Wilfley, D. E., Agras, W. S., Telch, C. F., Rossiter, E., Schneider, J., Cole, A. C., et al. (1993). Group cognitive-behavioral therapy and group interpersonal psychotherapy for the nonpurging bulimic individual: A controlled comparison. *Journal of Consulting and Clinical Psychology, 61*, 296–305.

Wilfley, D. E., & Eichen, D. M. [in press]. Interpersonal psychotherapy. In K. Brownell & T. B. Walsh (Eds.), *Eating disorders and obesity: a comprehensive handbook* (3rd ed.). New York: Guilford Press.

Wilfley, D. E., Mackenzie, K. R., Welch, R., Ayres, V., & Weissman, M. M. (Eds.). (2000). *Interpersonal psychotherapy for group.* New York: Basic Books.

Wilfley, D. E., Welch, R. R., Stein, R. I., Spurrell, E. B., Cohen, L. R., Saelens, B. E., et al. (2002). A randomized comparison of group cognitive-behavioral therapy and group interpersonal psychotherapy for the treatment of overweight individuals with binge-eating disorder. *Archives of General Psychiatry, 59*(8), 713–721.

Wilson, G. T. (2011). Treatment of binge eating disorder. *Psychiatric Clinics of North America, 34*(4), 773–783.

Wilson, G. T., Wilfley, D. E., Agras, W. S, & Bryson, S. W. (2010). Psychological treatments of binge eating disorder. *Archives of General Psychiatry, 67*(1), 94–101.

World Health Organization. (2015). *Guidelines Development.*

World Health Organization. (2016). *mhGAP Intervention Guide for mental, neurological and substance use disorders in non-specialized health settings.*

World Health Organization and Columbia University. (2016). *Group interpersonal therapy (IPT) for depression.* Geneva: WHO.

Young, J. F., Benas, J. S., Schueler, C. M., Gallop, R., Gillham, J. E., & Mufson, L. (2016). A randomized depression prevention trial comparing interpersonal psychotherapy—adolescent skills training to group counseling in schools. *Prevention Science, 17*(3), 314–324.

Young, J. F., Makover, H. B., Cohen, J. R., Mufson, L., Gallop, R. J., & Benas, J. S. (2012). Interpersonal psychotherapy—adolescent skills training: anxiety outcomes and impact of comorbidity. *Journal of Clinical Child and Adolescent Psychology, 41*(5), 640–653.

Young, J. F., Mufson, L., & Davies, M. (2006). Efficacy of interpersonal psychotherapy—adolescent skills training: an indicated preventive intervention for depression. *Journal of Child Psychology and Psychiatry, 47*(12), 1254–1262.

Young, J. F., Mufson, L., & Gallop, R. (2010). Preventing depression: a randomized trial of interpersonal psychotherapy—adolescent skills training. *Depression and Anxiety*, *27*(5), 426–433.

Young, J. F., Mufson, L., & Schueler, C. M. (2016). *Preventing adolescent depression: interpersonal psychotherapy—adolescent skills training*. New York: Oxford University Press.

Zanarini, M. C., Frankenburg, F. R., Reich, D. B., Wedig, M. M., Conkey, L. C., & Fitzmaurice, G. M. (2014). Prediction of time-to-attainment of recovery for borderline patients followed prospectively for 16 years. *Acta Psychiatrica Scandinavica*, *130*, 205–213.

Zhang, Y., Zhou, X., James, A. C., Qin, B., Whittington, C. J., Cuijpers, P., et al. (2015). Comparative efficacy and acceptability of psychotherapies for acute anxiety disorders in children and adolescents: study protocol for a network meta-analysis. *BMJ Open*, *5*(10), e008572.

Zlotnick, C., Capezza, N. M., & Parker, D. (2011). An interpersonally based intervention for low-income pregnant women with intimate partner violence: a pilot study. *Archive of Women's Mental Health*, *14*(1), 55–65.

Zlotnick, C., Johnson, S. L., Miller, I. W., Pearlstein, T., & Howard, M. (2001). Postpartum depression in women receiving public assistance: Pilot study of an interpersonal-therapy-oriented group intervention. *American Journal of Psychiatry*, *158*, 638–640.

Zlotnick, C., Miller, I. W., Pearlstein, T., Howard, M., & Sweeney, P. (2006). A preventive intervention for pregnant women on public assistance at risk for postpartum depression. *American Journal of Psychiatry*, *163*(8), 1443–1445.

Zuckerman, D. M., Prusoff, B. A., Weissman, M. M., & Padian, N.S. (1980). Personality as a predictor of psychotherapy and pharmacotherapy outcome for depressed outpatients. *Journal of Consulting and Clinical Psychology*, *48*, 730–735.

Zunner, B., Dworkin, S. L., Neylan, T. C., Bukusi, E. A., Oyaro, P., Cohen, C. R., et al. (2015). HIV, violence and women: unmet mental health care needs. *Journal of Affective Disorders*, *174*, 619–626.

ABOUT THE AUTHORS

Myrna M. Weissman, Ph.D., is Diane Goldman Kemper Family Professor of Epidemiology and Psychiatry, College of Physicians and Surgeons and the Mailman School of Public Health at Columbia University and Chief of the Division of Epidemiology at New York State Psychiatric Institute (NYSPI). She received her Ph.D. in Epidemiology from Yale University School of Medicine, where she also became a professor. Dr. Weissman is a member of the National Academy of Medicine, National Academy of Science. She has been the recipient of numerous grants from NIMH, NARSAD Senior Investigators Awards, grants from other private foundations, and numerous awards for her research. In April 2009, she was selected by the American College of Epidemiology as one of ten epidemiologists in the United States who has had a major impact on public policy and public health. The summary of her work on depression appears in a special issue of the *Annals of Epidemiology*, "Triumphs in Epidemiology." In January 2016 she was listed as one of the 100 highly cited researchers according to presence in Google Scholar Citation.

Early on in her career she began working with Gerald Klerman at Yale University on the development of IPT. Together they carried out this work, testing IPT in several clinical trials of maintenance and acute treatment of depression and a modification for primary care they called Interpersonal Counseling. They published the first IPT manual in 1984.

John C. Markowitz, M.D., received his medical degree from Columbia University and did his residency training in psychiatry at the Payne Whitney Clinic of Cornell Medical Center, where he was trained in IPT by the late Gerald L. Klerman, M.D. First at Cornell and then at Columbia University/New York State Psychiatric Institute, Dr. Markowitz has conducted a series of comparative studies of IPT, other psychotherapies, and medications, studying mood, anxiety, and personality disorders. He has received numerous grants from the National Institute of Mental Health and other organizations, has published several hundred articles and book chapters, and has taught and supervised IPT around the world.

Gerald L. Klerman, M.D., was the mentor of Dr. Weissman (his wife) and Dr. Markowitz. He was convinced that interpersonal relationships importantly influenced the course and recurrence of illness, and that psychotherapy could potentially stabilize interpersonal relations. Gerry was the force behind the original ideas in the first IPT manual (Klerman et al., 1984) and many of its adaptations. Gerry died young in April 1992. Even years after his death, his writing on IPT is pervasive. Out of respect for his contribution to the therapy, we are proud to continue to name him a posthumous author of this book.

Gerry held numerous prestigious positions in psychiatry and government. He graduated from New York University Medical School and did his residency at Harvard. He was professor at Yale University, Harvard Medical School, and, lastly, Weill Medical College of Cornell University. He was appointed by President Carter to lead the Alcohol, Drug Abuse, and Mental Health Administration, a position he held between 1977 and 1980.

Boxes, figures, and tables are indicated by *b*, *f*, and *t* following the page number.